SOCIETY FOR VETERINARY EPIDEMIOLOGY AND PREVENTIVE MEDICINE

Proceedings of a meeting held in

London, UK

1st - 3rd April 2009

Edited by J.R. Newton, D.U. Pfeiffer and the SVEPM Executive Committee

(Views expressed in these proceedings are not necessarily those of the Editors or the Executive Committee of the Society)

ISBN 978-0-948073-89-2

ACKNOWLEDGEMENTS

The following bodies provided financial support for the conference and the publication of these proceedings:

The Dog's Trust

European College of Veterinary Public Health

Veterinary Laboratories Agency

Palisade

DEFRA

Pfizer

Nordic Society for Veterinary Epidemiology

CIRAD

The Royal Veterinary College

Thanks are extended to INNTEL for their stationary contributions at this year's conference.

CONTENTS

EPIDEMIOLOGICAL METHODS

SCIENCE / POLICY INTERFACE

INFECTIOUS DISEASE MODELING

NETWORK ANALYSIS

***

ANTIMICROBIAL RESISTANCE

PATTERNS OF ANTIMICROBIAL RESISTANCE IN *SALMONELLA* TYPHIMURIUM DT104 IN ANIMALS AND HUMANS IN SCOTLAND: ARE THEY THE SAME?

A.E. MATHER*, D.T. HAYDON, D.J. MELLOR, L. MATTHEWS, D.J. BROWN, R.J. REID-SMITH, P. BOERLIN, S.A. MCEWEN, M.J. DENWOOD AND S.W.J. REID

SUMMARY

Antimicrobial resistance (AMR) is a public health matter of increasing concern. Antimicrobials used in veterinary medicine are, in many cases, the same, or of the same class, as drugs used in human medicine. Therefore, resistant bacteria in animals may play a role in the development of resistance in humans and *vice versa*. Phenotypic antimicrobial resistance data derived from human and veterinary *Salmonella* Typhimurium DT104 (DT104) isolates, collected in Scotland from 1990 to 2004, were analysed to identify potential differences in the epidemiology and evolution of AMR between human and animal populations in Scotland. Application of the eBurst algorithm (developed at Imperial College London) was used to visualise the estimated evolutionary history of AMR in the data. Simulation and bootstrapping methods were employed to explore associations between resistance in animals and humans. Bootstrapping was used to explore the extent to which random processes were driving the number of resistance profiles in animals and humans. Simulation techniques were assessed as means for investigating the factors influencing the number of profiles in each population, and to ascertain whether these factors were similar or different. Using the combined approach it was clear that different patterns were observed in humans and animals and different assumptions are necessary if the epidemiological relationships between the resistance phenotypes are to be successfully modelled. However, many similarities were also observed between the animal and human data in the estimated evolutionary history. Whilst there was more diversity in the human data, the similarities may be due to the clonal nature of DT104. Although the bootstrapping and simulation techniques can determine whether there are differences in the patterns of AMR in the two populations, they cannot, in isolation, determine the cause of such differences. There were significant advantages and disadvantages of each approach when applied in this manner to these data. These included ease of implementation and of interpretation, maximising information utility of the surveillance data and dependency on underlying assumptions and biological/molecular relationships. It was concluded that it was the combined approach that provided greatest epidemiological insight into the AMR evolution and relationships in the study data. Differences in AMR between the two populations may be due to differences in selection pressure, little mixing or transmission between the two populations, different DT104 subtypes infecting humans and animals, or bias in the sampling procedure.

* Alison Mather, Boyd Orr Centre for Population and Ecosystem Health, Institute of Comparative Medicine, Faculty of Veterinary Medicine, University of Glasgow, Glasgow, G61 1QH, UK. Email: a.mather@vet.gla.ac.uk

INTRODUCTION

Bacterial infections which are resistant to antimicrobial drugs are increasingly common phenomena, and represent a threat to animal and human health (Tenover, 2006). One of the most contentious issues is the use of antimicrobials in animals (Angulo et al., 2004; Bywater, 2004; Phillips et al., 2004; Wassenaar, 2005; Phillips, 2007), and how it contributes to resistance in human pathogens. Resistance that develops in animals may contribute to resistance in humans by several routes. Resistant bacterial infections can be transmitted to humans as zoonotic bacteria, either through direct contact or through environmental contamination. Meat or other animal food products can also be a conduit (Angulo et al. 2000; Anderson et al. 2003). Bacteria of animal origin can be a reservoir of broad-host range resistance determinants (Binh et al., 2008), as mobile resistance elements can transfer between bacterial species and genera (Kruse & Sørum, 1994; Sherley et al., 2004; Gebreyes & Thakur, 2005).

In order to develop effective control strategies, understanding the ecology of resistance in both animal and human populations and the respective impact of resistance in one population on the other are important prerequisites. Previous approaches have focused on assessing trends by examining changes in resistance to individual antimicrobials, and to measuring effects of interventions in the same way (Threlfall et al., 2003; Bywater et al., 2004; Alexander et al., 2008; Hendriksen et al., 2008). However, given many resistance determinants are genetically linked, such as the case with DT104 (Mulvey et al., 2006), it seems intuitive and sensible to consider the entire resistance spectrum of the organism (as determined by the specific testing method). The model system used in this analysis was *Salmonella* Typhimurium DT104 isolates collected from clinical infections of animals and humans in Scotland, over the period 1990 – 2004. The AMR patterns were compared and contrasted between the two populations, to assess the similarities and differences of the ecologies and system drivers for AMR in both animals and humans. To accomplish this, three techniques were employed: visualising reconstructions of evolutionary history, bootstrapping, and simulation.

MATERIALS AND METHODS

The datasets

Human DT104 isolates were submitted by medical diagnostic laboratories to the Scottish *Salmonella* Reference Laboratory (SSRL); veterinary DT104 isolates were submitted by veterinary laboratories to the SSRL. Both animal and human isolates were collected as part of an ongoing passive surveillance effort. Phenotypic antimicrobial susceptibility testing was performed by the SSRL on the isolates; the common resistances for which testing was carried out in both animals and humans were against ampicillin, chloramphenicol, ciprofloxacin, furazolidone, gentamicin, kanamycin, nalidixic acid, netilmicin, spectinomycin, streptomycin, sulphamethoxazole, tetracycline, and trimethoprim. Each isolate was identified as either susceptible (0) or resistant (1) to each antimicrobial.

The unit of interest was the resistance profile of an isolate. The profile was defined as the ordered combination of 0s and 1s that described the antimicrobials to which each isolate was resistant.

Visualising reconstructions of evolutionary history

There are several software packages available to estimate and graph the evolution of bacterial isolates. One such package is eBurst (eBurstv3, 2006). It estimates and graphs patterns of evolutionary descent for bacterial isolates (Feil et al., 2004), developed originally for multilocus sequence typing data. Based on this type of genotypic data, clonal complexes and the most probable founding genotype of each complex are estimated; bootstrapping is used as statistical support for the designations (Feil et al., 2004). These relationships are then graphically displayed in a radial diagram. Although originally designed to be used with genotypic data, the algorithms can also be applied to any type of data that is represented by a string of integers. For a full description of the algorithm, see Feil et al. (2004), Spratt et al. (2004) and the eBurst manual (eBurstv3, 2006).

The eBurst algorithm was applied to both the animal and human datasets. The most stringent definition of group (clonal complex) was used, with all members in a group having identical resistance outcomes for $\geq$ 12 of the 13 antimicrobials with at least one other member in the group. In the resulting diagrammatic representation, each line between dots represents either the loss or addition of resistance to a single antimicrobial.

Bootstrapping

In order to determine whether the numbers of different profiles found in humans and animals could have resulted from sampling from a single combined bacterial population, bootstrapping of the data was performed. The R statistical program was used for this purpose (R Development Core Team, 2008). The total numbers of resistance profiles found in animals only and in humans only were tabulated. The two datasets were combined, with consistent identifiers for the unique profiles and a variable indicating whether a particular isolate was originally from the animal or the human dataset. Datasets of the same size as the human and animal sets were then bootstrapped 1,000 times, without replacement from this combined data set. The number of profiles found only in animals, and only in humans, were tabulated for each of the bootstrapped datasets, and compared to those observed.

Simulation

In order to determine whether the observed AMR patterns in both populations could be recreated using the same structure of parameters and therefore whether it would then be appropriate to infer that AMR developed in a similar fashion in the two populations, simulation techniques were employed. Five hundred (500) simulated datasets each were created for animals and humans using R (R Development Core Team, 2008), containing the same number of isolates as in the original datasets. For each simulated isolate, resistance to each antimicrobial was determined using a Bernoulli distribution. The probability for each distribution was set as the prevalence of resistance to that antimicrobial within each dataset. The simulated data were plotted and compared to the observed data.

RESULTS

Over the period 1990 – 2004, there were 2,761 human DT104 isolates and 2,439 animal DT104 isolates. There were 65 unique resistance profiles overall; 52 profiles in the human dataset, and 35 in the animal dataset. There were 22 profiles that were found in both animals and humans.

Visualising reconstructions of evolutionary history

Figure 1A and B displays the predicted evolution of the isolates in the human dataset (A) and animal dataset (B), as determined by the eBurst algorithm.

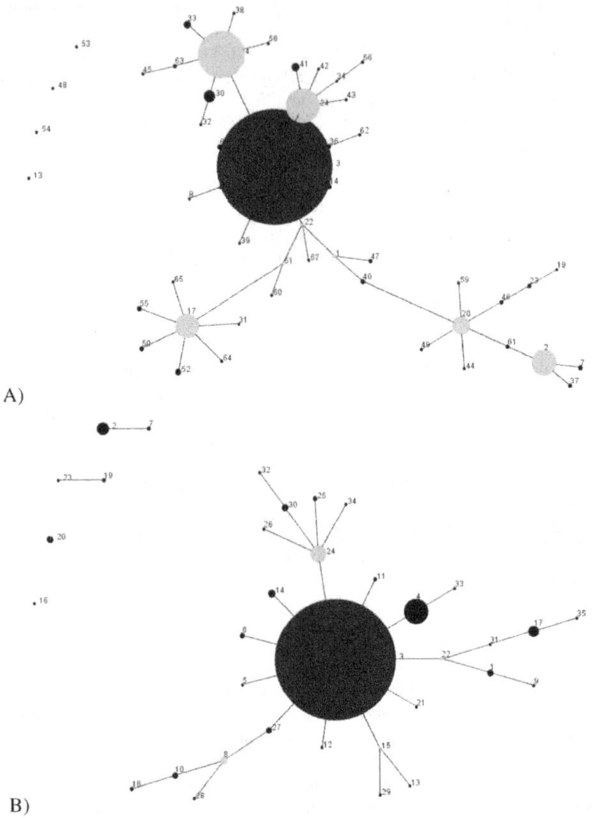

Fig. 1A and B. Estimated evolutionary history of profiles in the human dataset (A) and animal dataset (B) of S. Typhimurium DT104 in Scotland, 1990 to 2004. Numbers labelling the dots represent unique resistance profiles.

In the human data, 92% of the profiles were connected in the network by the addition or loss of resistance to a single antimicrobial. In the animal data, 83% of profiles were so connected. What was clear from inspection of the figures is that although there were some similarities between the two, there were also a number of differences. The same profile was predicted to be the founding, or ancestral, phenotype in both populations. On the other hand, the diversity of profiles and in particular the second tier of most prevalent types differed.

Bootstrapping

There were 30 profiles found only in humans, and 13 found only in animals. Figure 2A shows the distribution of the bootstrapped data for humans, and Fig. 2B shows the distribution of the bootstrapped data for animals.

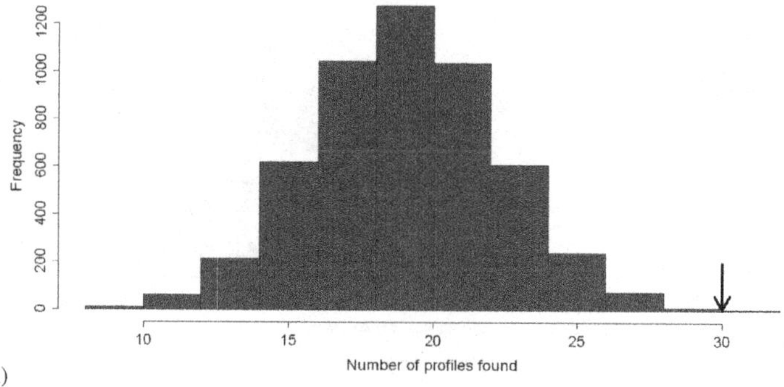

A)

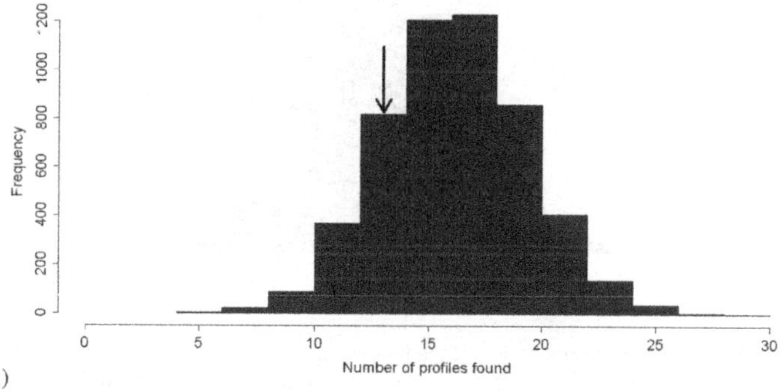

B)

Fig. 2A and B. Bootstrapping result for profiles found only in humans (A) and only in animals (B). Arrows represent the observed number of profiles in the original datasets.

There were differences between the animal and human populations. In the case of the human data, the observed number of human-only profiles (30) was in the extreme right end tail of the distribution of bootstrapped results; in the case of the animal data, the observed number of animal-only profiles fell well within the expected distribution.

Simulation

Figure 3 demonstrates output for the simulated human data (Fig. 3A) and animal data (Fig. 3B). In this case, the simulations again demonstrated differences between the animal and human populations. The observed number of profiles in the human data (52, including profiles found in both humans and animals), was much less than would be expected under the hypothesis that resistance to each antimicrobial are acquired independently of each other. Conversely, the number of profiles found in animals (35), again fell well within the expected distribution.

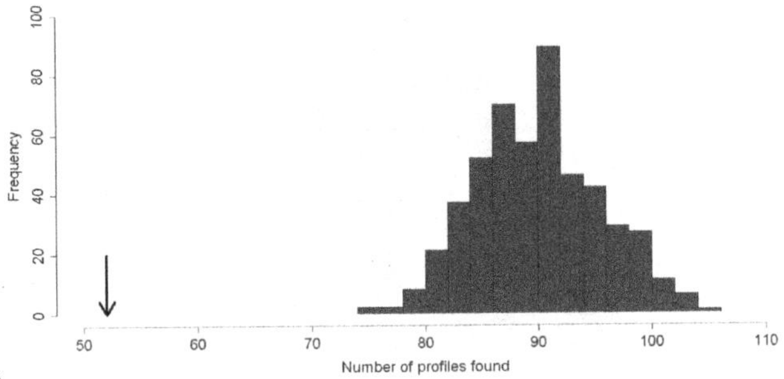

A)

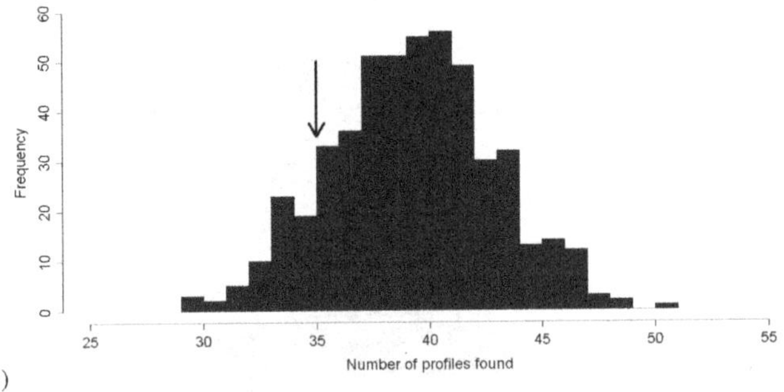

B)

Fig. 3A and B. Results of the simulation of the human dataset (A), arrow at the observed number of profiles (52). Results of the simulation of the animal dataset (B), arrow at the observed number of profiles (35).

Table 1 summarises the strengths and weaknesses, advantages and disadvantages of the various methods adopted in exploring these AMR data.

Table 1. Summary of advantages and disadvantages of each method

Method	Example	Purpose/advantages	Disadvantages
Visualising reconstruction of evolutionary history	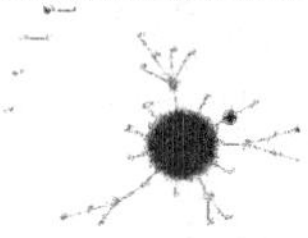	• Immediate • Connectivity • Attractive	• Real relationships? • Dependent upon assumptions • Not temporarily explicit
Bootstrapping	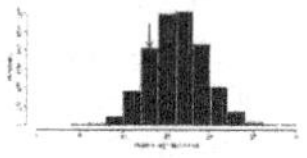	• Maximising value of data • Utilises real data	• Assumes random sample • Misses other *Salmonellae*
Simulation	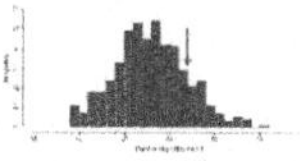	• Explore different hypotheses/rules in both populations • Not constrained by sample size	• Dependent upon assumptions • Misses other *Salmonellae*

DISCUSSION

The eBurst diagrams of Fig. 1A and B show animal and human data connected in a web generated by either an addition or loss of resistance to a single antimicrobial. Whilst there were similar shapes and connectivity within the diagrams, which may be due to the clonal nature of DT104, it is clear that the two are far from identical, suggesting the possibility of differing underlying ecologies and/or epidemiologies. The advantages of the eBurst approach are that it is simple and user-friendly, and creates a figure which is easier to interpret than typical phylogenetic trees. The use of the eBurst approach with phenotypic data is not without its limitations. Typically, there can be several different genetic mechanisms for any particular resistance phenotype. Therefore, the same phenotypic resistance in two isolates may have arisen through different evolutionary pathways. It is possible that if genotypic data had been available for these isolates and entered into eBurst, different diagrams may have been created. The utility of this approach is that it allows a snapshot overview of the estimated evolutionary history of the entire sample population to be visualised. Phenomena such as connectivity of isolates may not be detected by other approaches. Although a single evolutionary reconstruction is shown, the fact that it is an estimation of the evolutionary history, and not necessarily the true evolution, must be borne in mind.

Bootstrapping is a simple statistical technique that is used to resample datasets, thereby effectively taking multiple samples from a population, and is especially useful when dealing with small datasets. In this example, it was used to investigate whether the two samples can be regarded as having really come from a single combined sample. The important assumption in bootstrapping is that the data are a random, representative sample drawn from the population of interest; therefore, the definition of the population is very important. The isolates in both the animal and human datasets were obtained from clinical submissions. Clinically normal animals may also shed DT104 in faeces, but are not represented in the animal dataset. Furthermore, the isolates from both animals and humans were collected through passive surveillance. Therefore, it is unlikely that the datasets are representative of the entire population of DT104 from animals and humans in Scotland. Nevertheless, it is possible that they are a random sample from the clinical (ill) populations, although this is impossible to confirm. The advantages of bootstrapping techniques in the manner described here, besides the simplicity of the technique, are that real data are used, and therefore is not dependent upon assumptions of genetic linkage. In this example, the results suggest that the number of profiles appearing uniquely in animals and humans are unlikely to have resulted from animals and humans acquiring infections from a single well-mixed bacterial population, as the number of profiles in the bootstrapped human data did not match the observed data. This suggests that there may be different selection pressures in the two populations, or that how bacterial samples are acquired are importantly different in human and animal populations. Simulation techniques are useful tools for exploring patterns within complex datasets, and particularly for comparing datasets. Simulated datasets are created based on sets of assumptions about how the data may have been generated. If the simulated data have approximately the same properties as the observed data, then the assumptions made in the simulation process cannot be simply rejected. In the case presented here, the simulations suggest that different assumptions must be applied to the different populations if the models are to reflect the observed data, suggesting different epidemiologies. Simulations are only as good as the input parameters; the results are completely dependent on the assumptions built into the model. The next step of this work will be to refine the models by incorporating genetic linkage of resistance and other parameters. However, simulation techniques are an excellent way to explore relationships and test hypotheses, one that is not constrained by sample size.

A general limitation of comparing AMR in these populations is that only the patterns of AMR in DT104 were examined. The rest of the *Salmonella* genus, and other bacterial species, both Gram-negative and Gram-positive, were not included for consideration in this analysis. This has important implications when one considers the resistance determinant as the unit of interest – clearly the relationship between different bacterial populations will have an influence on the evolution of the profiles of all populations and is a factor that is worthy of further consideration.

In assessing the relative merits of each approach to the available data, there were significant advantages and disadvantages (Table 1). In summary these include, ease of implementation, ease of interpretation, maximising information utility of the surveillance data and the relative, differing dependency on underlying assumptions and biological/molecular relationships. However, it is the combined approach that provides greatest epidemiological insight into the AMR evolution and relationships in the study data.

Techniques such as the ones described above may play an increasingly important role in the development of mitigation strategies aimed at controlling or reducing AMR in both animals and humans. It is vital to determine the origins of resistance to antimicrobials, and where it is being amplified, if these essential pharmaceuticals are to remain available for the future control of bacterial disease.

REFERENCES

Alexander, T.W., Yanke, L.J., Topp, E., Olson, M.E., Read, R.R., Morck, D.W. and McAllister, T.A. (2008). Effect of subtherapeutic administration of antibiotics on the prevalence of antibiotic-resistant *Escherichia coli* bacteria in feedlot cattle. Appl. Environ. Microbiol. 74, 4405-4416

Anderson, A.D., Nelson, J.M., Rossiter, S. and Angula, F.J. (2003). Public health consequences of use of antimicrobial agents in food animals in the United States. Microb. Drug Resist. 9, 373-379

Angulo, F.J., Johnson, K.R., Tauxe, R.V. and Cohen, M.L. (2000). Origins and consequences of antimicrobial-resistant nontyphoidal *Salmonella*: implications for the use of fluoroquinolones in food animals. Microb. Drug Resist. 6, 77-83

Angulo, F.J., Nargund, V.N. and Chiller, T.C. (2004). Evidence of an association between use of anti-microbial agents in food animals and anti-microbial resistance among bacteria isolated from humans and the human health consequences of such resistance. J. Vet. Med. B Infect. Dis. Vet. Public Health 51, 374-379

Binh, C.T., Heuer, H., Kaupenjohann, M. and Smalla, K. (2008). Piggery manure used for soil fertilization is a reservoir for transferable antibiotic resistance plasmids. FEMS Microbiol. Ecol. 66, 25-37

Bywater, R.J. (2004). Veterinary use of antimicrobials and emergence of resistance in zoonotic and sentinel bacteria in the EU. J. Vet. Med. B Infect. Dis. Vet. Public Health 51, 361-363

Bywater, R.J., Deluyker, H., Deroover, E., de Jong, A., Marion, H., McConville, M., Rowan, T., Shryock, T., Shuster, D., Thomas, V., Valle, M. and Walters, J. (2004). A European survey of antimicrobial susceptibility among zoonotic and commensal bacteria isolated from food-producing animals. J. Antimicrob. Chemother. 54, 744-754

eBurstv3. (2006). eBurstv3. London, Department of Infectious Disease Epidemiology, Imperial College London

Feil, E.J., Li, B.C., Aanensen, D.M., Hanage, W.P. and Spratt, B.G. (2004). eBurst: inferring patterns of evolutionary descent among clusters of related bacterial genotypes from multilocus sequence typing data. J. Bacteriol. 186, 1518-1530

Gebreyes, W.A. and Thakus, S. (2005). Multidrug-resistant *Salmonella* enterica serovar Muenchen from pigs and humans and potential interserovar transfer of antimicrobial resistance. Antimicrob. Agents Chemother. 49, 503-511

Hendriksen, R.S., Mevius, D.J., Schroeter, A., Teale, C., Meunier, D., Butaye, P., Franco, A., Utinane, A., Amado, A., Moreno, M., Greko, C., Stark, K., Berghold, C., Myllyniemi, A.L., Wasyl, D., Sunde, M. and Aarestrup, F.M. (2008). Prevalence of antimicrobial resistance among bacterial pathogens isolated from cattle in different European countries: 2002-2004. Acta. Vet. Scand. 50, 28 doi: 10.1186/1751-0147-50-28

Kruse, H. and Sørum, H. (1994). Transfer of multiple drug resistance plasmids between bacteria of diverse origins in natural microenvironments. Appl. Environ. Microbiol. 60, 4015-4021

Mulvey, M.R., Boyd, D.A., Olson, A.B., Doublet, B. and Cloeckaert, A. (2006). The genetics of *Salmonella* genomic island 1. Microbes Infect. 8, 1915-1922

Phillips, I., Casewell, M., Cox, T., De Groot, B., Friis, C., Jones, R., Nightingale, C., Preston, R. and Waddell, J. (2004). Does the use of antibiotics in food animals pose a risk to human health? A critical review of the published data. J. Antimicrob. Chemother. 53, 28-52

Phillips, I. (2007). Withdrawal of growth-promoting antibiotics in Europe and its effects in relation to human health. Int. J. Antimicrob. Agents 30, 101-107

R Development Core Team. (2008). R: A language and environment for statistical computing. R Foundation for Statistical Computing, Vienna, Austria. ISBN 3-900051-07-0. http://www.R-project.org

Sherley, M., Gordon, D.M. and Collingnon, P.J. (2004). Evolution of multi-resistance plasmids in Australian clinical isolates of *Escherichia coli*. Microbiology 150, 1539-1546

Spratt, B.G., Hanage, W.P., Li, B., Aanensen, D.M. and Feil, E.J. (2004). Displaying the relatedness among isolates of bacterial species – the eBurst approach. FEMS Microbiol. Lett. 241, 129-134

Tenover, F.C. (2006). Mechanisms of antimicrobial resistance in bacteria. Am. J. Med. 119, S3-S10

Threlfall, E.J., Teale, C.J., Davies, R.H., Ward, L.R., Skinner, J.A., Graham, A., Cassar, C. and Speed, K. (2003). A comparison of antimicrobial susceptibilities in nontyphoidal salmonellas from humans and food animals in England and Wales in 2000. Microb. Drug Resist. 9, 183-189

Wassenaar, T.M. (2005). Use of antimicrobial agents in veterinary medicine and implications for human health. Crit. Rev. Microbiol. 31, 155-169

QUANTITATIVE RISK ASSESSMENT FOR THE ACQUISITION OF METICILLIN-RESISTANT *STAPHYLOCOCCUS AUREUS* (MRSA) IN DOGS

J. HELLER*, G.T. INNOCENT, L. KELLY, S.W.J. REID AND D.J. MELLOR

SUMMARY

Meticillin-resistant *Staphylococcus aureus* (MRSA) is an emerging companion animal infection with poorly described zoonotic potential. This study presents a quantitative risk assessment in the form of a second order stochastic simulation model with accompanying logistic regression sensitivity analysis that aims to define the most important factors for MRSA acquisition in dogs. Key findings are that both veterinary and non-veterinary routes of acquisition of MRSA are likely to be relevant for dogs. The most influential predictors for MRSA acquisition in dogs were found to be exposure to MRSA positive family members and attendance at veterinary clinics. Variations in the probability of transmission of MRSA from the (non-veterinary and veterinary) environment and from humans (family members and veterinary staff) were also found to be highly influential for MRSA acquisition in dogs.

INTRODUCTION

Meticillin-resistant *Staphylococcus aureus* is an important nosocomial and community-acquired pathogen with zoonotic potential. Although the relationship between MRSA in humans and companion animals is poorly defined, it is known that dogs may act as reservoirs of MRSA for humans and that the same strain is often found in dogs and humans inhabiting the same household, or veterinary workers in contact with infected dogs (Cefai et al., 1994; Manian, 2003; Leonard et al., 2006; Weese et al., 2006). MRSA found in dogs are indistinguishable from the most common hospital acquired strains isolated from humans (predominantly EMRSA-15, but also EMRSA-16 in the UK) and as such, it has not been possible to describe the direction of transfer between humans and dogs thus far (Baptiste et al., 2005; Rich et al., 2005; Weese et al., 2006; Leonard & Markey, 2007). While it is commonly acknowledged that dogs are likely to be the recipients of MRSA from humans and act as a secondary reservoir for potential reinfection or colonisation, rather than providing their own host-adapted source (Duquette & Nuttall, 2004; Rich et al., 2005), no conclusive evidence exists to support this. Consequently, while it is assumed that humans are the most important source of MRSA for dogs, it is not clear where the greatest risk for acquisition in dogs originates. Similarly, the potential contribution of dogs that carry or are infected with MRSA to the burden of disease in humans and conversely, the potential contribution of carrying, colonised and infected humans to canine disease, has not been directly quantified. Risk analysis is widely accepted and prescribed as a set of technical approaches that can be used to explore the combined effects of multiple factors implicated in a

* Jane Heller, Boyd Orr Centre for Population and Ecosystem Health, Institute of Comparative Medicine, Faculty of Veterinary Medicine, University of Glasgow, Bearsden, G61 1QH, UK. Email:j.heller@vet.gla.ac.uk

risk pathway. Critically, it is claimed that the first purpose and greatest strength of risk assessment is its ability to rank the effect of multiple inputs on a single output and thus identify high priority data gaps (or priority candidate mitigation targets) (Saltelli, 2000; Vose, 2000). In order to begin to quantify the contributions of dogs and humans to zoonotic transfer of MRSA, an initial assessment of the risk of acquisition of MRSA in dogs will allow the identification of important sources of the pathogen and the overall risk of acquisition of MRSA. Given the data-sparse nature of this field a secondary aim was to assess the ability of risk assessment to identify priority data gaps for future research.

While qualitative risk assessment is often used as the first step in assessing the risk from a putative hazard such as MRSA, an initial qualitative risk assessment in this area proved unsatisfactory due to a) failure of conformity of the specified model to sequential stepwise progression through defined events or modules and b) numerous complex dependencies between parameters and permutations that required consideration. In the absence of a rigorous qualitative assessment, a quantitative risk assessment was specified with the aim of defining important data gaps and influential areas for future research in this data-sparse field.

MATERIALS AND METHODS

Simulation model

A stochastic simulation model was developed to simulate the proportion of dogs that would acquire MRSA (as carriage, colonisation or infection) over a 24 hour period. The model structure was based on a pre-defined conceptual model that outlined the likely pathways of acquisition of MRSA for a single dog over a 24 hour time period. This model is presented elsewhere (Heller et al, submitted for publication) but, briefly, seven pathways for acquisition were specified and stratified to represent human (family member, non-family member or veterinary worker), animal (limited to dogs in the community or at veterinary clinics) and environmental sources of MRSA that could be accessed through community and veterinary hospital routes. The seven separate pathways for acquisition that were specified were considered to be non-sequential and not mutually-exclusive. The pathways available for each of the dogs that were simulated in the model depended on the result of an initial simulation of whether the dog in question attended a veterinary clinic or not in the 24 hours under consideration. All of the identified potential routes of acquisition of MRSA were accessible if a veterinary clinic was attended in the 24 hours under consideration but pathways were restricted to the community routes only if a veterinary clinic had not been attended during this period. Two sub-steps were considered within each pathway: first the risk of exposure to a positive source of MRSA (human, animal or environmental) and, secondly, the risk of transmission of MRSA from that source, given that exposure has occurred.

The simulation model was structured as a second-order nested stochastic model, accounting for uncertainty and dog-dependent variability. Variability was accounted for by the use of binomial distributions that were run for each dog using probabilities drawn from independent uncertainty distributions based on prior data (published, unpublished and expert opinion) and specified as beta or modified beta (PERT) distributions, run over a number of iterations. The probability of transmission (over 24 hours) was calculated using a scenario tree approach and defined by Eq. (1) as follows:

$$P(t_{24h}) = 1-(1-P(t_{contact}))^{contacts} \quad (1)$$

Where $P(t_{24h})$ is the probability of transmission per 24 hours, $P(t_{contact})$ is the probability of transmission per contact and contacts is the number of contacts per 24 hours.

The model was repeated, using the same input values, to obtain probabilistic results for colonisation of each dog over a number of days with no variation in environmental factors. As veterinary attendance is a rare event, the model was also re-run in full with the probability of a dog attending a veterinary clinic specified as 1 to obtain results for this population of animals separately.

Assumptions

In the current assessment, the hazard was defined as MRSA. A generalisation of 'MRSA positive' or 'MRSA negative' was used for human, animal and environmental status and refers to a source from which MRSA can be cultured directly and that has the ability to contaminate, colonise or infect others. This definition encompasses any limitations in test sensitivity and specificity that may be reflected in the real world.

Parameterisation

As this is a data-sparse area an expert opinion elicitation technique was undertaken to obtain data for model inputs at all steps within the simulation model where experimental or observational studies were unavailable. Briefly, useable opinions were obtained from 14 experts using a written questionnaire that followed previously defined techniques (Dillman, 1983; Vose, 2000) and the results for each parameter under consideration were combined with equal weightings. Experts were selected with varied backgrounds and experiences, spanning areas of medical and veterinary microbiology, antimicrobial resistance and epidemiology.

Sensitivity Analysis

A sensitivity analysis was undertaken using logistic regression to identify the steps of the simulation model associated with the greatest risk of MRSA acquisition. Two separate logistic regression models were run, assessing exposure and transmission explanatory variables respectively, for each of the simulation models, modelling all animals irrespective of veterinary attendance and only animals that had attended a veterinary clinic over the 24 hours in question, resulting in a total of four regression models. For all regression models, outcome was specified as MRSA positive or negative and explanatory variables considered for inclusion in each model are presented in Table 1. The regression models were fitted using a combined forwards and backwards stepwise algorithm, with improvement in Akaike's Information Criterion (AIC) used as the criterion for inclusion in the model.

Convergence

Prior to model implementation, convergence analyses were undertaken to define the number of simulation samples required to be taken: from the expert opinion distributions specified by each expert; for the combination of expert opinion elicited for each question, and for the uncertainty distributions to reach convergence. These analyses were undertaken by plotting the running mean for each iteration against the number of iterations used and convergence was assessed by visual comparison with the overall mean.

All simulation and statistical models were specified, implemented and analysed using R (R Development Core Team, 2008) and statistical significance was set at $P < 0.05$.

Table 1. Explanatory variables considered for logistic regression models used in the sensitivity analysis for acquisition of meticillin-resistant *Staphylococcus aureus* (MRSA) in dogs (all for a 24 hour time period)

Simulation model	Regression model	
	Exposure Model	Transmission model
All dogs	Number of MRSA contaminated environmental sites	P(transmission from environment)
	Number of MRSA positive family members	P(transmission from family member)
	Number of MRSA positive non family members	P(transmission from non family member)
	Number of MRSA positive dogs	P(transmission from dog)
	Attendance at veterinary clinic	P(attendance at veterinary clinic)
Dogs attending veterinary clinics only	Number of MRSA contaminated environmental sites	P(transmission from environment)
	Number of MRSA positive family members	P(transmission from family member)
	Number of MRSA positive non family members	P(transmission from non family member)
	Number of MRSA positive dogs	P(transmission from dog)
	Number of MRSA positive veterinary staff	P(transmission from veterinary staff)
	Number of MRSA contaminated veterinary environmental sites	P(transmission from environment at veterinary clinic)
	Number of MRSA positive dogs at veterinary clinic	P(transmission from dog at veterinary clinic)

RESULTS

Convergence analysis

The results of the convergence analysis showed that, for expert opinion results, convergence was reached for all experts and for the combination of all experts for all questions by 2000 iterations (examples presented in Fig. 1 and 2). Similarly, for the full simulation model, adequate convergence was reached by 1000 iterations (Fig. 3).

Overall uncertainty analysis

The model was run for 200 at-risk dogs over 1000 iterations, using 2000 samples to obtain and combine expert opinion distributions, as defined by the convergence analyses. While the model was specified as a second order model to take into account both variability (modelled between dogs) and uncertainty (modelled over iterations), it was not possible to differentiate between these two components of overall uncertainty within the outcome. The outcome of the model predicted the mean proportion of dogs that become positive for MRSA over any given 24 hour period to be 0.043 (95% simulation interval 0.042 – 0.044), represented by the distribution in Fig. 4.

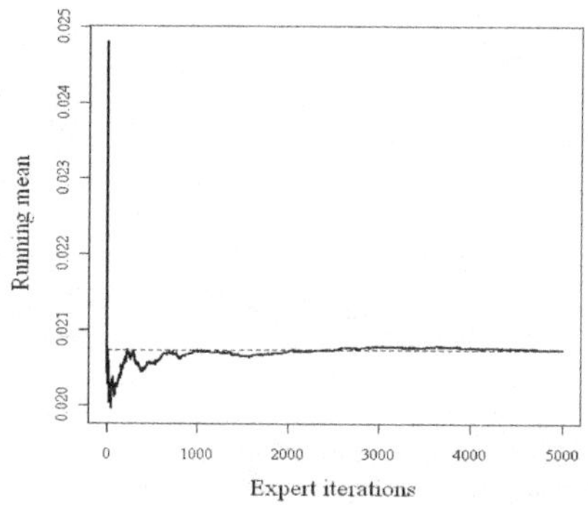

Fig. 1 Convergence analysis for the number of iterations required to obtain a representative distribution for a single expert and a single question from the Expert Opinion questionnaire for meticillin-resistant *Staphylococcus aureus* acquisition in dogs

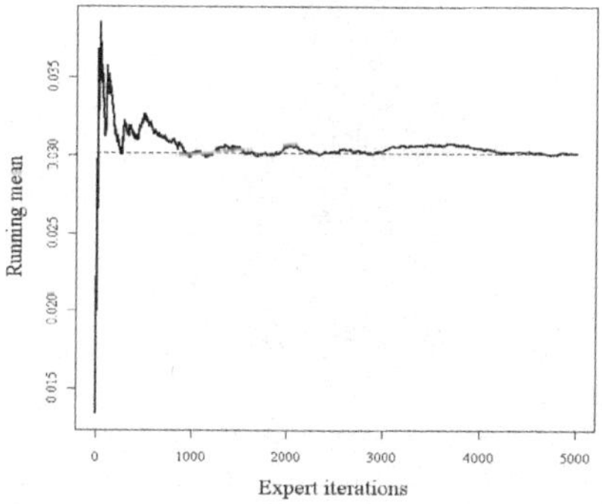

Fig. 2 Convergence analysis for the number of iterations required to obtain a representative distribution for the combination of the results of all experts for a single question in the Expert Opinion questionnaire for meticillin-resistant *Staphylococcus aureus* acquisition in dogs

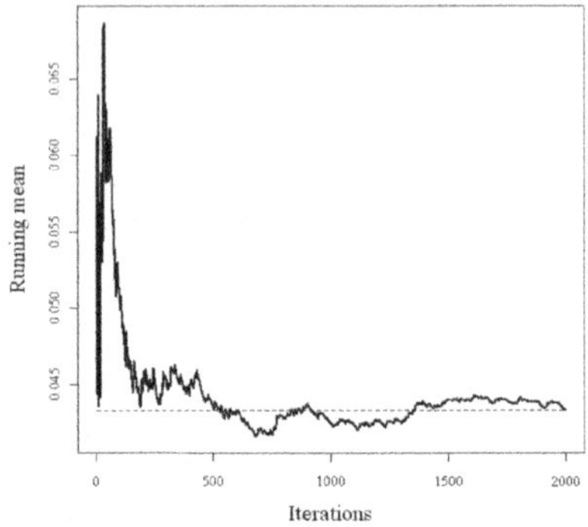

Fig. 3 Convergence analysis for number of iterations (samples from uncertainty distributions) required for the overall simulation model for meticillin-resistant *Staphylococcus aureus* acquisition in dogs

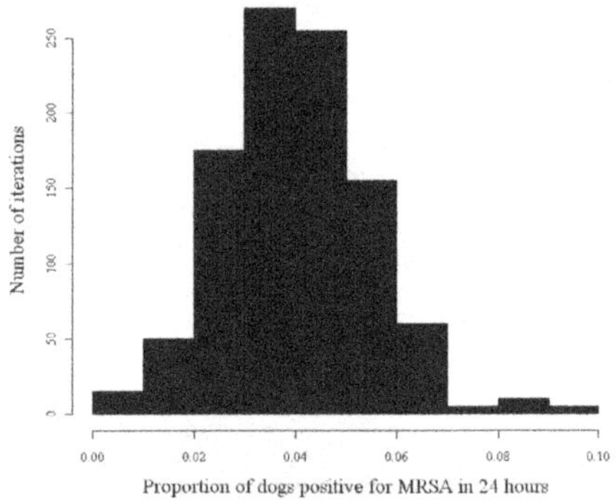

Fig. 4 Proportion of dogs positive for meticillin-resistant *Staphylococcus aureus* (MRSA) in 24 hours for a single model run with 1000 iterations of the simulation model for MRSA acquisition in dogs

Figure 5 shows the result of repeating the model over 50 iterations using static input parameters for each independent dog, for all 200 simulated dogs. Figure 6 shows the results of the same analysis but for a single dog over 50 repeats.

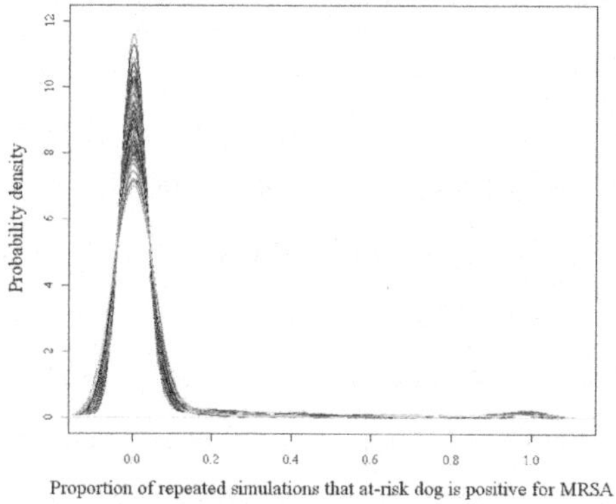

Fig. 5 Proportion of model repeats (N=50) that each dog (N=200) is positive for meticillin-resistant *Staphylococcus aureus* (MRSA) in a simulation model (1000 iterations) for MRSA acquisition in dogs

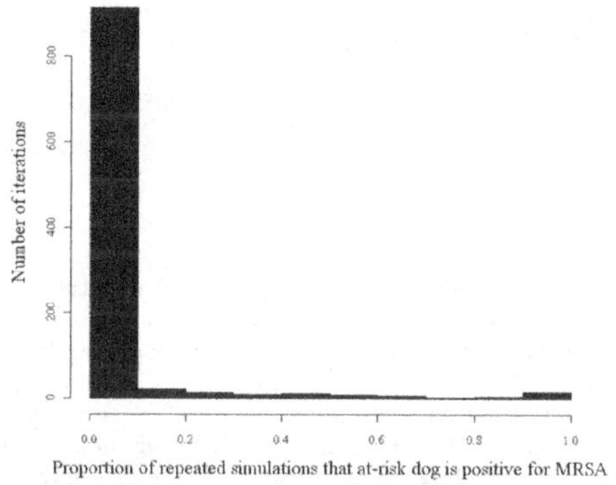

Fig. 6 Proportion of model repeats (N=50) that a single dog is positive for meticillin-resistant *Staphylococcus aureus* (MRSA) in simulation model (1000 iterations) for MRSA acquisition in dogs

Sensitivity analysis

The results of the separate exposure and probability of transmission logistic regression models that were specified for all dogs (irrespective of veterinary attendance) are presented in Table 2 and the regression models for dogs that attended a veterinary clinic over the 24 hours are presented in Table 3. The probability of transmission variables were categorised into five levels, the first of which represents a probability of 0 and the other four representing quartiles of the remaining observations.

Table 2. Results of logistic regression models run for all dogs under consideration in the simulation model for acquisition of meticillin-resistant *Staphylococcus aureus* (MRSA) in dogs

Model	Explanatory variable	Odds Ratio	95% Confidence Interval	P value
Exposure model	Number of MRSA contaminated environmental sites	1.16	1.15 – 1.17	<0.001
	Number of MRSA positive family members	10.30	9.11 – 11.64	<0.001
	Number of MRSA positive non family members	3.54	3.15 – 3.97	<0.001
	Number of MRSA positive dogs	4.41	3.72 – 5.22	<0.001
	Attendance at veterinary clinic	8.04	5.47 – 11.52	<0.001
Transmission model	P(transmission from environment)	7.86	7.32 – 8.47	<0.001
	P(transmission from non family member)	2.45	2.32 – 2.58	<0.001
	P(transmission from family member)	3.38	3.09 – 3.70	<0.001
	P(transmission from dog)	2.51	2.34 – 2.69	<0.001
	Attendance at veterinary clinic	22.80	15.10 – 33.55	<0.001

DISCUSSION

The results of this simulation study should be interpreted with care, given the lack of data, reliance on expert opinion estimates and complexity of the simulation model required to represent a largely undocumented biological process. Although iterative communication was maintained with experts in MRSA and risk analysts throughout the model-building process to ensure that any assumptions and parameterisations were well justified, caution in interpretation of model outputs is still required. However, the aim of the study in this instance was not to rely heavily on the absolute values of the outputs, but to use the results of the sensitivity analysis to define the most important and influential inputs with respect to the acquisition of MRSA in dogs and to inform the direction of future research activity in what might be considered a priority area.

Table 3. Results of logistic regression models run for dogs who have attended a veterinary clinic in the simulation model for acquisition of meticillin-resistant *Staphylococcus aureus* (MRSA) in dogs

Model	Explanatory variable	Odds Ratio	95% Confidence Interval	P value
Exposure model	Number of MRSA contaminated veterinary environmental sites	1.79	1.75 – 1.82	<0.001
	Number of MRSA positive veterinary staff	4.75	4.48 – 5.04	<0.001
	Number of MRSA contaminated environmental sites	1.09	1.08 – 1.10	<0.001
	Number of MRSA positive dogs at veterinary clinic	2.63	2.45 – 2.83	<0.001
	Number of MRSA positive family members	3.00	2.70 – 3.34	<0.001
	Number of MRSA positive non family members	1.39	1.28 – 1.52	<0.001
	Number of MRSA positive dogs	1.21	1.04 – 1.41	0.014
Transmission model	P(transmission from environment at veterinary clinic)	2.85	2.78 – 2.92	<0.001
	P(transmission from veterinary staff)	2.60	2.52 – 2.69	<0.001
	P(transmission from environment)	3.86	3.61 – 4.13	<0.001
	P(transmission from dog at veterinary clinic)	2.19	2.10 – 2.27	<0.001
	P(transmission from family member)	1.84	1.69 – 2.00	<0.001
	P(transmission from non family member)	1.28	1.23 – 1.33	<0.001
	P(transmission from dog)	1.28	1.20 – 1.38	<0.001

The output of the full simulation model shows that, on average, 4.3% of dogs (95% simulation interval 4.2% – 4.4%) will become positive for MRSA on any given day. It also predicts that, while most dogs will be negative on most occasions, a small proportion will be positive all of the time, depending on their input parameters, that is, there are some parameters (corresponding to exposures to and transmissions from certain sources) that are highly associated with the acquisition of MRSA. While it is not possible to corroborate or repudiate these results using data collection, given the temporal specification of the model along with the definition of 'MRSA positive' to encompass intermittent carriage, it is possible that this is an overestimation of reality, given previous cross-sectional estimates of MRSA nasal carriage in dogs of <1% (Rich & Roberts, 2006; Vengust et al., 2006; Hanselman et al., 2008). The structure of the simulation model used is dependent on individual estimation of contact and transmission information that is, for some parameters, collected by expert opinion and subsequently likely to encompass marked uncertainty. While this uncertainty is modelled to the best of our ability, the possibility of expert estimates to deviate from reality largely remains and, in the case of probability of transmission, is likely to continue to be unquantifiable given the inability to perform further data collection in this area due to ethical restrictions. Notwithstanding this, the output of the model presented herein is biologically plausible and allows the implementation of a sensitivity analysis, the output of which is the focus of this work.

The results of the logistic regression models show that the most influential predictors for MRSA acquisition in dogs include exposure to MRSA positive family members and veterinary clinic attendance. The number of MRSA positive family members that the at-risk dog is exposed to was also the second most important exposure variable for dogs that attended veterinary clinics, following exposure to MRSA positive veterinary staff. For exposures within a veterinary clinic, the greatest level of influence was found for exposure to veterinary staff, followed by exposure to dogs at a veterinary clinic and then exposure to the veterinary clinic environment. Within the regression models fitted to assess transmission parameters, the most influential variable was found to be attendance at a veterinary clinic. For animals that attended veterinary clinics, the probability of transmission from the community environment was the most influential variable (similarly reflected in the model specified for all dogs) followed by the probability of transmission from the veterinary clinic environment and from a veterinary staff member, respectively.

While the sensitivity analysis that has been undertaken is informative in defining the inputs to which the output of the model is most sensitive, and therefore most deserving of accurate quantification (Helton & Davis, 2000), it is incomplete insofar as many of the input variables of the simulation model have not been included in their primary form. This type of analysis does not facilitate inclusion and analysis of distributional or other basic input assumptions and while the effect of all variables are accounted for in the regression models through the inclusion of variables that are composites of many inputs, these inputs themselves cannot be examined. For example, in this study it is not possible to define whether the effect of a variable such as exposure to MRSA positive family members (to which the output is highly sensitive) is evenly distributed across all family members, whether it is greater for the primary owner, or whether it is dependent on owner risk group, all of which are included in the simulation model but cannot easily be included in the logistic regression sensitivity analysis due to their fine resolution, collinearity and potential for confounding. Similarly, interactions between input variables in the logistic regression have not been assessed in this analysis. Further research will be directed towards expanding the sensitivity analysis presented herein by assessing biologically plausible interactions between the variables in the logistic regression model and by implementing alternative sensitivity analysis techniques, such as factorial analysis, to account for a greater number and finer resolution of input variables. Consideration of the application and results of the current analysis highlights the practical complexity that limits the application of a truly global sensitivity analysis to a biological model such as this.

In addition, one must consider the usefulness of the results of a sensitivity analysis such as this. In this case, the finding that both veterinary and non-veterinary routes of acquisition are highly influential for MRSA acquisition in dogs is relevant and highlights the importance of continued research into the interaction between dogs and humans with respect to the zoonotic potential for MRSA. The exposure variables to which the output is highly sensitive provides information about where mitigation strategies might best be targeted, but the use of information about influential transmission parameters in the model provides a more difficult problem. While these variables (e.g. probability of transmission from the environment and from a veterinarian) are likely to benefit from further study and more accurate quantification, one must consider the practicality of undertaking these studies. The use of expert opinion, on which many of the input distributions for probabilities of transmission are based, resulted in marked uncertainty, reflected in large variation in expert responses, low confidence estimates and written comments imparting low assurance in the validity of the observations and is confirmed with the results of the logistic regression models. Given the expert comments, it is unlikely that this uncertainty is reducible by refinement of expert opinion technique. Furthermore, observational studies are likely to be inadequate for obtaining microorganism transfer data and experimental studies are not ethically tolerated and rarely represent real world situations with respect to this biological area. As such, the question is raised: does the identification of highly influential transmission variables merely quantify our unresolvable lack of knowledge?

The quantitative risk assessment and attendant sensitivity analysis that have been undertaken in this data-sparse area have improved on a previous qualitative risk assessment which returned unsatisfactory results due to the complexity of the specified model and lack of modular, sequential form. The approach that has been taken has identified veterinary and non-veterinary routes as important for the acquisition of MRSA in dogs and has also allowed the identification of influential exposure and transmission variables, but has raised many questions with respect to the subsequent use of this information.

ACKNOWLEDGEMENTS

This work was funded by DEFRA and SFC on the VTRI 0101 project. We also thank Matthew Denwood for his help in model coding.

[#] In this document, 'meticillin' has been used in place of 'methicillin' in accordance with the International Pharmacopoeia guidelines.

REFERENCES

Baptiste, K.E., Williams, K., Williams, N.J., Wattret, A., Clegg, P.D., Dawson, S., Corkill, J.E., O'Neill, T. and Hart, C.A. (2005). Methicillin-resistant staphylococci in companion animals. Emerg. Infect. Dis. 11(12), 1942-1944

Cefai, C., Ashurst, S. and Owens, C. (1994). Human carriage of methicillin-resistant *Staphylococcus aureus* linked with pet dog. Lancet. 344, 539-540

Dillman, D.A. (1983). Mail and other self-administered questionnaires, In: Rossi, P.H., Wright, J.D. Anderson, A.B., Eds. Handbook of survey research. Academic Press, New York, pp. 359-377

Duquette, R.A. and Nuttall, T.J. (2004). Methicillin-resistant *Staphylococcus aureus* in dogs and cats: an emerging problem? J.Small Anim. Pract. 45(12), 591-597

Hanselman, B.A., Kruth, S. and Weese, J.S. (2008). Methicillin-resistant staphylococcal colonization in dogs entering a veterinary teaching hospital. Vet. Microbiol. 126(1-3), 277-281

Helton, J.C. and Davis, F.J. (2000). Sampling-based methods. In: Saltelli, A., Chan, K., and Scott, E.M., Eds. Sensitivity Analysis. Chichester, John Wiley and sons Ltd, pp101-153

Leonard, F.C., Abbott, Y., Rossney, A., Quinn, P.J., O'Mahony, R. and Markey, B.K. (2006). Methicillin-resistant *Staphylococcus aureus* isolated from a veterinary surgeon and five dogs in one practice. Vet. Rec. 158(5), 155

Leonard, F.C. and Markey, B.K. (2007). Meticillin-resistant *Staphylococcus aureus* in animals: A review. Vet. J. 175(1), 27-36

Manian, F.A. (2003). Asymptomatic nasal carriage of mupirocin-resistant, methicillin-resistant Staphylococcus aureus (MRSA) in a pet dog associated with MRSA infection in household contacts. Clin. Infect. Dis. 36(2), e26-28

Saltelli, A. (2000). What is sensitivity analysis? In: Sensitivity Analysis, Saltelli, A., Chan, K. and Scott, E.M. (Eds.) John Wiley and Sons, Chichester, pp. 3-13

Rich, M. and Roberts, L. (2006). MRSA in companion animals. Vet. Rec. 159(16), 535-536

Rich, M., Roberts, L. and Kearns, A. (2005). Methicillin-resistant staphylococci isolated from animals. Vet. Microbiol. 105(3-4), 313-314

R Development Core Team (2008). R: A language and environment for statistical computing. Vienna, Austria

Vengust, M., Anderson, M.E., Rousseau, J. and Weese, J.S. (2006). Methicillin-resistant staphylococcal colonization in clinically normal dogs and horses in the community. Lett. Appl. Microbiol. 43(6), 602-606

Vose, D. (2000). Risk analysis: A quantitative guide, Second edition. John Wiley and Sons, Chichester

Weese, J.S., Dick, H., Willey, B.M., McGeer, A., Kreiswirth, B.N., Innis, B. and Low, D.E. (2006). Suspected transmission of methicillin-resistant Staphylococcus aureus between domestic pets and humans in veterinary clinics and in the household. Vet. Microbiol. 115(1-3), 148-155

GENETIC EPIDEMIOLOGY

SUSCEPTIBILITY TO PARATUBERCULOSIS IS ASSOCIATED WITH SINGLE NUCLEOTIDE POLYMORPHISMS IN BOVINE TOLL-LIKE RECEPTOR 2

A. KOETS*, W. SANTEMA, H. MERTENS, D. OOSTENRIJK, M. KEESTRA, M. OVERDIJK, R. LABOURIAU, P. FRANKEN, A. FRIJTERS, M. NIELEN AND V. RUTTEN

SUMMARY

Paratuberculosis is a chronic intestinal infection in ruminants, caused by Mycobacterium avium subspecies paratuberculosis (Map). To study the role of host genetics in disease susceptibility the Toll-like receptor 2 (TLR2) gene, selected based on its potential role in immunity to mycobacterial infections, was analysed for single nucleotide polymorphisms (SNP) and disease association.

Sequence analysis of the TLR2 gene and SNP discovery in a case-control study with 12 paratuberculosis infected animals, and 12 age-matched healthy herd-mates, revealed 21 different SNP. The TLR2-1903T/C SNP was significantly associated with resistance to Map. The allelic distribution of the TLR2-1903T/C SNP was subsequently confirmed to be significantly different between the infected and non-infected animals in a cohort study with 553 cows from farms with paratuberculosis.

In conclusion, this study identified genetic polymorphisms in bovine TLR2 which are associated with susceptibility to paratuberculosis in the Dutch Holstein-Frisian cattle population.

INTRODUCTION

Paratuberculosis (Johne's disease) is a chronic progressive infection of the intestinal mucosa in ruminants. It is caused by Mycobacterium avium subspecies paratuberculosis (Map), an intracellular pathogen, residing in host macrophages. The bacteria are excreted in faeces and milk of infected animals in later stages of the disease. The disease constitutes a worldwide threat to dairy cattle health. In addition, the presence of living bacteria in milk is a potential public health risk as Map has been implicated in the aetiology of human Crohn's Disease (Greenstein, 2003). In humans, host genetic variation has been known to influence resistance to infection and substantially influence the phenotype of infection following exposure to mycobacteria (Casanova and Abel, 2002). While in mice and humans several genes involved in resistance to mycobacterial infections have been studied in detail the data regarding cattle are scarce. Koets et al. (2000) indicated the presence of genetic variation in the susceptibility to paratuberculosis. Recent studies pointed at various chromosome regions or quantitative trait loci (QTL) associated with paratuberculosis (Gonda et al., 2006; Gonda et al., 2007). Two genes associated with innate

* Ad Koets, Department of Farm Animal Health, Epidemiology Division, Faculty of Veterinary Medicine, Utrecht University, Marburglaan 2, 3584 CL Utrecht, The Netherlands. Email: a.p.koets@uu.nl

immune responses, Nramp1 (Estonba et al., 2005) and Card15 (Pinedo et al., 2008), are highlighted as potentially involved in the mechanism of resistance to Map infection.

Infection of young calves mostly occurs after oral uptake of Map from food or the environment. After Map has crossed the intestinal barrier by M-cell-uptake, it is recognized by phagocytes, such as macrophages and dendritic cells (DCs) as part of the first line of defence against pathogens. Toll-like receptors (TLR) and cytosolic Nucleotide-binding Oligomerization Domain (NOD) receptors are, among other receptors, involved in the recognition of mycobacteria, as well as in stimulating phagocytosis and the development of cell mediated immunity (Quesniaux et al., 2004). Inefficient recognition of Map and failure in the subsequent innate and adaptive immune responses can be caused by defects in genes coding for TLR. TLR2 has been described as one of the main receptors for mycobacteria, and in humans, mutations in TLR2, have been detected and associated with higher susceptibility to tuberculosis (Kang and Chae, 2001; Ogus et al., 2004). After uptake, Map is able to evade the destructive processes by inhibition of phagolysosome fusion and is able to replicate inside the macrophages and possibly also inside DC (Hostetter et al., 2003; Weiss et al., 2004). These antigen presenting cells play a crucial role in the induction of adaptive immune responses and the polarization of T-helper-cells (Kalinski et al., 1999).

Resistance to intracellular pathogens such as Map predominantly depends on a T helper 1 (Th1) induction and effector phase of the acquired immune system. Production of interferon γ (IFNγ) by natural killer (NK) and T-cells is one of the first detectable signs of infection, indicating activation of cell mediated immunity (CMI). During the first stages of paratuberculosis (latent phase), a high level of CMI is present. Some cows remain in this stage for years; others rapidly progress to the subclinical and clinical stages of disease (Alzuherri et al., 1997). In these later phases, the Th1 cell mediated immune response declines to an undetectable low level and the amount of apparently non-protective antibodies increases. Loss of Th1-cells, i.e. potentially protective $CD4^+$ T cells, through apoptosis may be induced by macrophages and DCs via signalling mechanisms during cell to cell contact or via cytokines (Mustafa et al., 2001; Koets et al., 2002). The loss of protective CMI leads to a widely disseminated infection and uncontrolled growth of mycobacteria in macrophages, causing the clinical manifestation of paratuberculosis. Hence, following a prolonged period of chronic diarrhoea, weight loss and a decreased milk production, cows get emaciated and die from a protein losing enteropathy (Coussens, 2004). Regulatory T-cells may also play a role in suppression of Th1 activity, amongst others via the production of the immunosuppressive IL-10 (Weiss et al., 2005), and TLR2 may play a role in this process (Weiss and Souza, 2008). In cattle, TLR2 has been found to be expressed by myelomonocytic cells (monocytes, DC, macrophages and polymorphonuclear cells) and it is undetectable in resting or activated lymphoid subsets (Werling et al., 2004; Werling et al., 2006). Therefore, TLR2 may play a role in the recognition of intestinal pathogens, like mycobacteria, when these pathogens have crossed the intestinal epithelial barrier. Expression of TLR2 on bovine macrophages is eight times higher than that on DC (Werling et al., 2004). As bovine macrophages are the primary target cells in which Map is able to survive and replicate the TLR2 function may be critically important in paratuberculosis which is supported by recent studies by Weiss and Souza (2008).

The aim of the present study was to identify polymorphisms in TLR2 genes and to associate these SNP with different phenotypes of bovine paratuberculosis, as an indicator for high and low susceptibility to disease. Existence of genetic variants of TLR2 related to differences in resistance to paratuberculosis may enable marker assisted selection for MAP resistance.

MATERIALS AND METHODS

Study design and sources of bovine DNA

The DNA used in the case-control study was derived from 24 Holstein Friesian cows which originated from 12 different Dutch farms. The study population was divided into cases and controls; 12 cows in each group. Data from routine semi-quantitative faecal culture diagnostic tests (Jorgensen, 1982), conducted by the Dutch Animal Health Service, were used for primary classification. The cases shed Map in their faeces and showed clinical signs of paratuberculosis, which were confirmed by histopathology. The control cows were healthy age-matched herd-mates of the cases. Although the control cows had been kept in the same environment and were exposed to Map similar to the cases, they did not get infected, or cleared the infection. The clinical cows were defined as cows with a high susceptibility to paratuberculosis; the non-clinical control herd mates were defined as having a low susceptibility.

For confirmation studies following the SNP discovery in the case-control study, blood samples were collected from 553 adult cattle originating from an additional 8 farms with endemic paratuberculosis. These farms participated in a national program and their paratuberculosis status had been monitored for the last 4 years. Data from routine diagnostic tests for paratuberculosis conducted by the Dutch Animal Health Service, i.e. semi-quantitative faecal culture and absorbed ELISA (Institute Pourquier, France), were used to group animals by infection status. Data from 5 to 7 consecutive samplings over the period between January 2001 and November 2004 were analysed. Animals were only considered negative (uninfected) when all tests at all time points were negative. All other animals were considered to be infected with Map. Due to the nature of the Dutch Animal Health Service survey, no data were recorded regarding the clinical signs of paratuberculosis in these animals.

In 2007 an additional 50 animals were identified as being infected with paratuberculosis on 27 different farms (other than the farms used for previous studies) using a commercially available diagnostic ELISA (Pourquier) and confirmed by semi quantitative fecal culture by the Dutch Animal Health Service as described above.

Preparation of genomic DNA

As a source for genomic DNA peripheral blood mononuclear cells (PBMC, 22 cows) and whole blood (2 cows in the case control study and 553 cows in the confirmation study) were used. The PMBC had been obtained from whole blood earlier by density gradient centrifugation as published previously (Koets et al., 2002). The DNA from purified PBMC or whole blood was isolated using the DNA-Wizard-Kit (Promega, Madison, WI, USA), according to instructions provided by the manufacturer, and spectrophotometrically tested for yield and purity.

TLR2 primer design and DNA amplification

For SNP discovery in the case-control study primers were designed using Primer 3 web based software on the published sequence of TLR2 (AF368419). The coding (mRNA) sequence of TLR2 (2354 nucleotides (nt)) is located in one exon (exon 2) of the TLR2 gene which is located on chromosome Bta17. Five sets of primers were designed to generate amplicons by PCR between 526 and 822 nt in size from genomic DNA and covering the exon 2 completely. The primers used in this study are listed in Table 1.

Table 1. TLR2 primer sequences used for PCR amplification of TLR2 gene segments.

Primer	Sequence	Start Position	Amplicon (bp)
TLR2-1F	GGA CAA TGC CAC GTG CTT	192	552
TLR2-1R	GCA CTG ATC TCA AGC TCC TCA AG	744	
TLR2-2F	TGA GGA GCT TGA GAT CAG TG	724	822
TLR2-2R	ACT GTG TAT CCT TGT GCT GG	1546	
TLR2-3F	CCT AGG TAA TGT GGA GAC G	1111	574
TLR2-3R	AAG GAG GCA TCT GGT AGA G	1686	
TLR2-4F	CCA GCA CAA GGA TAC ACA GT	1527	526
TLR2-4R	CTT CAT GTA CCA CAG TCC GT	2053	
TLR2-5F	TTC CTG TTG CTC CTG CTC AC	1991	599
TLR2-5R	GAC CAC CAC CAG ACC AAG AC	2590	

PCR reactions were performed in a total volume of 40 µL containing 100 ηg of genomic DNA, 1.0 U pfu-polymerase (Promega, Madison, WI, USA), 10 x reaction buffer with MgSO4 (Promega, Madison, WI, USA), and final concentrations of 200 µM dNTPs (Invitrogen, Carlsbad, CA, USA) and 0.2-0.8 µM of forward and reverse primer (Invitrogen, Carlsbad, CA, USA). The PCR reaction mix was subjected to 30 cycles of amplification in an iCycler PCR system (Bio-Rad, Hercules, CA, USA). The cycling profile started with a 2-min step at 95 °C, followed by 30 cycles of 30 sec at 95 °C denaturation, 30 sec at 41–56 °C annealing (primer dependant) and 30 sec at 72 °C extension. The PCR products were analyzed by electrophoresis in 1% agarose gels, stained with ethidium bromide, and expected size was checked using appropriate molecular weight DNA standards (Massruler, Fermentas, Burlington, Ontario, Canada)

SNP Discovery

PCR products were bidirectionally sequenced by VIB Genetic Service Facility, Antwerp, Belgium, using ExoSAPIT (USB, Cleveland, OH, USA) for PCR cleanup and BigDye Terminator v3.1 Cycle sequencing reaction on an automated DNA Analyzer (Applied Biosystems, Foster City, CA, USA). Primers used for sequencing were the same as used for DNA amplification (table 1). The reference sequence was chosen based on the available Genbank sequence AF368419. The sequences of the PCR products were compared with this reference sequence by novoSNP software, which allowed detection of sequence variations, like SNP (Weckx et al., 2005).

SNP detection

Selected SNP (non monomorphic variants with a frequency larger than 10%) of TLR2 were selected for analysis in the larger cattle population (n=553). The SNP genotyping was again outsourced to the VIB Genetic Service Facility, Antwerp, Belgium and performed using a mass-spectrometry based SNP genotyping technique (Mass-array SNP genotyping, Sequenom, San Diego, CA, USA).

Measurement of bovine TLR2 induced NFκB activity

To study the functional consequences of different haplotypes of TLR2, an NFκB driven luciferase reporter assay was used. Primers were designed on the coding region of bovine TLR2 (GenBank accession no AF368419), downstream of the region coding for the signal peptide (first 60 bases of the coding sequence). The forward and reverse primers were TLR2F 5'-GAATTCGGCTGTCATCATCCTGCTCA-3', containing an enzyme-restriction site (EcoRI), and TLR2R 5'-GACCACCACCAGACCAAGAC-3', respectively. The amplified TLR2 DNA was ligated into a pGEMTeasy-vector (Promega, Madison, WI, USA) and E. coli DH5α-cells (Invitrogen, Carlsbad, CA, USA) were transformed with this vector. The TLR2-containing plasmid was isolated from confirmed DH5α-clones, and digested using the enzymes EcoRI and BamHI. This fragment was isolated and ligated in the p-FLAG-CMV-1 expression-vector (Sigma-Aldrich, St. Louis, MO, USA). Insert identity of the cloned genes in the pFLAG-CMV-1 vector was confirmed by sequencing.

The human embryonic kidney cell line 293 (HEK293 cells) was obtained from American Type Culture Collection (ATCC), USA and grown according to instructions provided. HEK293 cells were plated at $3.8x10^5$ cells/well in a 24-well plate (Costar, Cambridge, MA, USA) on the day before transfection. The cells were transfected using Lipofectamine 2000 (Invitrogen, Carlsbad, CA, USA) with 0,1μg NFκB-Luciferase reporter construct (Stratagene, La Jolla, CA, USA), 0.14 μg PDM-LacZ plasmid and 0.26 μg of the p-FLAG-CMV-1-vector, containing the relevant TLR2 DNA insert. For mock-transfection, the HEK293 cells were transfected with the 1μg NFκB-Luciferase reporter construct, 0.14 μg LacZ as well and 0.26 μg of the p-FLAG-CMV-1-vector, without the TLR2 DNA insert.

Forty-eight hours after transfection, the cells were stimulated with various final concentrations of synthetic tripalmitoylated lipopeptides PAM3CSK4 (palmitoyl-3-cysteine-serine-lysine-4) (200 and 500 ηg/ml), PAM2CSK4 (200 and 500 ηg/ml), Map ($0.7x10^6$, $1.4x10^6$ and $2.8x10^6$ bacteria/ml, multiplicity of infection (moi) of 2, 4 and 8 respectively) and recombinant Map Hsp70 (1, 5 and 10 μg/ml) in 500 μl medium for 5 hours. The cells were then lysed and luciferase activity was measured, using the luciferase assay system (Promega, Madison, WI, Madison, USA) according to the manufacturer's instructions, in relative light units (RLU) in a luminometer (Turner Design, Sunnyvale CA, USA). Luciferase activity was corrected via co-transfected LacZ-activity to account for differences in transfection efficiency. LacZ-activity was measured spectrophotometrically (Ultrospec 2000 UV/vis spectrophotometer, Amersham Pharmacia Biotech Ltd, Buckinghamshire, England). Relative luciferase activity is defined as the ratio of the luciferase activity measured in cells after stimulation and cells without stimulation.

Flowcytometric evaluation of TLR2 expression in HEK293 cells

TLR2 protein expression levels, prior to and after stimulation of the TLR2 protein with the ligands described above, were determined on single cell level by flowcytometry. In short, transfected HEK293 cells and mock transfected controls were stained with the M2 antibody which recognizes the N-terminal expressed FLAG epitope, present on the N-terminus of the extracellular LRR of expressed TLR2 molecules, according to instructions provided by the manufacturer (Sigma-Aldrich, St. Louis, MO, USA). Alexa-633 labeled goat-anti-mouse antibodies were used for indirect staining according to instructions provided the manufacturer (Molecular Probes - Invitrogen Carlsbad, CA, USA). Fluorescence of 20,000 cells per treatment was acquired on a FacsCalibur (BD Biosciences, San Jose, CA, USA) and analyzed using Cellquest software (BD Biosciences, San Jose, CA, USA).

Statistical analyses

Statistical analyses were done using the R software package (R Development Core Team, 2008).

To determine whether an association between genotype and susceptibility to paratuberculosis could be identified, we investigated the allelic association of SNP in the case-control group. Fisher exact tests with correction for multiple comparisons were used to compare the SNP-distribution in both groups. Several tests were performed, therefore the p-value of each test was corrected for the effect of test using a FDR (False Discovery Rate) (Benjamini and Hochberg, 1995). After adjusting for multiple comparisons, tests with (adjusted) p-values smaller than 0.05 were considered significant (Wright, 1992).

The cohort (confirmation) study was analysed using binomial logistic models (i.e. a generalized linear mixed model for binary response defined with a logistic link function) with the response variable given by a binary indicator of the paratuberculosis diagnosis. Several combinations of the five informative SNP markers were used as discrete explanatory variables, as described below. The SNP markers entered in the model as dominant markers, that is, each factor had two levels: homozygous of wild type or a genotype containing at least one variation allele (i.e. heterozygous or homozygous of variation type). All the logistic regressions contained a normal random factor representing the farm.

A global simultaneous association test was performed by comparing, via the likelihood ratio test, a full model containing simultaneously factors representing each of the five informative SNP markers (and a factor representing the farm) against a null model containing only a factor representing the farm (and none representing the five SNP markers).

Following the methodology described in Labouriau et al., (2008) we fitted a series of logistic models containing combinations of the five informative SNP markers, in order to identify possible associations with complex haplotypes. The model with smaller BIC (Bayesian Information Criterion or Schartz Information Criterion) was chosen among all the possible models formed with combinations of the five SNP markers. According to the general theory of model selection for generalized linear models, this procedure finds the model that best represent the data (Haughton, 1988). Similar results were obtained when using the AIC (Akaike Information Criterion) as the selection criteria.

Functional response differences between animals with the different TLR2 haplotypes in the luciferase reporter assay, were analyzed using a Students T-test. A p-value of <0.05 was considered significant.

RESULTS

Identification of disease associated SNP in the case-control population

In total 5 PCR amplicons from exon 2 of the TLR2 gene were sequenced from each of the 24 animals in the case-control study. Using the novo-SNP program, 82 polymorphisms were identified in 21 unique positions in the coding sequence (exon 2) of bovine TLR2 from 12 clinical (cases) and 12 non-clinical (controls) cows. The results are summarized in table 2. The 21 different SNP were detected in 5 amplicons, each amplicon contained 4 (n=4) or 5 (n=1) SNP. As 15 of the detected SNP were only found in one of 24 animals these were considered non-informative for the present study. Except for one SNP (827A/G), the animals were heterozygous for the SNP (97.6% heterozygosity). The majority of these SNP are transitions (64 out of 82 SNP (78%), largely determined by G>A and T>C substitutions). Fifteen T↔G transversions were identified (18.3%). In this study, the ratio transitions: transversions was 78.0:18.3 (4:1). Fifty-six of the 82 (68.3%) SNP are non-synonymous and caused an amino acid substitution (table 2). The ratio non-synonymous:synonymous is 56:26 (2.2:1). Eighty-two SNP give an average SNP frequency of 3.4 SNP per TLR2 gene sequenced (1 SNP per 689 bp).

Seventy-five SNP (91%) were located in the extra cellular leucine rich repeat (LRR) domain, which is used for ligand recognition. In one non-clinical animal 2 SNP were detected in the transmembrane domain and 5 in the TIR-domain, the intracellular signalling domain. The average SNP frequency per domain indicated that the LRR- domain had one SNP per 545 bp; the transmembrane domain one SNP per 756 bp and the TIR-domain one per 2098 bp.

Fifty-six non-synonymous SNP were found (10 different ones), 55 of 56 were located in the LRR-domain, none in the transmembrane- and 1 in the TIR-domain. The average frequency of non-synonymous SNP per domain was one SNP per 730 bp regarding the LRR-domain and one SNP per 10488 bp in the TIR-domain. In summary, the SNP at basepair position 385, 651, 798, 1828 and 1903 were seen frequently in the case-control study. Based on the Fisher exact test the 1903T/C SNP showed significantly different allelic distribution (p=0.045) between cases and controls, in addition the 1828C/T SNP showed a trend (p=0.097) (Table 2).

Table 2. SNP detected in bovine TLR2

SNP Position	Codon Change	Amino Acid **Change**	SNP frequency		p-value	**TLR2 Domain**
			Case	Control		
382	aat→aac	N=N	0	1	n.s.	putative LRR
385	*gat→gag*	*D→E*	*5*	*8*	*n.s.*	putative LRR
398	*ggc→agc*	*G→S*	*0*	*1*	*n.s.*	putative LRR
651	*cgg→cag*	*R→Q*	*4*	*7*	*n.s.*	putative LRR
798	*agc→aac*	*S→N*	*4*	*7*	*n.s.*	putative LRR
827	*att→gtt*	*I→V*	*7*	*8*	*n.s.*	putative LRR
1141	cgg→cgt	R=R	0	1	n.s.	putative LRR
1174	*cat→caa*	*H→Q*	*0*	*1*	*n.s.*	putative LRR
1206	*aga→aaa*	*R→K*	*0*	*1*	*n.s.*	putative LRR
1446	*aac→agc*	*N→S*	*0*	*1*	*n.s.*	putative LRR
1504	gga→ggc	G=G	0	1	n.s.	putative LRR
1828	ttc→ttt	F=F	2	6	0.097	putative LRR
1884	*cgc→cac*	*R→H*	*0*	*1*	*n.s.*	putative LRR
1903	**cat→cac**	**H=H**	**2**	**7**	**0.045**	putative LRR
1975	gct→gcc	A=A	0	1	n.s.	transmembrane
1978	gcg→gct	A=A	0	1	n.s.	transmembrane
2191	*cac→cag*	*H→Q*	*0*	*1*	*n.s.*	*TIR*
2221	cat→cac	H=H	0	1	n.s.	TIR
2251	att→atc	I=I	0	1	n.s.	TIR
2410	gag→gaa	E=E	0	1	n.s.	TIR
2491	ccc→cct	P=P	0	1	n.s.	TIR

Confirmation of SNP disease associations in the cohort study

The 5 SNP potentially associated with susceptibility to paratuberculosis were studied in 553 cattle originating from 8 farms with endemic paratuberculosis. Analysis of age distribution between paratuberculosis negative (average age 5.5 ± 1.8 years at final sampling) and positive (average age 5.2 ± 1.8 years at final sampling) cattle showed no significant differences. The average prevalence of paratuberculosis positive animals at the farm level at the last sampling time point was 32.2% and ranged from 22.2 – 56.0%. In these 8 farms the prevalence of infection was increasing in the 4 years of observations. The results from the binomial logistic model indicated a significant effect of farm and therefore results were corrected for herd of origin by introducing this factor in all the subsequent analyses. No statistically significant interactions between farm and the SNP markers were found. The SNP analysis on DNA from blood taken from the 553 animals present at the last sampling is summarized in Table 3.

Table 3. SNP typing and disease association in the cohort study

	MAP TEST NEGATIVE		MAP TEST POSITIVE		
TLR2 SNP ID	**CC+CT**	**TT**	**CC+CT**	**TT**	**P-VALUE**
SNP01-1903 T/C	58	248	68	176	0.0093
SNP03-1828 C/T	57	251	63	181	0.07
SNP05-385 G/T	71	228	82	159	0.06
SNP06-651 G/A	66	242	69	174	n.s.
SNP08-798 G/A	66	242	66	177	n.s.

The global simultaneous association test (i.e. a likelihood ratio test comparing a model containing factors representing all the SNP markers and a model where the markers are not represented) presented a p-value of 0.00024, indicating that at least one marker or one combination of markers was associated with resistance/susceptibility to paratuberculosis. The model with smallest BIC among all the possible models containing combinations of the five SNP markers was a model containing only the marker SNP01 TLR2-1903 T/C, confirming the preliminary association found in the case-control study. The allelic distribution and disease association of the SNP01 TLR2-1903 T/C was confirmed (p=0.0093), minor effects were found for the SNP03 TLR2-385 T/G (p=0.07) and the SNP05 TLR2-1828 C/T SNP (p=0.06). However the latter 2 were conditional on the presence of TLR2-1903 T/C (Table 3). For the remaining 2 SNP no significant allelic distribution between infected and non-infected animals was observed. In addition, none of the possible combinations for the 5 SNP indicated a significant association for a single combination. For the SNP01 TLR2-1903 T/C the Odds Ratio (O.R.) was calculated, similar to the dominance model used for the association the TT genotype was compared to CT and CC genotypes. That comparison lead to an O.R. of 1.64 (95% CI: 1.13<O.R.<2.43) for animals to be Map infected given the presence of the TLR2-1903 T/C mutation (i.e. the CT and CC genotypes).

Functional consequences of SNP in bovine TLR2

The three genes that were selected to study functional effects of SNP, had SNP in the extra cellular LRR domain of the molecule only; the transmembrane and intracellular parts of these TLR2 molecules were identical. One TLR2 gene was cloned from a healthy animal (no disease association, identical to the reference sequence), additionally 2 genes were selected from an animal with clinical signs of disease (TLR2K_S) and a healthy control animal (TLR2K_R) respectively, based on the SNP01 TLR2-1903T/C SNP types of these animals, respectively CC and TT. The results of resequencing of the genes which were cloned into the pCMV-FLAG expression vector indicated that the genes of the diseased and the healthy cow were different with respect to SNP01 TLR2-1903T/C and three additional, previously identified, positions leading to 3 non-synonymous point mutations as indicated in Fig. 1. It was also confirmed that all mutations were in extra cellular parts of the TLR2 molecules, the transmembrane and intracellular signalling parts were identical at protein level (not shown).

		1 50
	TLR2K_S	*MPRALWTAWV W*AVIILLTEGA SDQASSLSCD PTGVCDGHSR LNSIPSGLT
	TLR2K_R	*MPRALWTAWV W*AVIILLTEGA SDQASSLSCD PTGVCDGHSR LNSIPSGLT
		51 100
	TLR2K_S	AGVKSLDLSN NDITYVGNRD LQRCVNLKTL RLGANEIHTV EEDSFFHLRN
	TLR2K_R	AGVKSLDLSN N**E**ITYVGNRD LQRCVNLKTL RLGANEIHTV EEDSFFHLRN
t385g (D-E)		
		101 150
	TLR2K_S	LEYLDLSYNR LSNLSSSWFR SLYVLKFLNL LGNLYKTLGE TSLFSHLPNL
	TLR2K_R	LEYLDLSYNR LSNLSSSWFR SLYVLKFLNL LGNLYKTLGE TSLFSHLPNL
g651a (R-Q)		
		151 200
	TLR2K_S	RTLKVGNSNS FTEIHEKDFT GLTFLEELEI SAQNLQIYVP KSLKSIQNIS
	TLR2K_R	**Q**TLKVGNSNS FTEIHEKDFT GLTFLEELEI SAQNLQIYVP KSLKSIQNI**N**
g798a (S-N)		
		201 250
	TLR2K_S	HLILHLKQPV LLVDILVDIV SSLDCFELRD TNLHTFHFSE ASISEMSTSV
	TLR2K_R	HLILHLKQPV LLVDILVDIV SSLDCFELRD TNLHTFHFSE ASISEMSTSV

Fig. 1 Differences at protein level between the cloned TLR2 molecules from an cow with clinical signs of paratuberculosis (TLR2K_S) and resistance to paratuberculosis infection (TLR2K_R). The first 250 amino acids of the TLR2 protein (773 amino acids) are shown; from amino acid 12 onwards the sequence was cloned into the pCMV-FLAG expression plasmid and confirmed by sequencing for each cloned molecule. Differences at amino acid level between resistant and susceptible genetic variants are indicated by bold-underlined amino acids in the resistant TLR2. The corresponding nucleotide SNP is indicated on the left. In addition these two molecules differed at nucleotide level at position 1903 (SNP01 TLR2-1903T/C). TLR2K_S had a CC genotype, TLR2K_R had a TT genotype. The SNP01 TLR2-1903T/C does not lead to a change in amino acid sequence.

There was no detectable difference in the level of expression of the 3 cloned TLR2 genes in both stimulated and unstimulated pCMV-FLAG transfected HEK293 cells, as measured by flow cytometric detection of the N-terminal FLAG tag. (data not shown)

Transfection of HEK293 cells with the TLR2 gene cloned from the healthy animal resulted in NFκB-driven luciferase activity that was up-regulated in a dose-dependent manner after stimulation of the cells with PAM3CSK4, and PAM2CSK4 (Fig. 2).

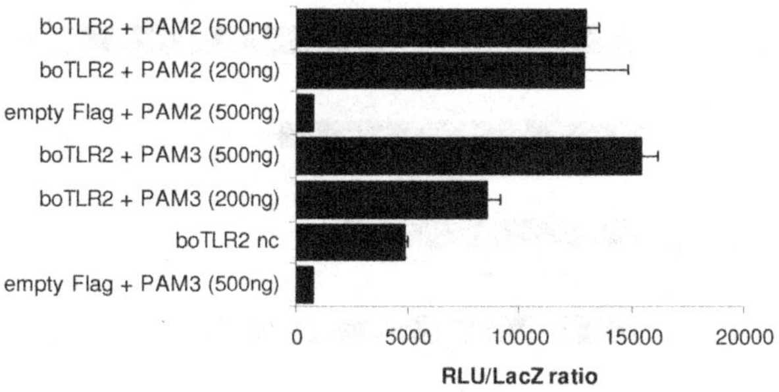

Fig. 2 TLR2-NFkB-Luciferase reporter system. The functionality of bovine TLR2 molecules in HEK293 cells transfected with the pFLAG-CMV-1-boTLR2 (boTLR2) or empty pFLAG vector (empty Flag), luciferase and LacZ reporter vectors is shown. Transfected cells were stimulated with ligands PAM2CSK4 (PAM2) or PAM3CSK4 (PAM3) at indicated concentrations, or not stimulated (bo TLR2 nc). A representative example of 3 independent experiments is shown. Luciferase activity was measured as Relative Light Units (RLU) and corrected for transfection efficacy based on the LacZ reporter gene activity (RLU/LacZ ratio).

In addition responses were also observed upon stimulation of cells with Map and recombinant Map Hsp70 protein (data not shown). No activation was observed in the mock-transfected HEK293 cells. We next investigated the effect of the disease associated haplotypes on the functionality of TLR2 i.e. NFκB activity. Stimulation with PAM3CSK4 resulted in NFκB activation with both haplotypes tested. The resistant haplotype showed significantly ($p<0.05$) higher responses to PAM3CSK4, which was also observed upon stimulation with 3 tested Map concentrations (Fig. 3). The recombinant Map Hsp70 protein did induce NFκB activation, but although the resistant haplotype had consistently higher average responses no significant differences were observed (data not shown).

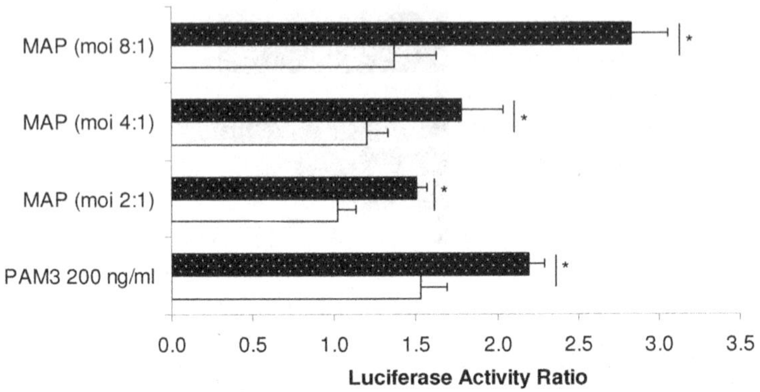

Fig. 3 Functional effects of TLR2 polymorphisms. The functional effects of disease associated (light bars) and resistant (dark bars) TLR2 haplotypes is shown when stimulated with indicated concentrations of the ligands PAM3CSK4 (PAM3), and Mycobacterium avium ssp paratuberculosis (Map) (at 3 multiplicities of infection (moi) indicating the number of Map cfu per cell). The luciferase activity was measured in Relative Light Units, corrected for transfection efficiency (LacZ) and related to unstimulated controls and the ratio is expressed as the luciferase activity ratio. Results of 3 independent experiments were combined. Differences which were tested as significantly different ($p<0.05$) between sensitive and resistant haplotypes using students t-test are indicated (*).

DISCUSSION

The results of the current study indicate that polymorphisms in the TLR2 gene, are likely to be involved in susceptibility to bovine paratuberculosis. In the case-control study the cases were cows with positive faecal culture that also showed symptoms of clinical paratuberculosis and as such were an extreme phenotype of the disease. In the farm level cohort study no records were available regarding the presence or absence of symptoms and classification of animals was exclusively done combining ELISA and faecal culture results. Nevertheless significant differences in allelic distribution of genetic polymorphisms in TLR2, in particular SNP01 TLR2 1903 T/C, associated with disease status were found that confirmed results of the case-control study. In the cohort study a significant farm effect was found. This was attributable to differences in prevalence of infection on these different farms. On one hand a higher prevalence may signify a relative abundance of susceptible animals. The lack of statistically significant interactions between farm and the SNP markers indicated that genetic differences between these populations were unlikely to be cause of the differences observed. On the other hand a difference between farm prevalence may be a result of management differences, a factor not taken into account in this study. Infection prevalence is an important issue in these studies as the chance of misclassifying faecal culture negative animals as 'resistant' increases if the overall infection pressure on a farm is lower and not all animals are (equally) exposed to Map as young stock.

The ratio non-synonymous:synonymous SNP indicates whether non-synonymous polymorphisms have caused a negative selection (ratio<1), a positive selection (ratio>1) or whether they are neutral (ratio=1) (Park et al., 2000). The ratio of 2.2:1, which we found with respect to TLR2 SNP, indicates a positive selection for non-synonymous polymorphisms in bovine TLR2. Average frequencies of one SNP per 689 bp regarding all SNP, and one non-synonymous SNP per 1009 bp were found. These are lower frequencies than reported in previous studies of other genes in cattle: an average of one SNP per 143 bp (± 62 bp) (Heaton et al., 2001) and one SNP per 90 bp (White et al., 2003) have been described. However, our data are consistent with SNP frequencies, described in humans (Bronte et al., 1998; Del Prete, 1998). These data are in line with studies in bovine, human and mouse TLR4 (Smirnova et al., 2001; Smirnova et al., 2000; White et al., 2003). In addition, the small number of non-synonymous SNP in the transmembrane and TIR-domain, confirms data about those conserved domains.

Previous studies in humans have shown that two mutations in TLR2, an Arg753Gln polymorphism and an Arg677Trp polymorphism, were associated with susceptibility to disease (Kang and Chae, 2001; Lorenz et al., 2000). Both mutations are located at the C-terminus of the TLR2, in the TIR-domain, and could affect the intracellular signalling function of the TLR. This is in contrast with the mutations observed in bovine TLR2 which are predominantly located in the extracellular ligand recognition domain. The Arg753Gln polymorphism has been associated with a negative influence on TLR2 signalling, increasing the risk to among others mycobacterial infections (Mycobacterium leprae and Mycobacterium tuberculosis) (Lorenz et al., 2000; Ogus et al., 2004). Bochud et al., (2003) have shown that the Arg677Trp mutation prohibits the Toll-pathway and production of NFkB.

A recent study of Pinedo et al., (2008) revealed SNP in the innate immune response CARD15/NOD2 gene in cattle which were associated with susceptibility to paratuberculosis. The associations observed in that study are similar to the associations observed in the TLR2 SNP. The O.R. of the CARD15 C733R is 3.35 in the study of Pinedo et al., (2008) and approximately twice as high as the O.R. for the TLR2 1903T/C, estimated in the current study. The TLR2 SNP 1903T/C, 1828T/C are both synonymous and do not lead to amino acid changes, however the 385T/G mutation leads to an amino acid change in the extra cellular ligand recognition domain of TLR2 and may lead to functional changes.

Our data on the function of TLR2 with synthetic lipopeptides confirm that PAM3CSK4 is recognized by bovine TLR2 (Aliprantis et al., 1999) and, that PAM2CSK4 is able to signal via TLR2, without TLR6 (Buwitt-Beckmann et al., 2005). Stimulation with Map, of which some cell wall components are ligands for TLR2, resulted in a lower response, compared to the response to the synthetic lipopeptides. This difference may be due to the concentrations used as PAM3CSK4 and PAM2CSK4 are purified, synthetic ligands in contrast to Map. Comparing the responses of cells transfected with TLR2, derived from cows with SNP associated with a susceptible versus a resistant phenotype, the latter showed the highest activity, after stimulation with PAM3CSK4 and especially after stimulation with Map. The other 3 common SNP in TLR2 represented in this susceptible versus resistant phenotype comparison are non-synonymous and despite the fact that no significant association was found with infection status these SNP lead to functional changes. These SNP are in the extracellular LRR part of TLR2 and lead to attenuation of NFκB signalling. The mutation CARD15 C733R, identified in the study of Pinedo et al., (2008) in this intracellular bacterial receptor may lead to attenuated NFκB signalling, as has been reviewed by Strober et al., (2006), although this has not been studied in cattle.

The current functional studies support the hypothesis that an attenuated TLR2 function is a risk factor for developing clinical paratuberculosis. Recent studies by Weiss et al., (2007) suggest an important role for TLR2 in regulating the intracellular fate of Map and our macrophage data support differential handling of Map vs. Maa organisms in terms of cytokine gene transcription.

In conclusion, cows with a susceptible haplotype may start the clinical phase of paratuberculosis at a younger age, or the clinical phase will be more severe, as a consequence of decreased cell mediated immune responses. However, more research into the functional effects of SNP and the downstream effects on protective Th1 type responses is needed. As suggested by other studies combined polygenic effects are likely involved in the pathogenesis. Particularly a combined study of the CARD15 and TLR2 polymorphisms should be considered, since they clearly point to functional differences in innate immune responses of macrophages in which mycobacteria manage to survive bacteriocidal mechanisms. Ultimately, the TLR2 and additional SNP may be useful in marker assisted breeding strategies, screening for risks for disease and improving the genetic resistance of cattle to paratuberculosis. Breeding of more resistant animals can be used as an additional method to control paratuberculosis in cattle populations besides management, test and cull and vaccination strategies.

ACKNOWLEDGEMENTS

This study was supported by a grant from the Technology Foundation (STW) of the Dutch Research Council (NWO), grant number STW-UDG5589.

REFERENCES

Aliprantis, A.O., Yang, R.B., Mark, M.R., Suggett, S., Devaux, B., Radolf, J.D., Klimpel, G.R., Godowski, P., Zychlinsky, A., 1999, Cell activation and apoptosis by bacterial lipoproteins through toll-like receptor-2. Science 285, 736-739.

Alzuherri, H.M., Little, D., Clarke, C.J., 1997, Altered intestinal macrophage phenotype in ovine paratuberculosis. Res Vet Sci 63, 139-143.

Benjamini, Y., and Hochberg, Y. (1995). Controlling the false discovery rate: a practical and powerful approach to multiple testing. Journal of the Royal Statistical Society Series B, 57, 289–300.

Bochud, P.Y., Hawn, T.R., Aderem, A., 2003, Cutting edge: a Toll-like receptor 2 polymorphism that is associated with lepromatous leprosy is unable to mediate mycobacterial signaling. J Immunol 170, 3451-3454.

Bronte, V., Wang, M., Overwijk, W.W., Surman, D.R., Pericle, F., Rosenberg, S.A., Restifo, N.P., 1998, Apoptotic death of CD8+ T lymphocytes after immunization: induction of a suppressive population of Mac-1+/Gr-1+ cells. J Immunol 161, 5313-5320.

Buwitt-Beckmann, U., Heine, H., Wiesmuller, K.H., Jung, G., Brock, R., Akira, S., Ulmer, A.J., 2005, Toll-like receptor 6-independent signaling by diacylated lipopeptides. Eur J Immunol 35, 282-289.

Casanova, J.L., Abel, L., 2002, Genetic dissection of immunity to mycobacteria: the human model. Annu Rev Immunol 20, 581-620.

Coussens, P.M., 2004, Model for Immune Responses to Mycobacterium avium Subspecies paratuberculosis in Cattle. Infect. Immun. 72, 3089-3096.

Del Prete, G., 1998, The concept of type-1 and type-2 helper T cells and their cytokines in humans. Int Rev Immunol 16, 427-455.

Estonba, A., Iriondo, M., Oyanguren, O., Garrido, J.M., Geijo, M.V., Sevilla, I., Juste, R.A., 2005, Bovine 3'-UTR (GT11) variant of the NRAMP1 gene under-represented among paratuberculosis seropositive cattle. . Proceedings of the 8th International Colloquium on Paratuberculosis.

Gonda, M.G., Chang, Y.M., Shook, G.E., Collins, M.T., Kirkpatrick, B.W., 2006, Genetic variation of Mycobacterium avium ssp. paratuberculosis infection in US Holsteins. J Dairy Sci 89, 1804-1812.

Gonda, M.G., Kirkpatrick, B.W., Shook, G.E., Collins, M.T., 2007, Identification of a QTL on BTA20 affecting susceptibility to Mycobacterium avium ssp. paratuberculosis infection in US Holsteins. Anim Genet 38, 389-396.

Greenstein, R.J., 2003, Is Crohn's disease caused by a mycobacterium? Comparisons with leprosy, tuberculosis, and Johne's disease. Lancet Infect Dis 3, 507-514.

Haughton, D.M.A., 1988, On the choice of a model to fit data from an exponential family. The Annals of Statistics 16, 342-355.

Heaton, M.P., Grosse, W.M., Kappes, S.M., Keele, J.W., Chitko-McKown, C.G., Cundiff, L.V., Braun, A., Little, D.P., Laegreid, W.W., 2001, Estimation of DNA sequence diversity in bovine cytokine genes. Mamm Genome 12, 32-37.

Hostetter, J., Steadham, E., Haynes, J., Bailey, T., Cheville, N., 2003, Phagosomal maturation and intracellular survival of Mycobacterium avium subspecies paratuberculosis in J774 cells. Comparative Immunology, Microbiology and Infectious Diseases 26, 269-283.

Jorgensen, J.B., 1982, An improved medium for culture of Mycobacterium paratuberculosis from bovine faeces. Acta Vet Scand 23, 325-335.

Kalinski, P., Hilkens, C.M., Wierenga, E.A., Kapsenberg, M.L., 1999, T-cell priming by type-1 and type-2 polarized dendritic cells: the concept of a third signal. Immunol Today 20, 561-567.

Kang, T.J., Chae, G.T., 2001, Detection of Toll-like receptor 2 (TLR2) mutation in the lepromatous leprosy patients. FEMS Immunol Med Microbiol 31, 53-58.

Koets, A., Rutten, V., Hoek, A., van Mil, F., Muller, K., Bakker, D., Gruys, E., van Eden, W., 2002, Progressive bovine paratuberculosis is associated with local loss of CD4(+) T cells, increased frequency of gamma delta T cells, and related changes in T-cell function. Infect Immun 70, 3856-3864.

Koets, A.P., Adugna, G., Janss, L.L., van Weering, H.J., Kalis, C.H., Wentink, G.H., Rutten, V.P., Schukken, Y.H., 2000, Genetic variation of susceptibility to Mycobacterium avium subsp. paratuberculosis infection in dairy cattle. J Dairy Sci 83, 2702-2708.

Labouriau, R., Sørensen, P., Juul-Madsen, H.R., 2008, An efficient strategy to characterize alleles and complex haplotypes using DNA-markers. arXiv:0804.1690v1 [Stat.AP].

Lorenz, E., Mira, J.P., Cornish, K.L., Arbour, N.C., Schwartz, D.A., 2000, A novel polymorphism in the toll-like receptor 2 gene and its potential association with staphylococcal infection. Infect Immun 68, 6398-6401.

Mustafa, T., Bjune, T.G., Jonsson, R., Pando, R.H., Nilsen, R., 2001, Increased expression of fas ligand in human tuberculosis and leprosy lesions: a potential novel mechanism of immune evasion in mycobacterial infection. Scand J Immunol 54, 630-639.

Ogus, A.C., Yoldas, B., Ozdemir, T., Uguz, A., Olcen, S., Keser, I., Coskun, M., Cilli, A., Yegin, O., 2004, The Arg753GLn polymorphism of the human toll-like receptor 2 gene in tuberculosis disease. Eur Respir J 23, 219-223.

Park, Y.H., Yoo, H.S., Yoon, J.W., Yang, S.J., An, J.S., Davis, W.C., 2000, Phenotypic and functional analysis of bovine gammadelta lymphocytes. J Vet Sci 1, 39-48.

Pinedo, P.J., Buergelt, C.D., Donovan, G.A., Melendez, P., Morel, L., Wu, R., Langaee, T.Y., Rae, D.O., 2008, Association between CARD15/NOD2 gene polymorphisms and paratuberculosis infection in cattle. Vet Microbiol.

R Development Core Team, 2008, R: A language and environment for statistical computing. R Foundation for Statistical Computing, Vienna, Austria. ISBN 3-900051-07-0, URL http://www.R-project.org.

Quesniaux, V., Fremond, C., Jacobs, M., Parida, S., Nicolle, D., Yeremeev, V., Bihl, F., Erard, F., Botha, T., Drennan, M., Soler, M.N., Le Bert, M., Schnyder, B., Ryffel, B., 2004, Toll-like receptor pathways in the immune responses to mycobacteria. Microbes Infect 6, 946-959.

Smirnova, I., Hamblin, M.T., McBride, C., Beutler, B., Di Rienzo, A., 2001, Excess of rare amino acid polymorphisms in the Toll-like receptor 4 in humans. Genetics 158, 1657-1664.

Smirnova, I., Poltorak, A., Chan, E.K., McBride, C., Beutler, B., 2000, Phylogenetic variation and polymorphism at the toll-like receptor 4 locus (TLR4). Genome Biol 1, RESEARCH002.

Strober, W., Murray, P.J., Kitani, A., Watanabe, T., 2006, Signalling pathways and molecular interactions of NOD1 and NOD2. Nat Rev Immunol 6, 9-20.

Weckx, S., Del-Favero, J., Rademakers, R., Claes, L., Cruts, M., De Jonghe, P., Van Broeckhoven, C., De Rijk, P., 2005, novoSNP, a novel computational tool for sequence variation discovery. Genome Res 15, 436-442.

Weiss, D.J., Evanson, O.A., de Souza, C., Abrahamsen, M.S., 2005, A critical role of interleukin-10 in the response of bovine macrophages to infection by Mycobacterium avium subsp paratuberculosis. Am J Vet Res 66, 721-726.

Weiss, D.J., Evanson, O.A., Deng, M., Abrahamsen, M.S., 2004, Gene Expression and Antimicrobial Activity of Bovine Macrophages in Response to Mycobacterium avium subsp. paratuberculosis. Vet Pathol 41, 326-337.

Weiss, D.J., Souza, C.D., 2008, REVIEW PAPER: Modulation of Mononuclear Phagocyte Function by Mycobacterium avium subsp. paratuberculosis. Vet Pathol 45, 829-841.

Weiss, D.J., Souza, C.D., Evanson, O.A., Sanders, M., Rutherford, M., 2007, Bovine monocyte TLR2 receptors differentially regulate the intracellular fate of Mycobacterium avium subsp. paratuberculosis and Mycobacterium avium subsp. avium. J Leukoc Biol.

Werling, D., Hope, J.C., Howard, C.J., Jungi, T.W., 2004, Differential production of cytokines, reactive oxygen and nitrogen by bovine macrophages and dendritic cells stimulated with Toll-like receptor agonists. Immunology 111, 41-52.

Werling, D., Piercy, J., Coffey, T.J., 2006, Expression of TOLL-like receptors (TLR) by bovine antigen-presenting cells--Potential role in pathogen discrimination? Veterinary Immunology and Immunopathology Innate Immunity and Vaccination 112, 2-11.

White, S.N., Taylor, K.H., Abbey, C.A., Gill, C.A., Womack, J.E., 2003, Haplotype variation in bovine Toll-like receptor 4 and computational prediction of a positively selected ligand-binding domain. Proc Natl Acad Sci U S A 100, 10364-10369.

Wright, S. P. (1992). Adjusted P-values for simultaneous inference. Biometrics, 48, 1005–1013.

OVERWINTERING OF VESICULAR STOMATITIS VIRUS IN THE UNITED STATES

A.M. PEREZ*, S.J. PAUSZEK, D. JIMENEZ, W.N. KELLEY, Z. WHEDBEE AND L.L. RODRIGUEZ

SUMMARY

From 2004 through 2006, 751 outbreaks caused by vesicular stomatitis virus (New Jersey serotype) (VSNJV) were reported in nine Southwestern U.S. states. Outbreaks occurred during late spring and summer and it has been hypothesized that over-wintering VSNJV strains caused the 2005 and 2006 epidemics (Rainwater-Lovett et al., 2007). The Euclidean distance to the nearest vesicular stomatitis virus (VSV) outbreak reported at the previous or following year (*d*), whichever was shorter, was recorded for each of the 751 outbreaks. The normal model of the time-space scan statistic identified two clusters of outbreaks with values of *d* significantly ($P<0.01$) smaller than the country's background. The clusters were centered in Colorado and Wyoming, respectively. Results were supported by the phylogenetic analysis of samples.

In conclusion, a combination of genetic epidemiology and techniques for identification of time-space clustering provided evidence that VSV-overwintering was likely to occur in 2005 and 2006 in a limited geographical region of the U.S. affected by the epidemic.

INTRODUCTION

Vesicular stomatitis (VS) is a zoonotic disease of horses, cattle, swine, and certain wild life species caused by the vesicular stomatitis virus (VSV). Two VSV serotypes, New Jersey (VSNJV) and Indiana, are responsible for the endemic presentation of the disease in certain regions of The Americas.

In addition to the potential zoonotic nature and direct economic impact of the disease, VS is important because its clinical signs in ruminants and pigs resemble those caused by foot-and-mouth disease (FMD) virus infection (Letchworth et al., 1999). Because the United States are FMD-free, there is a reasonable concern that early signs of a potential FMD epidemic in the country may be erroneously confused with VS.

The southwestern United States has been incidentally affected by VSV epidemics during the last 100 years (Rainwater-Lovett et al., 2007). VS epidemics follow a seasonal pattern and it has been hypothesized that the ability of the virus to over-winter explains the re-emergence of the disease frequently observed during the years that follow an initial introduction of the virus (Rodriguez, 2002). Mechanisms of VSV transmission are, however, not fully understood. Nevertheless, transmission between premises and over large geographical areas is believed to be

* Andres M. Perez, Center for Animal Disease Modeling and Surveillance, University of California in Davis, One Shields Avenue, Davis, CA 95616, USA. Email: amperez@ucdavis.edu

mediated by certain species of insects, which may provide a biological support to the reported ability of the VSV to over-winter.

Knowledge on epidemiological aspects of VSV infection in the United States is important in order to develop effective prevention and control strategies for the disease. In the study here, space clustering and phylogenetic techniques were used to test the hypothesis that the 2005 and 2006 VS outbreaks may have been associated with VSNJV over-wintering in certain regions of the United States affected by the disease in the previous year.

MATERIALS AND METHODS

From 2004 through 2006, 751 outbreaks caused by the VSNJV were laboratory-confirmed in the United States southwestern states of Arizona, Colorado, Idaho, Montana, Nebraska, New Mexico, Texas, Utah, and Wyoming. The geographic location (latitude, longitude) and susceptible species (bovine, equine, other) at the 751 VSNJV-infected premises was recorded by the United States Department of Agriculture's Animal & Plant Health Inspection Service (APHIS).

The Euclidean distance (km) to the nearest VSNJV outbreak reported at the previous or following year (d), whichever was shorter, was recorded for each of the 751 outbreaks. The normal model of the scan statistic was used to identify clusters of outbreaks for which the value of d was shorter than the background value of d estimated in the region affected by the epidemic. Circular windows of candidate clusters were alternatively placed over each infected premises with the size of window varying up to a maximum of 50% of the outbreaks (Kulldorff and Nagarwalla, 1995; Kulldorff et al., 1998). The value of d was computed for premises located within each candidate cluster c (d_c). The value of d_c was compared with the mean value of d estimated throughout the study region (d_m), which represents the null-hypothesis of uniform distribution of d. A Monte Carlo simulation process was used to estimate the probability that each candidate cluster c represents a true cluster of disease at $P<0.05$. Clusters with a value of d_c significantly ($P<0.05$) smaller than d_m were considered geographical regions where VSNJV over-wintering was likely to occur.

Fifty-nine VSNJV isolates were included in the phylogenetic analysis. Ten of the VSNJV were isolated from Mexican outbreaks from 2000 through 2004, whereas the remaining 49 isolates were obtained from the southwestern United States (29 in 2004; 14 in 2005; 6 in 2006). Isolates collected from 2000 through 2005 (n=53) have been previously described (Rainwater-Lovett et al 2007). The 6 VSNJV isolates collected in 2006 originated from Wyoming, the only state with confirmed infection in 2006, and were processed using previously described methods (Rainwater-Lovett et al 2007).

The scan statistic was run using SatScan (Kulldorff and Nagarwalla, 1995). Sequences were aligned using Clustal_X (Thompson et al., 1997). Phylogenetic analysis was performed using a maximum likelihood algorithm implemented in PAUP* version β10 (Swafford, 1998). Parameters of nucleotide substitution were estimated using Modeltest, version 3.7 (Posada and Crandall, 1998).

RESULTS

Two clusters of VS outbreaks with values of d_c significantly (P<0.01) smaller than the country's background (d_m = 1.36) were identified (Figure 1). The average value of d_c was 2.47 times smaller than d_m in a cluster of 375 outbreaks reported in Colorado and New Mexico. A cluster centered in Wyoming included 21 outbreaks for which the value of d_c was 11.3 times smaller than the value of d_m.

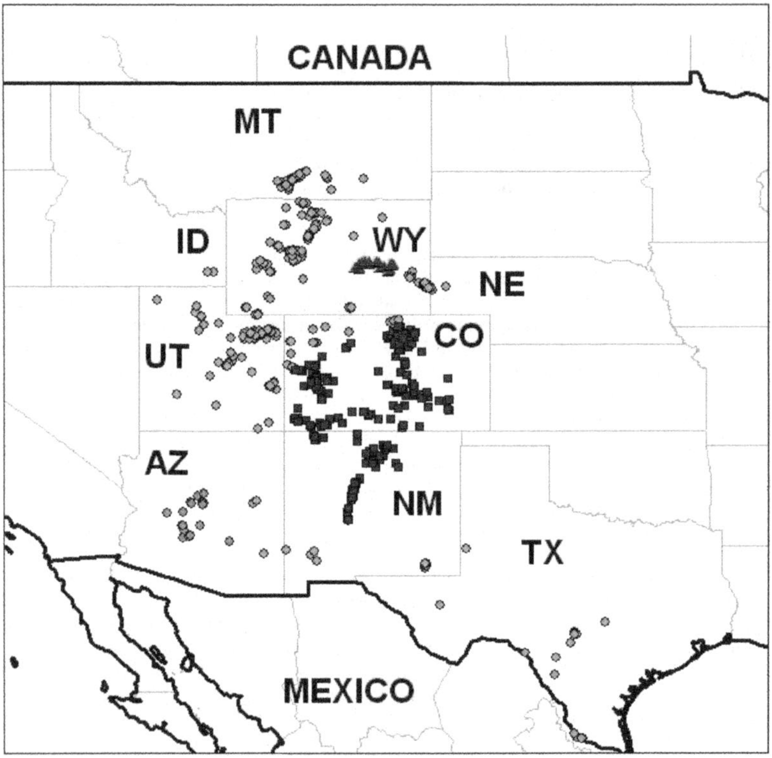

Fig 1. Geographical location of vesicular stomatitis virus reported in the United States from 2004 through 2006. Triangles and squares show the location of two clusters of outbreaks for which the Euclidean distance to the nearest outbreak reported in the previous or following year, whichever was shorter, was significantly (P<0.01) smaller than the epidemics mean. Outbreaks located outside the clusters are indicated with a gray circle. The acronyms correspond to the names of the nine States affected by the epidemics (AZ: Arizona; CO: Colorado; ID: Idaho; MT: Montana; NE: Nebraska; NM: New Mexico; TX: Texas; UT: Utah; WY: Wyoming).

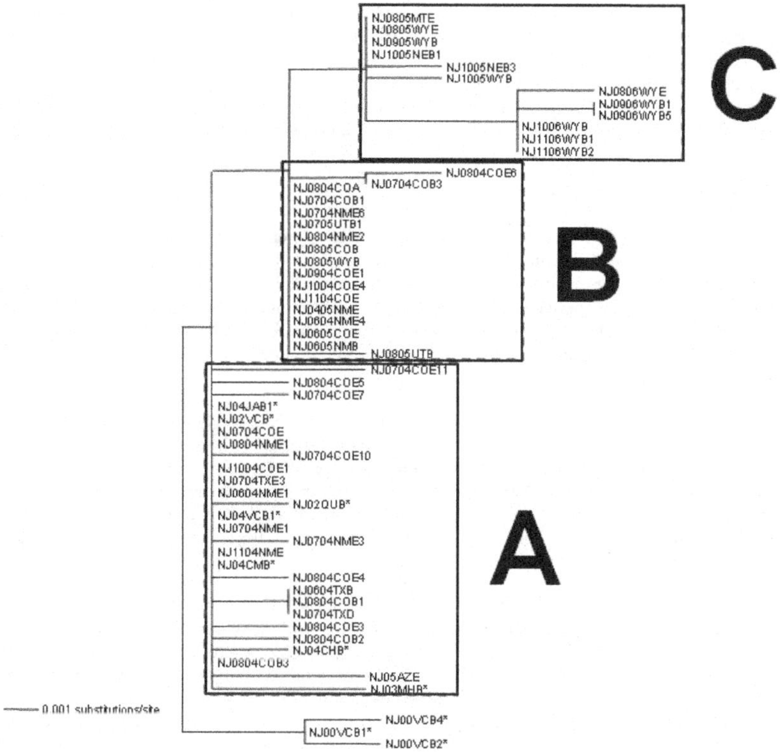

Fig 2. Phylogenetic tree constructed using a maximum-likelihood algorithm and genetic seqeunces of vesicular stomatitis viruses (VSV) isolated in the southwestern United States and Mexico. Sequence names indicate the serotype (NJ), the month (when available) and year of isolation, two-letter abbreviation indicating the U.S. or Mexican state of origin [AZ, Arizona; CH, Chihuahua; CM, Colima; CO, Colorado; JA, Jalisco; MH, Michoacan; MT, Montana; NE, Nebraska; NM, New Mexico; QU, Queretaro; TX, Texas; UT, Utah; VC, Veracruz; WY, Wyoming], and species affected (A, alpaca; B, bovine; D, donkey; E, equine). Isolates originating in Mexico are indicated with an (*). Group A: VSV isolated from Mexico in 2000-2004 and from the United States in 2004. Group B: VSV isolated from the United States in 2004 and 2005. Group C: VSV isolated from the United States in 2005 and 2006.

Sequencing and phylogenetic analysis suggested the presence of at least three different groups of VSNJV. The first group encompassed 27 viruses, which included 19 and 1 United States viruses isolated in 2004 and 2005, respectively, and 7 viruses from Mexico isolated from 2002 through to 2004. The sequences of 4 of the 7 Mexican viruses were identical to those from isolates collected in Texas, Colorado, and New Mexico in 2004 (Figure 2, A). The second group included 10 isolates from 2004 and 7 isolates from 2005 (Figure 2, B); 14 of those 17 isolates (82.35%) were part of the spatial cluster centered in Colorado and New Mexico (Figure 1). The third group encompassed 6 isolates from 2005 and the 6 isolates from 2006 (Figure 2, C), from which 9 (69.2%) were obtained from outbreaks located within the spatial cluster centered in Wyoming (Figure 1). The second and third groups did not include viruses from Mexico.

DISCUSSION

Over-wintering has been proposed as a possible biological mechanism associated to the re-emergence of VSV during consecutive years in the southwestern United States following initial introduction of the virus from endemic areas (Rainwater-Lovett et al., 2007). The study here presents results of the application of phylogenetic analysis and techniques for identification of time-space clustering that are consistent with the hypothesis that VSV-over-wintering was likely to occur in 2005 and in 2006 in two discrete geographical regions of the southwestern United States affected by the epidemic.

Two clusters of outbreaks were located significantly closer ($P<0.01$) to outbreaks that occurred during the previous or following year (Figure 1). Spatial clusters of outbreaks that took place in consecutive years suggest the presence of factors that facilitate or promote disease infection or spread. One would expect that if over-wintering occurs, premises close to the place where the virus over-winters will be more likely to be infected during consecutive years than herds located further away. Thus, the space clusters detected here may represent geographical locations where over-wintering is likely to occur.

Phylogenetic analysis of the isolates provides additional support for the hypothesis of over-wintering. Two of the three genetic lineages or groups of VSV identified at the epidemics (Figure 2 B and C) mostly overlap with the geographical location of the two space clusters identified. Isolates from the space cluster of herds located in Colorado and New Mexico correspond to a specific group of genetically-related VSV identified in 2004 and 2005 (Figure 2 B). This group seems to be phylogenetically closely related, yet different, to the group of VSV detected early in 2004, which was similar and in some cases identical to viruses originating in Mexico. Viruses from the space cluster of herds located in Wyoming were isolated in 2005 and 2006 and corresponded to a lineage phylogenetically distant to the Mexican and early 2004 United States isolates.

Previously, it was shown that two distinct genotypes existed in spatially disparate areas of Wyoming in 2005 (Rainwater-Lovett et al., 2007) with an isolate from western Wyoming belonging to Group B (Figure 2) and those isolated in eastern Wyoming belonging to Group C. It is likely that viruses from the Group C genotype, found in eastern but not in western Wyoming, gave rise to the 2006 viruses that were isolated only in eastern Wyoming, and not on any other part of the southwestern United States.

Combined interpretation of the phylogenetic and space clustering analyses suggest that VSV may have over-wintered in 2004-2005 in certain regions of New Mexico and Colorado and in 2005-2006 in a limited area of eastern Wyoming. Moreover, results also suggest that over-wintering may have resulted in evolution of the virus into a distinct genetic lineage derived from that detected in the previous year.

In total, these results suggest that certain regions of Colorado, Wyoming, and New Mexico may offer ecological, epidemiological, or demographic conditions that facilitate over-wintering, adaptation and evolution of the VSNJV. Specific factors associated to conditions that favour over-wintering are still to be elucidated. One may hypothesize, however, that if insect-borne transmission plays a role in the spread of the disease, then persistence, latency or maintenance of the virus in biotic or abiotic substrates may occur during winter, followed by reactivation of the mechanisms of infection at the next warm season. Thus, a possible explanation for the geographical and genetic association detected here could be the selective presence of such factors or forces on the geographical regions where space clusters were detected. Noteworthy is the observation that genetically similar VSV were identified from outbreaks that affected Colorado and New Mexico in 1995 and 1997 (Rodriguez et al., 2000), supporting the hypothesis that this particular region may offer conditions that favour over-wintering of the VSV.

In conclusion, this study presents evidence supporting the hypothesis that VSV overwintering was likely to occur in certain regions of the Southwestern United States affected by the VSV epidemics in 2004-2006. These results will help the development and application of disease prevention strategies in the event of another VS epidemic.

ACKNOWLEDGEMENTS

This paper was funded in part by the United States National Center for Medical Intelligence, by the United States Department of Agriculture (USDA) Agricultural Research Service (ARS), and by the United States Department of Energy Oak Ridge Institute for Science and Education (ORISE).

REFERENCES

Kulldorff, M., Athas, W.F., Feurer, E.J., Miller, B.A., and Key, C.R. (1998). Evaluating cluster alarms: a space-time scan statistic and brain cancer in Los Alamos, New Mexico. Am J Public Health 88, 1377-1380.

Kulldorff, M., and Nagarwalla, N. (1995). Spatial disease clusters: detection and inference. Stat Med 14, 799-810.

Letchworth, G.J., Rodriguez, L.L., and Del cbarrera, J. (1999). Vesicular stomatitis. Vet J 157, 239-260.

Posada, D., Crandall, K.A., 1998. MODELTEST: testing the model of DNA substitution. Bioinformatics (Oxford, England) 14, 817-818.

Rainwater-Lovett, K., Pauszek, S.J., Kelley, W.N., and Rodriguez, L.L. (2007). Molecular epidemiology of vesicular stomatitis New Jersey virus from the 2004-2005 US outbreak indicates a common origin with Mexican strains. J Gen Virol 88, 2042-2051.

Rodriguez, L.L. (2002). Emergence and re-emergence of vesicular stomatitis in the United States. Virus Res 85, 211-219.

Rodriguez, L.L., Bunch, T.A., Fraire, M., and Llewellyn, Z.N. (2000). Re-emergence of Vesicular Stomatitis in the Western United States Is Associated with Distinct Viral Genetic Lineages. Virology 271, 171-181.

Swafford, D.L., 1998. PAUP*. Phylogenetic Analysis Using Parsimony. Version 4. In: Sunderland (Ed.) Sinauer Associates., Massachussetts.

Thompson, J.D., Gibson, T.J., Plewniak, F., Jeanmougin, F., Higgins, D.G., 1997. The CLUSTAL_X windows interface: flexible strategies for multiple sequence alignment aided by quality analysis tools. Nucleic acids research 25, 4876-4882.

ANIMAL HEALTH ECONOMICS

IMPACT OF INDIVIDUAL DECISIONS OF FARMERS ON THE EFFICIENCY OF VACCINATION AT A REGIONAL LEVEL: A MODELLING APPROACH

O. RAT-ASPERT*, E. PETIT AND C. FOURICHON

SUMMARY

Control strategies for infectious diseases at a regional level can rely on vaccination. When the decision to vaccinate is made by each farmer on a voluntary basis, a farmer vaccinates to protect his own herd. If the vaccinated herds are protected against infection, the risk for other herds is reduced, creating a positive externality (i.e. an impact on a third party that is not directly involved in an economic decision). The two main objectives of this study were to evaluate the efficiency of voluntary vaccination at a regional level and to analyze the effect of financial incentives, considering the externalities due to vaccination. A dynamic model was developed, coupling an epidemiologic model with an economic model. It gave the proportion of farms that vaccinated, and the evolution of the prevalence. Assuming the farmers were fully informed on prevalence and the decision to vaccinate was made each year, the model showed that voluntary vaccination could not eradicate the disease, even in the presence of incentives for vaccination.

INTRODUCTION

Animal diseases can be classified in two categories depending on whether they are or are not regulated. For regulated diseases, such as foot-and-mouth disease, farmers should follow the predefined rules. But when a disease is not regulated, the choice of control measures is left to farmers. In the latter case, farmers make choices to protect their own herds. Decisions are made comparing the constraints of control measures to their potential benefit. For transmissible diseases, when a farmer protects his own herd, he also protects other herds by reducing the probability for other herds to be infected.

The control of BVD (Bovine Viral Diarrhoea), an endemic bovine disease in many countries, illustrates this. Different methods of management are practiced in different regions, depending on the local constraints of production. In France, farmers organizations, the GDS (*Groupements de Défense Sanitaire*) are supporting control plans for endemic diseases. In Burgundy for example, a cow-calf production region with high between-farm contact, vaccination is the principal means of limiting the virus spread (Petit, 2005). Thus, the GDS communicate about the protection of herds by vaccination. To improve the health status of herds in this region, financial incentives could be implemented to promote the adoption of vaccination by farmers. However, even if communication and incentives can influence his individual

*Olivier Rat-Aspert, UMR1300 Bioagression, Epidemiology and Risk Analysis, ENVN-INRA, Atlanpole-Chantrerie, B.P. 40706, 44307 NANTES CEDEX 03
Email: rat-aspert@vet-nantes.fr

decisions, the farmer has the choice to vaccinate his herd or not, depending on the perceived risk, attitude toward risk, constraints of the vaccination, and its expected costs and efficiency.

This situation must be taken into account when considering the allocation of resources for collective disease management. Vaccination, that is used by the farmer for the protection of his herd, creates a positive externality: vaccination reduces the prevalence of the disease in the area and limits the exposure to the virus for the neighbourhood. In turn, this reduced risk may affect the willingness of farmers to vaccinate.

In the (human) health economics literature, the issue of individual behaviour in terms of vaccination has been previously studied. Brito et al. (1990), studied externalities caused by vaccination. This issue has not yet been addressed in the field of animal heath economics. Using a theoretical model, the present work aims to study the evolution of the disease and of the vaccinal coverage as well as the impact of incentives for vaccination when the final choice is left to the farmers.

MATERIALS AND METHODS

We developed a dynamic model, coupling an epidemiologic model with an economic one. The economic model provides the proportion of vaccinated herds to the epidemiologic model whereas the epidemiologic situation issued from the epidemiologic model is an input for the decision process of the economic model.

Epidemiologic model

A classical SIR epidemiological model is considered, where the unit of interest is the herd. The states of herds are *S* Susceptible, *I* Infectious and *R* Recovered (Fig. 1). A proportion of the susceptible herds are vaccinated. The vaccine is assumed to protect the herd for one year. For simulations, the model parameters were calibrated in accordance with the biology of BVD.

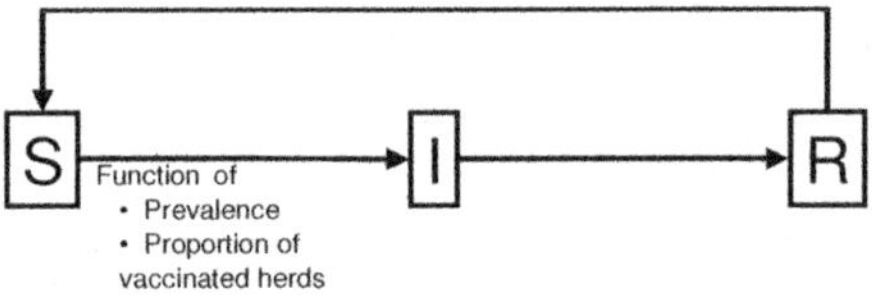

Fig. 1 Transition between epidemiologic states of herds *S* Susceptible, *I* Infectious and *R* Recovered.

Because the decision to vaccinate is taken each year and the protection of the vaccine is assumed to be one year, the time step used in the model was one year. The transition between epidemiologic states of herds was formulated by the following equations (Eq.1):

$$\begin{cases} S_{n+1} = S_n - S_n \beta I_n (1 - V_n \cdot e) + R_n / \gamma \\ I_{n+1} = I_n + S_n \beta I_n (1 - V_n \cdot e) - I_n / \delta \\ R_{n+1} = R_n + I_n / \delta - R_n / \gamma \end{cases} \qquad (1)$$

S_n, S_{n+1}, I_n, I_{n+1} R_n and R_{n+1} were respectively the proportion of *Susceptible*, *Infectious* and *Recovered* herds the years n and $n+1$. The proportion of herds that became infected during year n depended on the transmission rate β and the prevalence of the disease in the area (i.e. I_n, the proportion of infectious herds). A proportion βI_n of the herds which were susceptible became infected during the year n. Because of the protection induced by the vaccine, the proportion of susceptible herds infected in year n was equal to $1 - V_n \cdot e$, where V_n was the proportion of susceptible herds vaccinated during year n, given by the economic model, and e the effectiveness of vaccination at the herd level. The value of e (with $e \in]0;1]$), corresponds to the probability of having a protected herd when the farmer vaccinated his herd. It depends on the efficacy of the vaccine and the effectiveness of its use in farms. The *Infectious* herds became *Recovered*, after an average time δ and *Recovered* herds became *Susceptible* again after an average time γ. In the model, vaccination of *Infectious* and *Recovered* herds had no impact on γ and δ, so vaccination was of no value for *Infectious* nor *Recovered* herds. The total number of farms was assumed to be constant which means that the disease, despite its economic impact on farms, had no impact on their viability.

Decision model

The decision model calculated the proportion of farmers who vaccinated their herds for a given prevalence. The following hypotheses were made:

- The only control measure that differed between farmers was the vaccination, that protected the herd with an imperfect effectiveness.

- Vaccination protected the herd for one year. Consequently, vaccination had no effect on the protection of the herd nor the cost of the vaccination the following year (vaccination decision is fully reversible).

- Farmers had perfect information about the economic consequences of their choices.

The farmers were free to choose whether or not to invest in vaccination. Farmers are rational agents, motivated by a rational economic behaviour (they maximise their expected utility). Utility was used to compare, in terms of economic welfare, possible choices of the agents. Because agents are risk averse (prefer a certain outcome over an uncertain or risky outcome), the choice that maximises expected outcomes does not necessarily maximise their expected satisfaction. Utility here is a measure of this relative satisfaction from the outcome allowing the comparison of choices with regard to uncertain gambles. The measure of utility is done with a utility function. Following Reynaud (2008), the present theoretical model used a constant relative risk aversion (CRRA) utility function, which is widely used in agricultural economics. The function was defined as $U_\alpha(\Pi)$ for an outcome Π as shown in Eq. (2):

$$U_\alpha(\Pi) = \frac{1}{1-\alpha}\Pi^{1-\alpha} \qquad (2)$$

where α was the coefficient of relative risk aversion, specific to each agent. In the model, the coefficient of relative risk aversion was triggered according to a uniform distribution within a population of farmers, around an average value, 0.2, that reflects a rather risk adverse population. Two situations were considered with a wide or narrow range of variation of α, corresponding to heterogeneous or homogeneous attitude towards risks.

Each agent with a herd status *Susceptible* had a binary choice each year, n: to vaccinate or not. This choice had an impact on the possible outcome and the probability of infection. This choice is described in the following decision tree (Fig. 2):

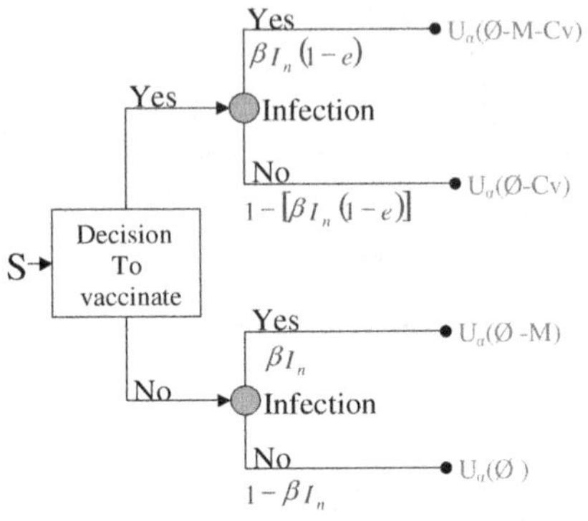

Fig. 2 Vaccination decision tree. The choice to vaccinate or not has an impact on the probability to be infected (function of I_n) and on the possible utility (U_α).

The outcome depended on *Ø*, the outcome of a farm that did not vaccinate and was not infected, *Cv*, the cost of the vaccine and *M*, the losses due to the disease. To simplify the model, losses due to the disease were assumed to be concentrated within the year of infection. The probability of having a herd infected during the year n was given by the epidemiologic model and was a function of the prevalence level I_n. The probability of infection and the utility provided by each situation allowed the calculation of the expected utility of choices.

The expected utility of an agent who decides to invest in vaccination is given by U^V_{α,I_n} (Eq.(3)):

$$U^V_{\alpha,I_n} = \beta I_n(1-e)U_\alpha(\text{Ø} - Cv - M) + [1-\beta I_n(1-e)]U_\alpha(\text{Ø} - Cv) \tag{3}$$

while the expected utility of an agent who does not invest in vaccination is given by U^O_{α,I_n} (Eq.(4)):

$$U^O_{\alpha,I_n} = \beta I_n U_\alpha(\text{Ø} - M) + (1-\beta I_n)U_\alpha(\text{Ø}) \tag{4}$$

Each year n, an agent decided to invest in vaccination if the excess of expected utility over the expected utility without vaccination was non-negative, according to the prevalence level (if $U^V_{\alpha,I_n} \geq U^O_{\alpha,I_n}$). The aggregation of agents' choices defined V_n, the proportion of herds vaccinated in year n.

Coupling

Epidemiologic and economic models are interdependent. Vaccination affects the prevalence level and in turn the prevalence level affects the decision to vaccinate (Fig. 3).

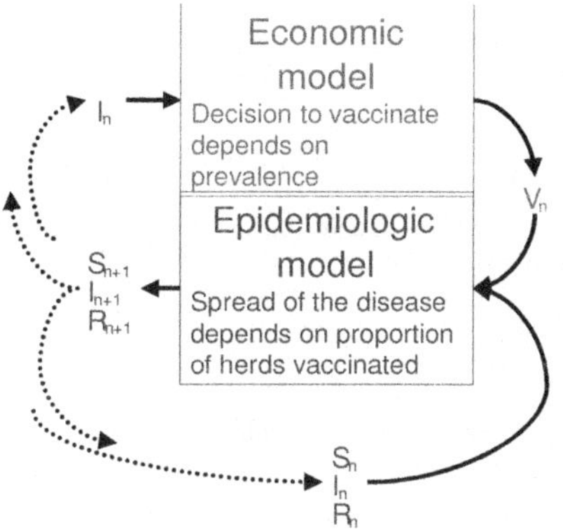

Fig. 3 Interrelationship between the economic and epidemiologic models, with S_n, S_{n+1}, I_n, I_{n+1} R_n and R_{n+1}, and V_n the proportion of *Susceptible*, *Infectious Recovered* and *Vaccinated* herds in years *n* and *n+1*.

The prevalence level I_n the year *n*, which was an output of the epidemiologic model was the input for the economic model in year *n*. In turn, an output of the decision model, the proportion of vaccinated herds in year *n*, was the input for the epidemiologic model in year *n+1*. The epidemiologic model provided data to itself from one year to the next, whereas for the decision model, decisions taken in year *n* had no direct impact on decisions taken in year *n+1*.

RESULTS

The coupling of the economic and epidemiologic models allowed us to follow the evolution of vaccination and the epidemiology of the disease over time. The initial epidemiologic conditions of the model were the epidemiologic condition at the equilibrium, without vaccination. The year zero of the model matches with the introduction of the possibility of vaccination.

An equilibrium of vaccination and prevalence

The observed vaccination situation led either to a single equilibrium or to oscillations around the equilibrium values. The first case was obtained when the heterogeneity of risk aversion was strong in the population of farmers (Fig 4a). The second case was met when risk aversion varied slightly across producers (Fig 4b).

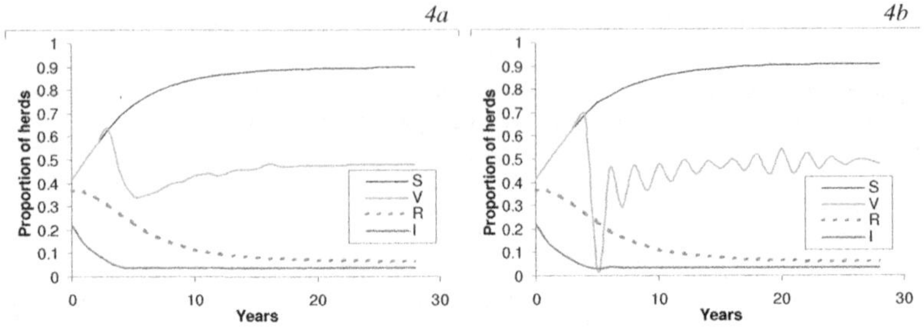

Fig. 4 Evolution the proportions of herds Susceptible S, Infectious I, Recovered R and Vaccinated V with heterogeneous risk aversion (4a) and with homogeneous risk aversion(4b).

<u>An impossible eradication</u>

The prevalence level $\hat{I}_\alpha$ for which the agent, characterised by a coefficient of relative risk aversion α , was indifferent to vaccination or non-vaccination (i.e. the value of I that verifies $U^V_{\alpha,I} = U^O_{\alpha,I}$) is given by Eq.(5).

$$\hat{I}_\alpha = \frac{U_\alpha(\emptyset) - U_\alpha(\emptyset - Cv)}{\beta\left[U_\alpha(\emptyset) - U_\alpha(\emptyset - M) - (1-e)\left(U_\alpha(\emptyset - Cv) - U_\alpha(\emptyset - Cv - M)\right)\right]} \tag{5}$$

For each agent, there was a positive value of the prevalence level below which the agent did not vaccinate, insofar as Cv, the cost of the vaccine, was positive. In fact, the value of $\hat{I}_\alpha$ was positive for every value of α because the utility function is an increasing function and $U_\alpha(\emptyset) - U_\alpha(\emptyset - M) \approx U_\alpha(\emptyset - Cv) - U_\alpha(\emptyset - Cv - M)$. Whether it was vaccinated or not, the losses and gains when a herd became infected were equal and so, the losses of utility were quasi equal. The proportion of farmers who vaccinated as a function of I were obtained from Eq.(5) applied to all farmers in the population. The shape of this function depended on the distribution of the risk aversion in the population. It is the economic condition $\hat{V}(I)$. The proportion of farmers that vaccinated decreased with the value of the prevalence I.

The epidemiologic model allowed the determination of the prevalence at the equilibrium as a function of the proportion of farmers that vaccinated. This function is the epidemiologic condition $I^*(V)$ Eq.(6).

$$I^*(V) = \frac{\beta\delta(1 - V \cdot e) - 1}{\beta(\gamma + \delta)(1 - V \cdot e)} \tag{6}$$

The unique equilibrium is given by the intersection of the two curves, economic condition and epidemiologic condition (Fig. 5). It gives the equilibrium values of the prevalence level I^* and the proportion of vaccinated herds V^*.

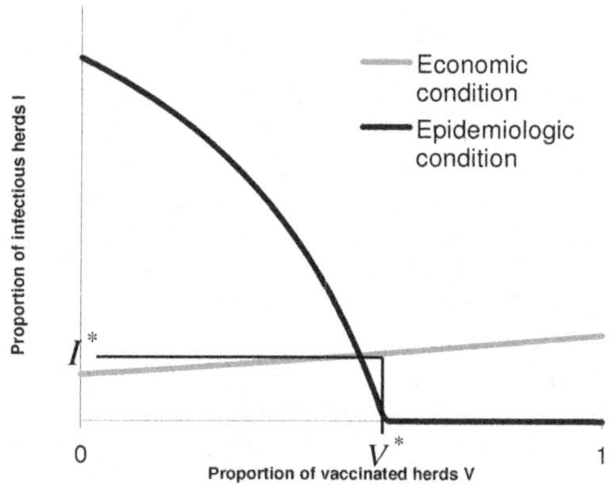

Fig. 5 Links between proportion of infectious herds and the proportion of vaccinated herds due to economic and epidemiologic conditions.

The equilibrium is not necessarily achieved. In the case of oscillations around the equilibrium, adjustment of the proportion of vaccinated herds was on a short term (one year), while the evolution of the epidemiological situation took place over a longer period. Under the assumptions of the model, vaccination could not eradicate the disease, unless the vaccination was of no cost. In this case, it was assumed that all of the agents vaccinated until the risk became null because of the eradication of the disease (from Eq.(5), $Cv = 0 \Rightarrow \hat{I}_\alpha = 0$ and $\hat{V}(I) = 1 \ \forall I \in [0,1]$).

Incentives

Two kinds of incentives were considered. The first consisted of subsidising vaccination. The second consisted of compensating for losses due to the disease in the case of a severe outbreak only in vaccinated herds. Subsidising vaccination in the model decreased the cost of the vaccine, Cv. Conditioning financial support on vaccination in the model decreased the losses M induced by the disease for the farmers who vaccinated.

Subsidising and compensating for losses led to a decrease of the threshold prevalence $\hat{I}_\alpha$ below which farmers did not vaccinate, decreasing *de facto* the prevalence level at the equilibrium. On the other side, subsidies for vaccination and compensating for losses have important costs. Whatever the level of subsidises, prevalence at the equilibrium was greater than zero, except when the costs of the vaccine were fully subsidised.

DISCUSSION

The results highlight the importance of taking into account individual decisions and externalities they generate in collective animal health control schemes. They are consistent with other models used in human health and concluded that vaccination coverage at the equilibrium does not allow the eradication of the disease (Coudeville, 2004)

The results depended weakly on decision-making and the epidemiological process modelled in this work. The strong assumptions of these models could have had an impact on the results obtained.

The epidemiological model is very simple. It can be applied to a specific disease by calibrating the SIR model or by adopting a more representative and more complex epidemiology of the disease. The model can also be adapted to represent more accurately the impact of vaccination (vaccination of recovered and infectious herds).

The decision model assumed that agents have perfect information. However, there might be some cognitive bias: the perception of risk associated with the disease, as well as with the effectiveness of the vaccine, might be biased according to available information (from GDS or veterinarians or more broadly the entire social network). The perception of risk is most likely shifted over time. Farmers do not have direct and immediate access to information about the prevalence of the disease. Overvaluation of risks might lead some farmers to vaccinate although they do not yet have concern, and thus lead to eradication.

The choice to vaccinate or not is probably more complex than a binary choice. First, the decision is related to other means of control implemented on a farm scale. Furthermore, this decision is not fully reversible. While some vaccines to protect livestock are administered each year, vaccination of livestock can be seen by a farmer as an investment to keep his herd healthy. The farmer may take his decision based on risk, but also on previous decisions. The labour constraint related to vaccination should also be taken into account in the choice of the farmer.

Finally, the farmer's rationale is probably more complex than the simple economic rationale considered in the model. The farmer adjusts his animal health decisions to the perceived health status of his herd and his aims are also a function of his economic and social environment (Brossier, 1980)

CONCLUSIONS

Based on a simple hypothesis, this work revealed that if vaccination is left to the initiative of farmers, it does not lead to the eradication of the disease because of the adjustment of farmers choices to an epidemiological situation that evolves with vaccination. The strong assumptions of the decision model necessitate that the results are treated with caution. But they raise new questions about risk perception and decision making of agents.

By introducing the impact of incentives on the management of the disease, this work is a first step towards the development of tools to optimise the means of collective management of animal health, thereby streamlining funds allocated to animal health management.

ACKNOWLEDGEMENTS

The authors would like to thank Anne-France Viet and Stéphane Krebs for their comments on the manuscript.

This work was carried out with the financial support of the ANR (Agence Nationale de la Recherche - The French National Research Agency) under the Programme Agriculture et Développement Durable, project ANR-05-PADD-014, (Action collective pour une maîtrise durable de la santé animale : qualification sanitaire en élevage de ruminants).

REFERENCES

Brito, D., Sheshinski, E. and Intriligator, M., (1990). Externalities and compulsory vaccination. Journal of Public Economics, 45, 69-90

Brossier, J., (1980). De la recherche sur les décisions des agriculteurs à la formation économique des agriculteurs. Pour la constitution de groupes de Recherche-Développement. Economie Rurale, 136, 111-113

Coudeville, L., (2004). Comportements individuels en matière de vaccination : Une approche bayésienne. Revue Economique, 55-4, 745-766

Reynaud, A., 2008, Revue d'Etudes en Agriculture et Environnement, forthcoming.

Petit, E., 2005, Mise en place d'un observatoire régional de l'infection par le virus de la Diarrhée Virale Bovine (B.V.D.) en Bourgogne. Rencontres Recherches Ruminants, 12, 276

ECONOMIC CONSEQUENCES OF THE DUTCH BLUETONGUE SEROTYPE 8 EPIDEMIC IN 2006 AND 2007

A.G.J. VELTHUIS*, H.W. SAATKAMP, M.C.M. MOURITS, A.A. DE KOEIJER AND A.R.W. ELBERS

SUMMARY

In this study the economic consequences of the bluetongue (BT) epidemic of 2006 and 2007 in the Netherlands were calculated. A deterministic economic model was constructed, reflecting the Dutch livestock production systems for cattle, sheep and goats. The net costs of the BT epidemic in 2006 (BT2006) has been valued at 32.4 million Euros and for the BT epidemic 2007 (BT2007) at 117-128 million Euros. The control measures constituted 91% of net costs of BT2006 and diagnosis costs, 7%. For BT2007, 90% of the net costs were production losses plus veterinary treatment, whereas only 9% was related to control measures. The cattle sector suffered 88% and 76% of the net costs for BT2006 and BT2007, respectively.

INTRODUCTION

Bluetongue (BT) is a viral disease among ruminants, transmitted by biting midges (*Culicoides*) (Verwoerd, 2004). Sheep, and less commonly cattle, can have severe clinical symptoms as a result of the infection and can even die (Elbers and van der Spek, 2008). The disease has been named after the swollen and sometimes cyanotic tongue, which is one of the symptoms of the disease. Because of the economic damage induced by bluetongue, it was listed as a notifiable disease in the 1960's by the World Organization for Animal Health (OIE).

In August 2006, the first BT virus serotype 8 (BTV8) outbreak ever in North-Western Europe was detected in the Netherlands. In that year, a total of 460 Dutch livestock farms were officially registered to be infected with BTV8. In the same period farms in Belgium, France, Germany, and Luxemburg became infected with BTV8 (Elbers et al., 2008a, b). Although a comprehensive set of control measures was put in place at national and at EU level in 2006, the infection reappeared and new outbreaks were reported in the Netherlands and the other originally infected countries in the summer of 2007. The epidemic developed quickly over a large part of North-Western Europe, resulting in the Netherlands in more than 6,000 outbreak farms.

It was clear that the BTV8 epidemic had a large impact, particularly in 2007. However, insight into the economic consequences of the epidemic and control measures was still missing. For the decision-making about the epidemic control it is important to know i) the losses due to BT, ii) the costs of control measures, and iii) the saved losses that resulted from the control

* Annet Velthuis, Business Economics, Wageningen University, Wageningen, the Netherlands. Email: annet.velthuis@wur.nl

measures. This economic analysis of the epidemic and the applied control measures contributes to bridging the information gap concerning the impact of the BTV8 epidemic.

A cost-benefit analysis (CBA) is the process of weighing the total expected costs against the total expected benefits of a project, or in this case epidemic control, to optimize control, i.e. choosing the best or the most profitable option to control. Cost-benefit analysis is typically used by governments to evaluate the desirability of a given intervention and the aim is to gauge the efficiency of the intervention. Based on the demographic, epidemiologic and economic information, the costs and expenditures due to the BTV8 epidemic and applied control measures for the different stakeholders can be calculated, but also the possible benefits. The net costs or losses that will be the output of the CBA include costs and expenditures that are corrected for possible profits.

In this paper a CBA of the BTV8 epidemic for the Netherlands is presented. It calculates the losses for different livestock production systems of the BTV8 epidemic from July 2006 to July 2007 (BT2006) and of the BTV8 epidemic from July 2007 to July 2008 (BT2007).

MATERIALS AND METHODS

To evaluate the economic impact of BT in the Netherlands a deterministic economic model was constructed, reflecting the Dutch livestock production systems. In this model the economic impact (the losses and expenditures, corrected for possible benefits) of BT was calculated by an integration of demographic, epidemiologic and economic data. Data from official sources were used as much as possible. Where information was lacking, experts were asked to make estimations. With respect to the model, assumptions and inputs, discussions with several parties from the sectors took place to secure the representativeness of the Dutch practice by the model.

Economic model

The economic consequences of the BTV8 epidemic included the impact on the production of animals due to the disease, the treatment of diseased animals, diagnostic costs, costs of control measures taken during the course of the epidemic (including price changes of animals and animal products due to transport restrictions)Eq.(1).

$$L = \sum_i \sum_j P_{i,j} + T_{i,j} + D_i + M_{i,j} \tag{1}$$

where L represents the total damage for the entire livestock population due to the epidemic, P the production losses at farm type i and for animal type j, T the corresponding treatment costs, D the diagnostic costs, M the cost of the control measures. The different farm and animal types are given in the section titled Model Input. The different cost categories are explained in more detail in the following paragraphs.

Production losses

The production effects that have economic consequences include mortality (MT), early culling (EC), reduced milk production (MP), weight losses (WL), no gestations (NG), postponed gestations (PG), abortions (AB), less fertile rams (RF), lower birth weight (BW) and stillbirth (SB) Eq.(2).

$$P_{i,j} = \sum_i \sum_j MT_{i,j} + EC_j + MP_j + WL_j + NG_j + PG_j + AB_j + RF_j + BW_{i,j} + SB_j \tag{2}$$

The losses due to mortality were calculated as shown in Eq.(3):

$$MT_{i,j} = mtr_{i,j} \cdot rp \cdot ar_i \cdot (v_j - sv_j + rc_j), \tag{3}$$

where *mtr* is the mortality rate (in number per 100 animal months), *rp* the period at risk, *ar* the number of animals at BTV8 infected farms, *v* the production value (for ewes it was the difference in the value of an ewe and the replacement lamb and for dairy cattle it was the retention pay-off (RPO value) (Houben, 1995)), *sv* the missed slaughter value and *rc* the costs made to send an animal for rendering.

The cost of early culling was calculated as shown in Eq.(4):

$$EC_j = pt_{EC,j} \cdot mbr_j \cdot rp \cdot ar_j \cdot v_j, \tag{4}$$

where pt_{EC} is the percentage of BTV8 infected cows culled early and *mbr* the morbidity rate (in number of animals per 100 animal months).

The lost revenues due to BTV8 related reduced milk production were calculated as ahown in Eq.(5):

$$MP_j = amp_j \cdot rmp_j \cdot 0.5 \cdot dd_j \cdot VM_j, \tag{5}$$

where *amp* equals the average daily milk production, *rmp* the relative reduction in milk production, *dd* the number of days that the animal was diseased (it was assumed that the milk production is reduced during the first half of this period) and *VM* the value of the milk that was lost.

If an animal is BTV8 infected, clinical symptoms occur that can lead to weight loss. The losses related to weight loss equal the costs of extra feed needed for compensatory growth (Eq.(6)):

$$WL_j = pt_{WL,j} \cdot EF_j, \tag{6}$$

where pt_{WL} is the proportion of animals with a weight loss and *EF* the costs for the extra feed needed for compensatory growth.

If a reproduction animal was not pregnant with a calf or lamb, the animal was culled. The economic consequences included therefore the production value (v), the lost value of the calf or lamb ($Price_{calf}$ or $Price_{lamb}$) corrected for the costs on feed and housing saved (*FC*) combined with an increased slaughter value (Δsv) in relation to the average cow or ewe going to slaughter Eq.(7):

$$NG_j = pt_{NG,j} \cdot (v_j + Price_j - FC_j - \Delta sv_j), \tag{7}$$

where pt_{NG} is the proportion of animals that was not pregnant with a calf or lamb.

If the number of cycles before gestation increased due to a BTV8 infection (*PG*) the losses for dairy cows equalled an extra insemination (AI_2) and the losses of a prolonged calving interval with one cycle (ΔCI_1). The latter included less milk returns, less calves, and a change in feeding costs (Jalvingh and Dijkhuizen, 1997) Eq.(8):

$$PG_{cow} = pt_{PG,cow} \cdot (AI_2 + \Delta CI_1). \tag{8}$$

The losses of having more cycles before gestation for ewes equalled the reduced slaughter value of lambs ($\Delta Price_{lamb}$), since they could not be sold in the right period Eq.(9):

$$PG_{ewe} = pt_{PG,ewe} \cdot \Delta Price_{lamb} \tag{9}$$

The losses of extra abortions due to a BTV8 infection equalled the losses due to a prolonged calving interval for dairy cows for 6 cycles (ΔCI_6) and the costs of two inseminations (AI_1+AI_2) Eq.(10):

$$AB_{cow} = pt_{AB,cow} \cdot (AI_1 + AI_2 + \Delta CI_6). \tag{10}$$

Hereby we assumed that the cows were not culled due to abortions and that two inseminations were needed for the following gestation. For ewes we assumed that they were culled due to abortion and the losses therefore equalled the losses of early culling ($C_{i,j}$) and the missed returns of an average of 1.5 the lambs that cannot be sold ($Price_{lamb}$) Eq.(11):

$$AB_{ewe} = pt_{AB,ewe} \cdot (C_{ewe} + 1.5 \cdot Price_{lamb}). \tag{11}$$

During the BT epidemic it was observed that BTV8 infected rams were less fertile or infertile for a certain period. The losses corresponding to this category equal the costs made to buy an extra breeding ram Eq.(12).

$$RF_{ram} = pt_{RF} \cdot Price_{ram} \tag{12}$$

Calves with lower birth weight (*BW*) and stillbirths (*SB*) were observed on BTV8 infected dairy farms. The losses due to a lower birth weight equalled the lower price the dairy farmer received for the calf from the veal calf farms ($\Delta Price_{calf}$). However, the losses for the veal calf farm equalled the costs of extra feed needed for compensatory growth (*EF*) minus the reduced price he had to pay for the calf Eq.(13):

$$\begin{aligned} BW_{dairyfarm} &= pt_{BW} \cdot \Delta Price_{calf} \\ BW_{vealcalffarm} &= pt_{BW} \cdot (EF_{calf} - \Delta Price_{calf}) \end{aligned} \tag{13}$$

The losses due to stillbirths equalled the missed price of a calf or lamb ($Price_{calf}$ or $Price_{lamb}$) corrected for the costs that were not made until the selling moment of a young calf, i.e. the feed costs (*FC*). For lambs these costs are zero since they are fed by the ewe, Eq.(14).

$$SB_j = pt_{SB,j} \cdot (Price_j - FC_j) \tag{14}$$

Treatment costs

BTV8 diseased animals could have been treated with pain killers (*pk*), antibiotics (*ab*) or corticosteroids (*cs*) to relieve the suffering of the diseased animal and to prevent secondary infections as a result of reduced immunity. However, a treatment to fight a BTV8 infection does not exist. The treatment costs included only the costs of the veterinary medicines and the application materials (*mt*). The costs of the veterinarian were not included, since most animals were treated at the first visit of the farm to make a BT diagnosis and those costs were included in the diagnostic costs. The treatments later in time were assumed to be applied by the farmer. The treatment costs were calculated as shown in Eq.(15):

$$T_i = mbr_j \cdot (pt_{pk,j} \cdot Price_{pk,j} + pt_{ab,j} \cdot Price_{ab,j} + pt_{cs,j} \cdot Price_{cs,j} + pt_{treated} \cdot Price_{mt}), \qquad (15)$$

where $pt_{pk}, pt_{ab}, pt_{cs}$ represent the proportion of diseased animals that are treated with pain killers, antibiotics and corticosteroids, respectively, and $pt_{treated}$ the total proportion of animals treated. The price of the veterinary drugs and materials are represented by $Price_{pk}, Price_{ab}, Price_{cs}$ and $Price_{mt}$, respectively. If a dairy cow was treated with antibiotics an additional loss due to the milk that couldn't be delivered for 5 to 8 days was included in the calculations.

Diagnostic costs

The diagnostic costs included the costs of the veterinarians (state and own or private veterinarian), the materials for taking blood samples, and the test costs (including the submission costs to the lab). All tested farms and animals were included, so also the test-negative farms, the (screening) farms that were monitored to follow the spread of the epidemic and the animals to be exported. Until September 2007, the diagnostic costs were calculated as shown in Eq.(16):

$$D_i = VET_{own} + VET_{state} + samples \cdot (Price_{mt} + pt_{PCR} \cdot Price_{PCR} + pt_{ELISA} \cdot Price_{ELISA}) + sc, \qquad (16)$$

where VET_{own} represents the costs of the own veterinarian, VET_{state} the costs of the state veterinarian, *samples* the number of samples taken, $Price_{mt}$ the price of the materials, pt_{PCR} the proportion of samples tested with the PCR, $Price_{PCR}$ the price of the PCR test, pt_{ELISA} the proportion of samples tested with the ELISA for the price of $Price_{ELISA}$, and *sc* the submission costs to the lab. As from September 2007, the official diagnosis of BT was allowed to be based entirely on the clinical inspection of a veterinarian, bringing the VET_{state} to zero. However, a number of samples were still submitted, that were included in the calculations.

Costs of control measures

During the BTV8 epidemic, control measures were put in place for animal holdings in different control zones around infected farms. The control measures included obligatory indoor housing of ruminants (*OH*), treatment of animals, stables and lorries for animal transport with insecticides (*TI*), extra testing and controls of animals for export (*EX*), and animal movement restrictions. The losses due to the animal movement restrictions were considered to be price changes of animals and animal products (*PC*) as an effect of market influences Eq.(17).

$$M_{i,j} = OH_{i,j} + TI_{i,j} + EX_{i,j} + PC_{i,j}. \qquad (17)$$

In a 20 kilometre area around infected farms (20km-zone) all ruminants had to be housed at all times from August 17 till September 26, 2006. These animals had to be housed indoors during the evening and night from September 26 till October 13, 2006. The costs of obligatory indoor housing included feed, water, bedding materials and the costs for spreading of the extra manure produced on the fields during the first 14 days and the costs of removing the manure from the farm for the last 42 days. The latter costs were due to the regulation on minerals, which indicate that from September 1st the manure cannot be spread over the fields. The calculation is shown in Eq.(18):

$$OH_{i,j} = pt_{outdoor,i} \cdot na_{i,j} \cdot ((40 + \tfrac{1}{2} \cdot 17) \cdot EF_j + EBM_j + MP_{1,i} \cdot CSM_j + MP_{2,i} \cdot CMS_j), \qquad (18)$$

where $pt_{outdoors}$ is the proportion of animals that is usually in the fields in between August and November, na the number of animals, EF the costs of extra feed per day, EBM the costs of extra bedding materials, MP_1 the extra manure produced during the first 14 days, CSM the costs of spreading the extra manure on the fields, MP_2 the extra manure produced during the last 42 days and CMS the costs of removing the extra produced manure.

The farms that had to house the ruminants indoors also had to treat their animals and stables with insecticides. During the BTV8 epidemic officials regulated that lorries and the animals to be transported also had to be treated with insecticides. The corresponding costs are calculated as shown in Eq.(19):

$$TI_{i,j} = pt_{IT} \cdot (sa_i \cdot Price_{IS} \cdot nsa + na_{i,j} \cdot Price_{IA,i,j} \cdot nna_j) + nl \cdot Price_{IL} + nat_j \cdot Price_{IA,j}, \qquad (19)$$

where pt_{IT} is the proportion of farmers that obeyed the insecticide control measures, sa is the stable area, $Price_{IS}$ the price of insecticides for stables, nsa the number of treatments needed in 56 days, na the number of animals treated, nna the number of treatments per animal in 56 days, $Price_{IA}$ the price of the insecticides for animal treatment, nl the number of lorries treated, $Price_{IL}$ the price of insecticides per lorry, and nat the number of animals transported and treated.

The extra testing related to the export of dairy heifers includes the testing needed to find BTV8 negative farms and the extra testing of heifers to be exported. These costs were calculated as shown in Eq.(20):

$$EX_{exporters} = NFT \cdot (price_{PCR2} + VFT_{own} + sc) + NEH \cdot Price_{testEH} + \Delta NEH \cdot REV_{EH}, \qquad (20)$$

where NFT is the number of farms tested, $price_{PCR2}$ the price of a PCR test at a non-accredited lab, sc the submission costs, NEH the number of export heifers, $Price_{testEH}$ the total test costs of an export heifer, ΔNEH, the decrease in number of export heifers due to the BTV8 epidemic, and REV_{EH} the revenues earned per exported heifer. The number of dairy farms tested increased during the epidemic, since more farms were positive and therefore not suitable for export. For the BT2007 epidemic it was assumed that for each farm that had exported two heifers, three farms were tested on BTV8. Furthermore, each exported heifer had been tested twice before export until October 2007, whereupon it was tested three times (to reduce the risk of exporting BTV8 positive animals). The cost of testing a BTV8 positive heifer on an export stable was also included. This situation happened 20 times and the costs included the decrease in value of the positive heifer, an extended quarantine period of the other heifers in the stable, and an extra test for the other heifers. The cost of testing a BTV8 positive heifer in the importing country was not included, since the probability of this situation was low (although it has happened) and the consequences were complex.

Price changes

Due to the BTV8 epidemic some export streams of animals (and animal products) were banned for set periods. Furthermore, movement restrictions within a country can disturb the supply and demand so that the price of animals can change for a certain period. To study the effects of the size of the 20km zone on the average market prices of production animals per month an Autoregressive Integrated Moving Average model was used. For export heifers no data were available and therefore experts on export heifers were asked to estimate the required input based on their experiences. The economic effect of price changes is calculated as shown in Eq.(21):

$$PC_{i,j} = NA_{i,j} \cdot \Delta Price_{i} \tag{21}$$

where NA is the number of animals sold or bought, and $\Delta Price$ the change in price.

Model input

Sector information

The CBA included the cattle, sheep and goat sector. For each sector different farm types with average herd or flock size were considered (Table 1). Since farm numbers and sizes differed between the Northern (the provinces Friesland, Groningen, Drenthe and North Holland), Middle (the provinces Overijssel, Flevoland and Utrecht) and Southern regions (the provinces North Brabant, South Holland, Zealand and Limburg) of the Netherlands and because of the fact that mortality and morbidity rates differed between these regions due to the spread of the BTV8 epidemic in 2006 and 2007 from the Southern to the Northern regions, the CBA model differentiated between these regions. The information for the goat sector about different farm numbers and sizes over the different regions was not available.

Table 1. Demographic data about the Dutch cattle, sheep and goat sectors

	# Holdings				Average # animals/year/farm	
	N[1]	M[1]	S[1]	Total	Total[2]	for reproduction
Cattle holdings						
Dairy farms	6,863	11,361	4,077	22,301	116	64
Veal calf farms	599	1,818	757	3,174	133	0
Other cattle farms	1,838	4,961	2,927	9,726	37	16
Total				35,201	3,745,000	2,991,000
Sheep holdings						
Dairy sheep farms	11	14	5	30	245	240
Traditional herding	15	19	6	40	2015	448
Breeding farms	3,820	4,952	1,660	10,432	147	51
Fattening farms	732	949	318	2,000	157	0
Hobby farms	18,999	24,625	8,256	51,881	8	4
Total				64,383	4,286,091	1,325,092
Goat holdings						
Dairy goat farms				351	612	447
Fattening farms				45	297	0
Hobby farms				74,824	4	3
Total				75,220	502,540	369,756

[1] North (N), Middle (M), South (S)

[2] At a farm count in May 2007 for cattle and in November 2004 for sheep and goats, excluding the new born lambs and calves that were born and slaughtered within one year.

Reconstruction of the restriction zones

During the BTV8 epidemic different restriction zones were put in place, where different control measures were applied. The area within a 20 kilometres radius around infected farms – reflecting the area where most control measures were applied - was called the 20km zone. The area between the radii of around 100 and 20 kilometres around the infected farm was called the protection zone. In this area fewer control measures were in place than in the 20km zone. The remainder of the Netherlands is called the free zone, in which no control measures were in place. Based on the press publications of the Dutch Ministry of Agriculture, Nature and Food Quality the size of the different zones per month per half a province was reconstructed. By multiplying the number of farms per province by the size of the different zones in time the number of farms affected by different control measures was determined per unit of time.

Epidemiological input

Since the first detection of BTV8 in the Netherlands, different epidemiological studies have been conducted. For our model we used epidemiological input from different studies. Table 2 summarizes the input. Due to different estimates of the morbidity and mortality rates for cattle from different studies, we distinguished two scenarios in our model for the BT2007 epidemic. The morbidity and mortality rates in the first scenario (BT2007-A) were based on a longitudinal study of 585 officially BTV8 infected cattle farms ((Elbers & van der Spek, 2008)). The rates in the second scenario (BT2007-B) were based on a longitudinal study on 72 dairy farms in the Netherlands ((Bartels et al., 2008; Berends, 2008)). The information needed to calculate the losses due to the effects of BTV8 on animal production is summarized in Table 3.

Table 2. Morbidity, mortality, percentage adult animals with clinical symptoms, period at risk, and percentage and number of infected farms for the different animal types, regions and years

Description	Var.	Cattle			Sheep			Goats
		N[1]	M[1]	S[1]	N[1]	M[1]	S[1]	-
Morbidity rate (#/100 animal months)	*Mbr*							
BT2006		-	-	0.42[2]	-	-	1.30[2]	-
BT2007-A		1.66[3]	6.48[3]	4.65[3]	3.24[3]	6.48[3]	7.99[3]	1.30[4]
BT2007-B		1.42[5]	0.81[5]	1.03[5]	3.24[3]	6.48[3]	7.99[3]	1.30[4]
Mortality rate (#/100 animal months)	*Mtr*							
BT2006		-	-	0.04[2]	-	-	0.70[2]	-
BT2007-A		0.03[3]	0.23[3]	0.17[3]	0.79[3]	1.23[3]	1.60[3]	0.00[4]
BT2007-B		0.28[8]	0.26[8]	0.40[8]	0.79[3]	1.23[3]	1.60[3]	0.00[4]
Diseased adult animals (%)	pl_{adult}	88[2]	88[2]	88[2]	80[2]	80[2]	80[2]	-
Period at risk (months)	*Pr*	6	6	6	6	6	6	6
% Infected farms								
BT2006		0.0[2]	0.0[2]	100.0[2]	0.0[2]	0.0[2]	100.0[2]	100.0[2]
BT2007		82.7[6]	99.4[6]	99.9[6]	70.0[7]	70.0[7]	70.0[7]	100.0[7]
Estimated # Infected farms								
BT2006		0	0	200	0	0	270	0[4]
BT2007		7196	16224	6997	16505	21391	7172	25

[1] North (N), Middle (M), South (S), [2] (Elbers et al., 2008), [3] (Elbers & van der Spek, 2008), [4] (Dercksen et al., 2007), [5] (Bartels et al., 2008), [6] A study of the Animal Health Service on screening farms, [7] (Elbers et al., 2008), [8] (Berends, 2008)

Input for the cost calculation on diagnostics

For the calculation of the diagnostic costs, data from the official BTV laboratory (i.e. the Central Veterinary Institute) were used to calculate the input. The model differentiated between the number of samples taken on positive and negative tested farms, and farms tested for export (Table 4). Not all samples were tested by PCR or ELISA, the proportion tested with the different tests differed between years and farm types (Table 4). The economic input for the calculation of the diagnostic costs of BTV8 is summarized in Table 4.

Table 3. Input for the cost calculations on the production effects caused by BTV8

Description	var.	Cattle		Calves		Sheep		Goats	
		2006[1]	2007[1]	2006	2007	2006	2007	2006	2007
Days diseased (#)	*Dd*	18	21	-	-	18	21	18	18
BT related early culling (%)	pt_{EC}	3	3	-	-	3	0	0	0
BT related no gestation (%)	pt_{NG}	5.2	9.9	-	-	5.0	9.8	-	-
BT related postponed gestation (%)	pt_{PG}	36.9	53.5	-	-	0.0	10.0	-	-
BT related abortion (%)	pt_{AB}	2.0	6.2	-	-	1.9	3.2	-	-
BT related reduced fertility rams (%)[2]	pt_{RF}	-	-	-	-	0.0	75.0		
BT related reduced birth weight (%)	pt_{BW}	2.6	6.7	-	-	-	-	-	-
Average daily milk production (kg/day)	*amp*		26.90		-		2.00		2.48
Relative reduction milk production (%)	*rmp*		20		-		20		80
Value missed milk (€/kg)[3]	*VM*		0.06		-		1.13		0.41
Feed costs related to weight loss (€/a)	*EF*		5.60		19.93		-		-
Costs 1st artificial insemination (€/a)	AI_1		23.75		-		-		-
Costs 2nd artificial insemination (€/a)	AI_2		13.85		-		-		-
Costs postponed gestation (1 cycle) (€/a)	ΔCI_1		9.00		-		6.00		-
Costs postponed gestation (6 cycles) (€/a)	ΔCI_6		101.90		-		-		-
Feed costs until sale (€/animal)	*FC*		-		3.57		-		-

[1] BT2006 or BT2007

[2] Percentage of sheep farms that need one extra ram

[3] Due to the quota system for dairy milk equals the value of dairy milk the variable costs of milk produced.

Table 4. Average # of samples taken per farm and average proportion of samples tested with PCR or ELISA for farms tested positive, negative or for export, and economic input for calculation of the diagnostics costs

Description	Var.	Cattle		Sheep		Goats	
		BT2006	BT2007	BT2006	BT2007	BT2006	BT2007
Number of samples taken (#/farm)	*Samples*						
		11	4	3	2	-	8
		12	4	13	3	24	3
		44	81	6	4	52	683
Proportion samples tested PCR (%)	pt_{PCR}						
		100	100	100	100	-	100
		58	88	91	100	12	55
		80	90	27	100	27	51
Proportion samples tested ELISA (%)	pt_{ELISA}						
		70	94	40	96	-	100
		100	100	100	78	100	100
		100	100	100	32	100	100

		BT2006	BT2007
Veterinary cost for BTV8 diagnosis			
Own veterinarian	VET_{own}	78.67	78.67
State veterinarian	VET_{state}	183.32	183.32
Price of PCR (€/sample)	$Price_{PCR}$	87.58	33.2
Price of ELISA (€/sample)	$Price_{ELISA}$	5.83	6.13
Price materials for sampling (€/sample)	$Price_{mt}$	0.02	0.02
Submission costs (€/farm)	*Sc*	9.52	9.52

Input for the cost calculation on control measures: The input used for the cost calculations of the obligatory indoor housing is based on a Dutch handbook on livestock production ((ASG, 2006)) (Table 5).

Table 5. Input for the cost calculations on obligatory indoor housing

Description	Var.	Farm type			
		Dairy	Other cattle	Sheep	Goat
Proportion animals outdoor	$pt_{outdoor}$	85%	75%	100%	0%
Manure produced (m^3/farm in first 14 days)	MP_1	*70*	37	-	-
Manure produced (m^3/farm in last 42 days)	MP_2	*164*	46	-	-
ANIMAL TYPE		COW	CALF	SHEEP	GOAT
Extra feed costs - obligatory indoor housing (€/animal/day)	*EF*	€ 0.53	-	€ 0.04	-
Extra bedding materials (€/animal/day)	*EBM*	€ 0.06	€ 0.03	€ 0.08	-
Costs spreading manure on own fields (€/m^3)	*CSM*	€ 4.30	€ 4.30	€ 0.00	-
Costs removal of manure from the farm (€/m^3)	*CMS*	14.00	€ 14.00	€ 0.00	-

For the cost calculations of the treatment of stables and animals with insecticides, input was based on internet information and prices of insecticides were suggested by the Dutch Ministry of Agriculture, Nature and Food Quality (Table 6).

Table 6. Input for the cost calculations on treatment of stables and animals with insecticides

Description	Var.	Value
Proportion farmers obeying insecticide treatment measure	pt_{IT}	75%
Stable area	*sa*	
Dairy, veal calf, traditional herding		500
Other cattle farm, dairy sheep and goat farm		250
Sheep breeding and fattening, goat fattening, hobby farms		50
Costs treatment stall (100 $m^{3)}$	$Price_{IS}$	€ 27.55
Number of treatments	*nsa*	1.5
Costs treatment animal	$Price_{IA\text{-}nna}$	
Cattle		€ 1.09
Sheep and goats		€ 0.58
Number of animal treatments	*nna*	
Cattle		2
Sheep and goats		4

<u>Sensitivity analysis</u>

A sensitivity analysis was performed on the variables that were assumed to be most influential, i.e. the number of BTV8 infected farms, the number of farms that had to obey the obligatory indoor housing in 2006, mortality rates, morbidity rates and the proportion of reproduction animals with a postponed gestation or an abortion.

RESULTS

Reconstruction of the restriction zones

Figure 1 shows the relative number of farms in the different BTV8 restriction zones. The 'free zone' disappeared within one month after the detection of the first outbreak farm. The number of farms in the 20km zones increased quickly to more than half of the farms in the period between January 2007 and August 2007, after which all farms were located in the 20km zone. From November 2007 the whole area of the Netherlands was officially a protection zone until July 2008.

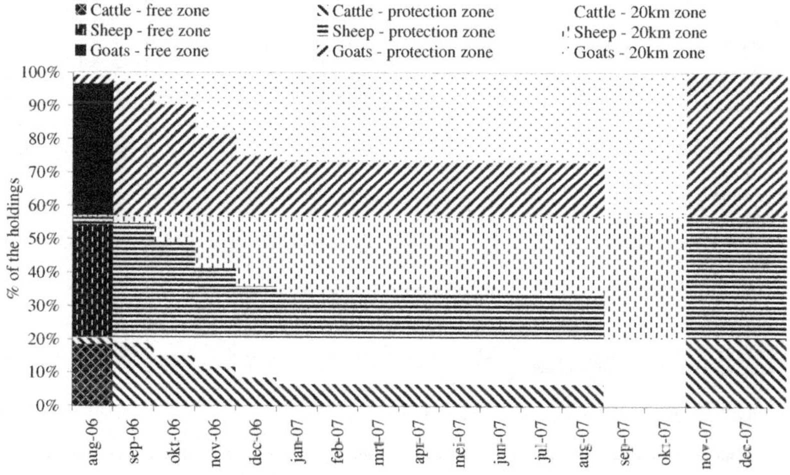

Figure 1. Relative number of cattle, sheep and goat farms in the different restriction zones.

Net costs BT2006 and BT2007 epidemics

The net costs of the Dutch BT2006 epidemic were more than 32 Million Euros and 117.1 to 128.4 million Euros for the BT2007 epidemic, depending on the applied epidemiological estimations (scenario A or B: Tables 5 and 6). The compulsory indoor housing determined 55% of total economic impact in 2006, transport restrictions 36%, diagnosis costs 7%, and the production losses plus treatment less than 2%. In 2007, 90% of total economic impact was caused by the production losses and treatments and only 9% by the transport restrictions. The distribution of the losses over the different components in 2007 differed from 2006. This is because the compulsory indoor housing did not take place in 2007, the rules of diagnosis were relieved from September 2007, and the higher number of farms and animals that were infected with BTV8 during the BT2007 epidemic.

Table 5. Net costs (*1000 Euros) of the BT2006 epidemic per farm type, sector and in total

FARM TYPE SECTOR	PRODUCTION LOSSES	DIAGNOSIS	TREATMENT	CONTROL MEASURES	TOTAL
Dairy	371.8	185.9	5.4	14,940.5	15,503.6
Veal calf	0.7	-	-	303.0	303.7
Other cattle	22.6	75.9	0.6	916.9	1,016.1
Susp. test neg[1]	-	196.8	-	-	196.8
Screening	-	1,313.8	-	-	1,313.8
Export	-	-	-	10,086.3	10,086.3
Cattle subtotal	395.0	1,772.5	6.1	26,246.7	28,420.3
Dairy sheep	0.1	0	0	9.5	9.6
Trad. Herding	0.5	0.2	0	97.8	98.5
Breeding	59.4	46.4	2.9	1,954.4	2,063.2
Fattening	4.3	8.9	0.5	414.7	428.4
Hobby	5.4	94.9	0.3	598.3	699.0
Susp test neg.	-	99.3	-	-	99.3
Screening	-	120.2	-	-	120.2
Export	-	-	-	19.4	19.4
Sheep subtotal	69.7	367.0	3.7	3,094.1	3,537.6
Dairy goat	0	0	0	54.8	54.8
Fattening	0	0	0	0.9	0.9
Hobby	0	0	0	225.8	225.8
Susp. test neg	-	6.2	-	-	6.2
Screening	-	120.2	-	-	120.2
Export	-	-	-	5.6	5.6
Goat subtotal	0	126.5	0	287.1	413.5
Transport subtotal				1.9	1.9
Total	464.8	2,268.9	9.8	29,629.8	32,373.3

[1] Suspected farm but tested negative

Comparison economic impact of subsectors

The cattle sector suffered the greatest economic impact, i.e. 88% of total economic impact in the 2006 epidemic and 76% of the impact in the 2007 epidemic. Within the cattle sector, the economic impact for the dairy farmers was highest (55% of the total economic impact for the cattle sector in 2006, and 77% in 2007). Thereafter, the exporters and the quarantine farms for export experienced most economic impact (35% of the total economic impact in the cattle sector in 2006 and 11% in 2007). Within the sheep sector, the sheep producers suffered most economic impact (58% of the total economic impact for the sheep sector in 2006 and 71% in 2007). The small-scale sheep farms experienced an economic impact that corresponded to 20% of the total economic impact for the sheep sector in 2006 and 5% in 2007.

Table 6. Net costs (*1000 Euros) of the BT2007 epidemic per farm type, sector and in total.

FARM TYPE SECTOR	PRODUCTION LOSSES		DIAGNOSIS	TREATMENT		CONTROL MEASURES	TOTAL	
	2007-A	2007-B		2007-A	2007-B		2007-A	2007-B
Dairy	55,463.3	71,621.9	354.5	8,821.5	2,123.8	1,493.4	66,132.6	75,593.6
Veal calf	257.2	257.2	-	-	-	0.1	257.2	257.2
Other cattle	8,100.6	11,253.3	158.0	1,641.6	314.5	0.1	9,900.3	11,725.9
Susp. test neg	-	-	154.1	-	-	-	154.1	154.1
Screening	-	-	182.2	-	-	-	182.2	182.2
Export	-	-	-	-	-	9,414.8	9,414.8	9,414.8
Cattle subtotal	63,821.0	83,132.3	848.8	10,463.1	2,438.4	10,908.3	86,041.3	97,327.8
Dairy sheep	5,344.2	5,344.2	0.0	12.8	12.8	0.2	5,357.2	5,357.2
Trad. Herding	327.8	327.8	1.2	419.4	419.4	0.5	749.0	749.0
Breeding	14,771.3	14,771.3	324.9	2,671.4	2,671.4	43.8	17,811.4	17,811.4
Fattening	2,408.8	2,408.8	62.3	1,980.8	1,980.8	15.7	4,467.7	4,467.7
Hobby	1,076.5	1,076.5	339.8	142.2	142.1	1.8	1,560.3	1,560.3
Susp. test neg.	-	-	91.7	-	-	-	91.7	91.7
Screening	-	-	26.0	-	-	-	26.0	26.0
Export	-	-	-	-	-	1.8	1.8	1.8
Sheep subtotal	23,928.7	23,928.7	846.0	5,226.5	5,226.5	63.9	30,065.1	30,065.1
Dairy goat	199.6	199.6	311.8	311.8	311.8	54.8	823.2	823.2
Fattening	0.0	0.0	0.0	4.9	4.9	0.9	4.9	4.9
Hobby	0.0	0.0	2.8	101.3	101.3	225.8	104.1	104.1
Susp. test neg	-	-	3.3	-	-	-	3.3	3.3
Screening	-	-	26.0	-	-	-	26.0	26.0
Export	-	-	-	-	-	18.1	18.1	18.1
Goat subtotal	199.6	199.6	344.0	418.0	418.0	18.1	979.7	979.7
Transp.subtotal						0.7	0.7	0.7
Total	87,949.4	107,260.6	2,038.9	16,107.6	8,082.9	10,991.0	117,086.8	128,373.4

<u>Sensitivity analysis</u>

The net costs of the BT2006 epidemic were most sensitive to a change in the number of farms that had to obey the indoor housing obligation (Table 7). The net costs of the BT2007 epidemic was most sensitive to the number of BTV8 infected farms, but was also sensitive to the mortality rate and less sensitive to the morbidity rate and fertility variables.

Table 7. Relative change in net costs due to a 10% change of an input variable.

VARIABLE	CHANGE	RELATIVE CHANGE IN NET COSTS	
		BT2006	BT2007
# BTV8 infected farms	-10%	-0.28%	-6.46%
# BTV8 infected farms	+10%	0.13%	5.92%
# Farms compulsory indoor housing	-10%	-5.43%	-
# Farms compulsory indoor housing	+10%	5.43%	-
Mortality cattle and sheep	-10%	-0.03%	-3.02%
Mortality cattle and sheep	+10%	0.03%	3.02%
Morbidity cattle and sheep	-10%	-0.01%	-1.44%
Morbidity cattle and sheep	+10%	0.01%	1.44%
Proportion animals postponed gestation	-10%	-	-1.51%
Proportion animals postponed gestation	+10%	-	1.44%
Proportion animals abortion	-10%	-	-2.05%
Proportion animals abortion	+10%	-	1.19%

DISCUSSION

This cost benefit analysis focussed on a sector point of view. Although the different farm types, the distribution of the farm types over the Netherlands, as well as the presence of unregistered hobby sheep and goat farms are taken into account, it calculated the average economic impact (net costs) due to a BTV8 infection for the average farm. This research is suitable to support decision-making at sector level on, for example, the retrospective evaluation of implemented control measures, like the transport restrictions. It can also be used to evaluate future control measures, like vaccination strategies. However, assumptions have to be made on the size of the epidemic in the future. An evaluation of vaccination strategies in the epidemic year of 2008 (July 2008 till July 2009) has been made and will be published soon.

The cost benefit analysis is not suitable to support decisions at individual farm level on, for example, voluntary vaccination or the treatment of animals for several reasons. Each farm is unique and is not described by the average farm demographics as used in this study. Moreover each farm has a specific financial situation that puts the losses due to BTV8 infection in a unique risk perspective. Furthermore, an individual farmer does not make decisions purely on economic criteria, but also on the BTV8 history of the farm in the previous year(s). Thereby, experienced emotional impact can influence the BTV8 related decisions at farm level.

The net costs related to the BTV8 epidemic (until July 2008) were between 150 to 160 million Euros. At the start of the epidemic (i.e. in BT2006) the majority of losses were due to control measures, whereas in the second year of the epidemic (i.e. in BT2007) the majority of the losses were due to the production losses and treatment of diseased animals.

Epidemiological variables (e.g. morbidity and mortality) had a relative big influence on the net costs, especially when the epidemic has affected a large number of farms (BT2007). This study used two scenarios of morbidity and mortality estimates for cattle. The net costs were 11 million Euros (about 10%) higher in scenario B than in scenario A. Looking more in detail it showed that the production losses in scenario A were 22% lower, whereas the treatment costs were 50% higher compared to scenario B. In scenario A the morbidity rates were higher causing higher treatment costs, whereas in scenario B the mortality rates were higher, which caused (even) higher production losses.

The results showed that the net costs for the cattle sector were much higher than for the sheep sector or the goat sector, while the number of sheep and goats were much higher and the morbidity and mortality rates of sheep were much higher. The difference in net costs was due to the fact that the value of cattle (and therefore also the losses in case of diseases) was much higher.

Summarizing, this study shows that an introduction of an exotic disease in the Netherlands can cause very high losses, due to the disease and due to the control measures taken.

ACKNOWLEDGEMENTS

This study was funded by the joint commission on cattle health and quality (DKR) of the Product Boards for Livestock and Meat and the Dutch Dairy Board. We gratefully acknowledge Chris Bartels, Inge Berends, Lammert Moll, Gerdien van Schaik and Piet Vellema (Animal Health Service) for their input.

REFERENCES

ASG (2006). Kwantitatieve Informatie Veehouderij 2006-2007. Animal Sciences Group van Wageningen UR Lelystad

Bartels, C., van Schaik, G. and Vellema, P. (2008). Bluetongue infecties op melkveebedrijven in de periode van mei 2007 - mei 2008. GD, Deventer, p. 51

Berends, I.B. (2008). Memo koppeling VWA data met data van de rundermonitor en vergelijking met de data van de sentinel bedrijven. Gezondheidsdienst voor dieren, p. 5

Dercksen, D., Groot Nibbelink, N., Paauwe, R., Backx, A., van Rijn, P. and Vellema, P. (2007). Eerste bluetongue-uitbraak bij geiten in Nederland: beschrijving van de klinische verschijnselen en differentieeldiagnose. Tijdschrift voor Diergeneeskunde, 786-790

Elbers, A.R.W.and van der Spek, A. (2008). De ernst van de BTV-8 epidemie in Nederland in 2007 en de verschillen met de situatie in 2006. CVI, Lelystad, p. 25

Elbers, A.R.W., Backx, A., Mintiens, K., Gerbier, G., Staubach, C., Hendrickx, G. and van der Spek, A. (2008a). Field observations during the Bluetongue serotype 8 epidemic in 2006. II. Morbidity and mortality rate, case fatality and clinical recovery in sheep and cattle in the Netherlands. Preventive Veterinary Medicine 87, 31-40

Elbers, A.R.W., Popma, J., Oosterwolde, S., van Rijn, P.A., Vellema, P. and van Rooij, E.M.A. (2008b). A cross-sectional study to determine the seroprevalence of bluetongue virus serotype 8 in sheep and goats in 2006 and 2007 in the Netherlands. BMC Veterinary Research 4, 1-5

Houben, E.H.P. (1995). Economic optimization of decisions with respect to dairy cow health management. Farm Management. Wageningen University, Wageningen, p. 144

Jalvingh, A.W. and Dijkhuizen, A.A. (1997). Dairy cow calving interval: optimum versus allowable length; theory and possible use in herd health programs. In, International

Symposium for Veterinary Epidemiology and Economics (ISVEE), Paris, pp. 10.16.11-10.16.13

A SIMPLE ECONOMIC DECISION SUPPORT TOOL FOR THE CONTROL OF PARATUBERCULOSIS IN A SUCKLER BEEF HERD

I. MCCLEMENT*, I.D. MCFARLANE AND R.M. BENNETT

SUMMARY

The dynamic, deterministic, economic model *'Suckler_Johnes_model_1.1'* was developed to estimate the costs and benefits of controlling *Mycobacterium avium* subspecies *paratuberculosis* (Johne's disease) in a suckler beef herd. The aim was not only to design a cost benefit disease control model but also to design a communication tool that could be used by veterinarians and advisors with their clients to discuss the costs and benefits of controlling Johne's disease within their herd.

The model simulates the impact of different control strategies on herd prevalence and shedding with total costs of disease over ten years. The control strategies were, 'no control', 'testing & culling of diagnosed animals', 'improving management measures' or a dual strategy of 'testing & culling with improving management measures'. Testing and culling alone did not reduce prevalence or total costs however, 'testing & culling with improving management measures' considerably reduced prevalence, severity of shedding and herd costs over ten years.

INTRODUCTION

The causative agent of Johne's disease *Mycobacterium avium* subspecies *paratuberculosis (MAP)* is typically transmitted from dam to young via the faecal-oral route or via contaminated colostrum and milk (Begg & Whittington, 2007). Johne's disease is characterised by a wasting, chronic enteritis, resulting in decreased production, reduced fertility, increased replacement rates (Chiodini et al., 1984) and loss of cull value because 'diagnosed' Johne's diseased animals cannot enter the UK food chain (FSA, 2001). In advanced cases the animal suffers diarrhoea, emaciation and submandibular oedema (Chiodini et al., 1984). Infection with Johne's disease therefore implies significant economic losses to the herd (Kudahl et al., 2007).

The disease has a chronic, progressive subclinical phase with a proportion of those animals becoming clinical between two and six years of age, though the range can be 4 months to 15 years (Caldow et al., 2001).

The disease can be split into four stages according to the severity of clinical signs and the potential for shedding organisms via faeces into the environment. The stages are often called the 'iceberg effect' which suggests that for every clinical case there can be up to 25 subclinical

* Isobel McClement, Dept. of Agricultural and Food Economics, University of Reading, Earley Gate, Whiteknights Road, Reading, RG6 6AR Email: i.mcclement@reading.ac.uk

cases (Whitlock & Buergelt, 1996). Furthermore, Johne's disease is suspected to cause Crohn's disease in humans (Collins et al., 2000) and has received significant attention from scientists and policymakers (FSA, 2001).

There have been many approaches to modeling and managing the cost effective control of Johne's in dairy cattle such as described in Collins & Morgan 1992, Groenendaal et al., 2002, Kudhal et al., 2007 and Caldow et al., 2001. There are however, far fewer approaches that attempt to model the cost effective control of Johne's in beef suckler cattle or that attempt to *'communicate'* the cost effectiveness of managing Johne's disease at the farm level to farmers and herd managers. For that reason this paper aims to deliver on two levels:

Part 1 describes the modeling process which enabled *estimation* of economic outcomes of different control strategies in a suckler herd on herd prevalence, performance parameters and total herd cost in terms of the sum of production losses and control expenditures (Bennett, 2003). The strategies examined were:

i) No control (no action taken).

ii) Testing & Culling mild (annual targeted testing and removal of high shedding animals).

iii) Testing & Culling severe (annual targeted testing and removal of low and high shedding animals).

iv) Improved management (husbandry measures aimed at reducing the milk and faecal routes of infection to the neonatal and young calf).

v) Improved management with testing & culling severe (husbandry measures aimed at reducing the milk and faecal routes of infection to the neonatal and young calf plus the annual targeted testing and removal of low and high shedding animals).

Part 2 describes the tools, techniques and methods used to develop a computer based decision support tool (DST) capable of estimating the costs and benefits of controlling Johne's in suckler cows.

MATERIALS AND METHODS

Background to the decision support model

This model was funded as part of the UK Department of Environment, Food and Rural Affairs (Defra) Farm Health Planning (FHP) project. The project facilitates stakeholder partnership through establishing industry-led-working groups in all farmed animal sectors. Farm Health Planning stakeholder groups were set up for the poultry, pig, sheep and cattle (dairy and beef) sectors and consisted of farmers, veterinarians, advisers, and a number of experienced people from across each sector. The groups worked together to encourage producers to introduce proactive measures to help manage disease and improve performance. Each stakeholder group was asked to suggest diseases or conditions they considered were of economic importance to their business. Twelve disease control models were commissioned (www.fhpmodels.reading.ac.uk) in total which include the control of: Bovine Viral Diarrhoea (BVD) and *M. avium* sub. *paratuberculosis* (Johne's disease) in dairy and suckler cows; Digital

Dermatitis in dairy cattle; Footrot, Ectoparasites (sheep scab and lice) and *Fasciolosis* (Liver Fluke) in sheep; *Mycoplasma hyopneumoniae* (Enzootic Pneumonia) and Porcine Reproductive and Respiratory Syndrome (PRRS) in finishing pigs; Coccidiosis in broiler chickens and Mycoplasma *gallisepticum* in laying hens.

The aim of the initial project was to make a set of cost-benefit disease control case study models available to each group in CD format. Each model was to be designed with advice and input from each stakeholder group. However, as the project progressed it became clear through regular meetings with the stakeholder groups that what was actually needed was 'a software tool that could be downloaded from a free-content website to help veterinarians, animal health consultants, advisors and professionals, communicate and discuss disease control measures with their clients.' This highlighted the need for a flexible design process, accommodating design iterations, model reviews and regular stakeholder and end-user group feedback during model and graphical user interface (GUI) development.

The systems simulation modelling package Stella 9 ® (www.iseesystems.com) was used to construct the model. The programme consisted of a set of interacting layers; a top GUI, a graphical mapping layer, a modelling layer with graphical stock and flow diagrams that model discrete and continuous processes over time and a final equations (logic) layer.

Part 1: Epidemiological & Economic model

Input variables to describe herd composition, herd management, acquisition and disposal values and veterinarian charges for diagnosis and treatment were supplied by the user. From this data, together with epidemiological characteristics of Johne's disease described in published scientific and technical publications and interviews with practising veterinarians and herd managers, the model calculated the probability of perinatal and subsequent infection.

The suckler cow system

The Suckler cow system modelled was assumed to be broadly representative of most UK systems. All the animals ran as one unit, cows had a default calving percent of 90% per annum (though this could have been changed by the model user), calves were kept within the herd until weaning at 6 – 7 months, a proportion were then sold for finishing elsewhere and a proportion of heifer calves were kept for replacements (the model adjusted the proportion kept based on the control measures chosen). If there were not enough replacements due to heavy culling the model then costed in the price of purchasing in–calf, certified Johne's free replacement heifers. Due to lack of data and structural constraints no attempt was made to differentiate between autumn and spring calving herds.

Epidemiological model structure

The model was split into two interconnecting systems, the epidemiological pathway of disease under different control scenarios and the economic consequences of those different scenarios. The model tracked the sequence of events happening to proportions of animals in the herd and not individual animals (i.e. the model was herd rather than individual animal based). The animals then either became infected or not and were culled, died or continued to live.

All the animals either progressed into an infected state or remained in the resistant state. The course of infection was defined by six states; susceptible (those animals younger than 1 year and not yet infected), resistant (animals over 1 year old and not infected are assumed resistant), latent (early asymptomatic stage of the disease), low shedding (asymptomatic stage of the disease), high shedding (potentially symptomatic), clinical (displaying severe symptoms).

Epidemiological model disease transition mechanisms

The key mechanism driving animals through each disease state was based on the current disease pressure (dictated by the number of shedding animals present in the herd) and the age of exposure, i.e., the number of shedding animals and the age of exposure to those shedding animals determined the probability of infection.

Table 1. Parameter values for infection routes

Infection route	Probabilities	Reference
Foetal infection (infected dams)	0.20	Groenendaal et al., 2002
Foetal infection (clinical dams)	0.70	Groenendaal et al., 2002
Perinatal infection	Varies with I(a,b)	Adjusted Kudhal et al., 2007
1-19 weeks infection	Varies with I(a,b)	Adjusted Kudhal et al., 2007

a) The numbers and shedding states of animals in the herd at that time (disease rate).
b) Shedding state associated contaminated milk and colostrum.

The probabilities used by the model were influenced by herd management choices, actual or hypothetical, suggested by the user (Table 1). Three infection paths were modelled, each with an associated probability: (1) infection passed directly from infected dam (2) infection passed by faeces in the calving area (3) infection passed in colostrum and milk. In addition, transmission and progression of the disease used six weekly time steps from birth to 19 weeks (Kudhal et al., 2007) to take account of the rate at which the probability of becoming infected diminishes during the year after birth. After 19 weeks the model updated herd demographics and a proportion of the herd moved into each shedding state – or not if considered resistant (i.e. over 1 year old) every six months (Humphry et al., 2006) this maintained a constant population size throughout the ten years.

Johnes infection develops slowly; it remains hidden or latent and is not easily detected until it has progressed to the stage where the animal has itself become a source of infection. This was represented in the model (and in the diagram) by parallel progression either via resistant heifer status to healthy adult status, or via latent status from which the animal may or may not reach a stage when its feces constitute a moderate or serious risk. By the time high shedding or clinical status is reached, the animal will show other visible symptoms.

The second part of the model represented the financial cash flow of the business during the period, chosen to be 10 years, over which the presence of the disease in the herd was simulated. The two parts of the model are illustrated in Fig. 1.

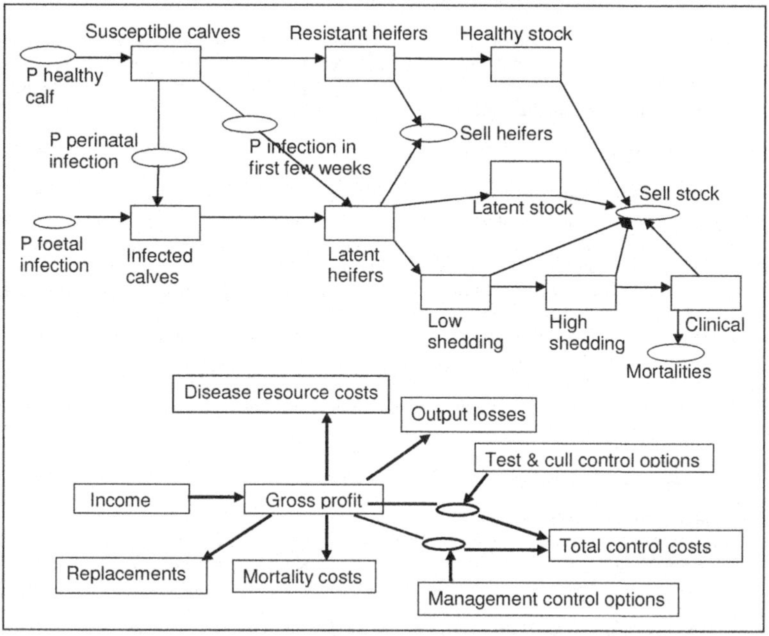

Fig.1. Johne's disease progression and cash flow impacts

Economic model structure

In the cash flow model, animals were represented as saleable up to the stage where risk of mortality was significant. The input parameters such as herd size, cull rate, calving percent, in calf heifer replacement value, calf value at weaning, cull cow value, national fallen stock charges (NFSS) had baseline default values, and the models were interactive so the users could enter herd details themselves (see Fig. 2).

Quantifying the economic impact of Johne's disease was based on McInerney's (1996) 'economic optimum level of the disease and disease control' method for measuring farm animal disease, and later defined by Bennett (2003) as direct disease cost, Eq.(1);

$$C = (L + R) + T + P \tag{1}$$

Where L is the value of loss in output due to disease, R are the increased expenditures on farm resources such as labour, T are the increased inputs to treat disease, P is the cost of disease prevention.

Economic Johne's control calculation mechanisms

The model output was split between information showing approximate numbers of animals in each disease state and information showing breakdowns of disease impacts (Fig. 2). The number of animals in each disease state was dictated by the control measure chosen which in turn drove the total cost calculations.

Johne's control details

No attempt was made to include a vaccination strategy. Vaccination only reduces and prolongs emergence of the number of clinical animals within the herd. Considerable disease pressure still exists due to the 'ice berg' effect of Johne's disease within the herd (Whitlock and Buergelt 1996). Furthermore, because Johne's disease cannot be cured control strategies focused on breaking transmission routes of infection and or a reduction of infection pressure by testing and culling infectious animals (Kennedy et al., 2001). In addition, supplementary on-farm labour costs were included as well as additional veterinary charges resulting from presence of Johne's disease in the herd. Further details included costs of management time associated with improved management procedures. All these costs were scaled to increase with herd size, but not in direct proportion. For example, some economy-of-scale applies to veterinary charges when many animals are tested together.

Control strategies

1. No control (no action taken)

This involved no attempt to break transmission and no attempt to identify or remove positive animals; therefore no control expenditure was assigned to this strategy.

Testing and Culling

Reduce infection pressure within the herd through a program of testing and culling, thereby removing the more infectious heavily shedding animals. Test accuracy was known to vary with parity and infection state. A test accuracy parameter was set within the model to reflect the herd factors affecting test accuracy.

2. Test & Cull 'mild'

This involved the annual targeted testing of high shedding, high parity animals. Positive animals were confirmed and then culled. Test and diagnostic charges per hour responded to scale, i.e. the more animals tested within an hour the cheaper the cost per animal. However this was highly farm and handling system specific. Default charges in the model shown were derived from interviews with practising veterinarians.

3. Test & Cull 'severe'

As per test & cull 'mild', plus the annual targeted testing and removal of low shedding animals. Additional farm labour costs when disease was present in the herd were from up to 10 hours per month for up to 10 animals in 'shedding' categories, and then on a smoothly varying scale up to maximum 50 hours per month if there were 250 in 'shedding' categories.

Management measures

Reduce the number of infected animals entering the herd through a combination of management steps, involving calf hygiene and clean environment husbandry measures.

4. Improve management

This involved reducing the number of infected animals entering the herd through a combination of management steps, involving calf hygiene and clean-environment husbandry measures (i.e. bio-security measures). The model assumed all risks of infection were reduced by 50% (based on Kudahl et al., 2007 & Pennsylvania State University, 2007). This was achieved firstly by calf hygiene and husbandry measures such as; ensuring a designated clean calving box, clean dam's udder and legs, rearing calves in separate age groups. Machinery and other feed/muck/bedding equipment are washed between young animals and older cows plus careful muck and slurry spreading is carried out which includes not allowing young stock on recently spread fields. Secondly by milk hygiene measures such as; no pooling of colostrum and no pooling of bulk tank or waste milk (suckled calves assumed to receive dam's milk only).

Valuing management measures where no formal data existed created a challenge. Therefore to enable some default 'estimation' of the costs involved, interviews were set up with farmers and veterinarians to estimate the per animal per week costs of implementing these changes. The result of the interviews suggested that a nominal cost could be £0.05 per animal per week. However a very strong caveat was attached to this estimate that the figure entered into this box was likely to be highly farm specific.

5. Improve management and testing & culling severe

As per 'improve management' the model assumed a reduction of 50% in the risk of infection plus the annual targeted testing and removal of low and high shedding animals.

Part 2: Designing and delivering a tool to assist decision making

Many DSS and DST that are developed are not widely adopted by users. Key reasons for failure to adopt have been excessive focus on technological factors (Mathews et al., 2008), surrendering decision makers to black box tools designed by others (McCown, 2002) and unclear DSS role definition i.e. implementation, how it will be used and by whom.

Decision support tool design factors

The *Suckler_ Johnes_model_1.1* is more of a decision support 'tool' than a decision support 'system' i.e. the latter is more data (supports the collection and analysis of a large data base) than information focused. However, it was considered appropriate to follow a DSS software development framework as it provided a disciplined structure to follow. Parker (1999) suggests developing DSS software can follow 'hard' methods which focus on system functionality, i.e. what the system is intended to do, in this case calculate the costs and benefits of controlling Johne's disease in suckler cows or 'soft' systems methodologies which still focus on system functionality but encourage more end user participation during development. The development issues raised above ensured the following factors were considered:

The decision support tool role

The software designed fulfils a decision support 'tool' role, making complex calculations that encapsulate knowledge that is difficult to derive from experiential learning (McCown, 2002).

Dangers: Successful in primary role but often discarded once facts gained (McCown, 2002).

Mitigation: By aiming the tool at veterinarians, animal health professionals and organisations with a multiple client base ongoing use could be better ensured.

Model Functionality

A tool capable of estimating the costs and benefits of controlling Johne's disease over 10 years and of displaying 'meaningful' output in the form of prevalence and financial data.

Dangers: Undue focus on 'techno-centric' functions. The tool becomes too 'black box' and users don't understand the relationships modelled which casts doubt on credibility (McCown, 2002).

Mitigation: Parallel focus on; i) the 'computer' programming work regarding the epidemiological factors and economic factors described in part 1 ii) managing the 'human' partnerships, interactions and end user's requirements.

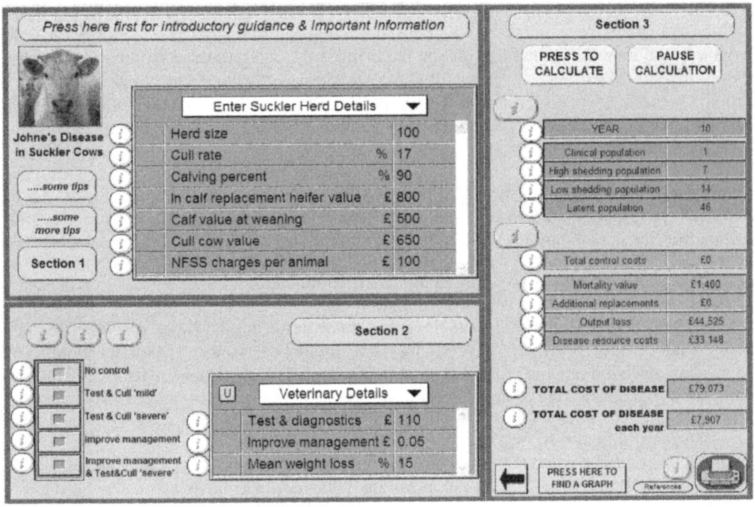

Fig.2. The Suckler_Johnes_Model_1.1 graphical user interface

Design process

A 'soft systems' flexible process based on a participatory design approach (Carbery et al., 2002) was used to allow design iterations based on FHP stakeholder groups and end user feedback. During the initial stages the groups met regularly and the modelling team presented conceptual models (Fig. 1) based on epidemiological and economic peer reviewed data to the groups for disease information feedback. Once the modelling work had started work began on the GUI particularly on how and what information the user considered useful.

By using Stella 9 ® the GUI could be constructed using the same programme as the model, and the interacting GUI and modelling layers allowed immediate changes and editing to the modelling layers if a different output format was required. The top interface layer (see Fig. 2) toolbar had many input devises such as List Input Devises (LIDs) to input farm/system specific information concerning herd/flock size, market values, performance parameters, husbandry practices, and costs of disease control methods, switches to turn binary decision variables 'on' or 'off', i.e. when choosing a control strategy or not and sliders to adjust constant values.

Communicating the severity of Johne's disease to herd owners and managers is notoriously difficult because test accuracy is dependent on the shedding state of the animal and production losses during the protracted asymptomatic phase are difficult to quantify. Therefore, a core advisory group of veterinarians in the field with experience and interest in Johne's disease in suckler cows was involved with the output format for the *Suckler_ Johnes_model_1.1*. This focused on showing prevalence details over the ten years, so that the 'iceberg' effect could be appreciated (see Fig. 2), breaking the costs and losses down into, control expenditure, mortality, replacements, output losses and resources costs and each output box needed a 'pop up' information box. A graphical function was also included via means of a clickable linked page; this showed prevalence details over the ten years. The group also highlighted important GUI features – it must not cover more than one page i.e., no scrolling down the page, as a) this took too long and b) users forgot, and importantly the whole process from data input to data output must not take more than a few minutes – time is money!

Model delivery

A survey carried out by Matthews et al., (2008) in 2000 suggested that preferred delivery mechanism of agricultural DSS were via software products, then via web-based services then via consultancies. It was suggested that the users preferred to have control over the software tool itself –empowering more user freedom with how and where the tool could be used. This confirmed model delivery via a dedicated website, where the model can be downloaded to the user's computer/disc/laptop with a link to install the free viewer version of the Stella software (ISEE Player). Access to the model (all the models) would be control free, i.e. anyone could access the models (though the modelling layer is locked to unauthorised access) and user details would not be collected. Explanation and analysis of web design is not within the scope of this paper however, Castaneda et al., (2007) developed a 'web acceptance model' (WAM) based on the social psychology model of the 'Theory of Reasoned Action'. This model suggests that factors influencing website use and acceptance focus on 'perceived ease of use' and 'perceived usefulness', therefore the website had to be simple in navigation with minimal unnecessary content and focus on the models and effective downloading procedure.

RESULTS

Part 1: epidemiological & economic model

An initial population was set with herd size plus heifers and their calves (set in calving percent). Next, according to whichever control was chosen, the model assumed 'a level' of residual disease (10 low shedding animals entered the herd) and progressed for the next 10 years (Table 2). The model would not eliminate Johne's (during the 10 year run), because it reduced but did not eliminate transmission routes.

The main output was in the form of tabulation of the disease costs and treatment costs (Table 3) and a graphical output is available via a linked page. The model described in this paper had herd and management default figures set at; 100 cow suckler herd with a calving rate of calves reared of 90%, a cull rate of 17%, an in-calf (Johne's free) replacement heifer value of £800, calf value at weaning of £500, a cull cow value of £650 and NFSS charges of £100 per animal. Veterinary default details and figures were set at: test and diagnostics £110 per hour, nominal farm specific per animal per week charge for implementing management changes £0.05 and mean weight loss set at 15% (see model for more details). All figures entered for default demonstration runs were adjustable (Fig. 2).

Table 2. Cumulative shedding populations in year 10.

Shedding populations	No Control	Test & Cull mild (m)	Test & Cull severe (s)	Improve management	Improve man. & Test & Cull (s)
Clinical	1	0	0	1	0
High	7	4	0	5	0
Low	14	14	8	7	5
Latent	46	47	46	24	27

Table 3. Cumulative values over 10 years (2nd quarter 2008 output and input prices).

Breakdown costs (£)	No Control	Test & Cull mild (m)	Test & Cull severe (s)	Improve management	Improve man. & Test & Cull (s)
Total control costs	0	990	990	351	2511
Mortality value	14	0	0	1200	0
Replacements	0	0	800	0	800
Output loss	44,525	42,155	39,304	24,013	24,015
Resource costs	33,148	31,764	27,899	22,562	19,808
Total cost of disease	79,073	74,909	68,993	48,125	47,134
Average total costs of disease (each year)	7907	7491	6899	4813	4713

DISCUSSION

Model merits

The work of Kudahl et al. (2007) claimed a similar benefit to that shown in Table 2 in terms of reducing prevalence when combining testing and culling with management steps. Furthermore, better hygiene management will benefit other diseases as will targeted testing and monitoring of herd health.

In terms of the first delivery level (the modelling of Johne's control epidemiology and economic relationships over time) there was general concurrence that the Johne's model recommended 'improve management' strategy avoided replacements after culling, and hence was a better option than 'test & cull'. This was supported by comments from users asked at the 2008 UK Dairy event if they considered the *Suckler_ Johnes_model_1.1.* to be useful when discussing Johne's or wider issues (costs, impacts etc.) with their client, 45% of those asked considered the model 'quite useful' and 55% considered the model 'very useful' with others adding that they liked the way the model allows the simulation of a combined strategy.

In terms of the second delivery level (designing and delivering a tool to assist decision making) the website usage statistics are favourable for a model and project with very limited formal marketing or publicity. The reporting of bounce rates (measurement of visitor views lasting 10 seconds or less or only visiting one page on the site) are a useful tool for e-commerce sites but it is of questionable value for free content sites such as this site. With free content sites visitors tend to find what they want immediately (e.g. a model), initiate download then bounce off the site. For free content sites, metrics (categories) such as returning visitors vs. new visitors might be more informative and this is somewhat confirmed by the model and ISEE viewer page bounce rates of 64% and 74% respectively. In addition, when users were asked at the 2008 UK Dairy event if they considered the use of computer based tools to be useful when discussing disease issues (costs, impacts etc.) with their client, 72% of those asked considered computer based tools as 'quite useful' and 28% considered computer based tools' very useful'.

McCown, (2002) suggests that a key factor in uptake success is credibility of the information provided. The comments from visitors suggested that references on the model to multiple data sources enhanced the credibility of the model and reputation was helped by using a more participatory approach (involving stakeholders, end users and funding providers). Veterinarians reported a favourable response from their clients largely through using the Johne's model as more of a discussion 'facilitator' and some reported that the very *process* of thinking about disease in their herd and entering their own farm data into the model was as useful as the output. Many herd managers regard their vet as a trustworthy source of information and knowledge, and the fact that the model was designed by an 'independent' rather than commercial model builder also claimed a more favourable response from their clients.

Model limitations

Placing a value on milk and environment (husbandry) management measures aimed at reducing neonatal calf infection posed a big challenge. The interviews with veterinarians and a few herd managers were rather ad hoc and lacked scientific rigour however, in the absence of any other data this method was considered sufficient but not ideal, however, the user can enter their own 'improve management' estimate.

Though a more participative development approach was used for this project and model, the second delivery level could have been helped more by employing more software and systems design evaluation tools. For example users reported difficulty with the downloading procedure namely editing file extensions and a useful function could be a tool to save and compare outcomes. By using more software design observational approaches, involving one-way glass to better assess GUI use and better observe more vet and client interactions, these problems could possibly have been averted. This project aimed to deliver the model and assess model use intentions. There are plans for evaluating implementation of the strategies suggested in the models and ongoing uptake issues.

ACKNOWLEDGEMENTS

The authors would like to thank the Defra Farm Health Planning team, John Sumner and the Farm Health Planning Cattle group, Keith Cutler of Endell Veterinary Group, Matt Dobbs of Westpoint Veterinary Group, Peter Orpin of Park Veterinary Group, Neil Blake of Charter Veterinary Group, George Caldow, (SAC) Alistair Stott, (SAC) members of the Johnes Initiative Group. Any errors or omissions of the paper are the responsibility of the authors.

REFERENCES

Bennett, R. M. (2003). The 'Direct costs' of livestock disease: The development of a system of models for the analysis of 30 endemic livestock diseases in Great Britain. Journal of Agricultural Economics. 54, 55-71

Begg, D. J., and Whittington, R.J., (2007). Experimental animal infection models for Johne's disease, an infectious enteropathy caused by *Mycobacterium avium* subsp. *paratuberculosis*. The Veterinary Journal. 176, 129-145

Caldow, G., Greig, A., Gunn, G.J., Humphry, R., Low, C.J., Ashworth, S.W., Jones, G.M., Sott, A.W., Cranwell, M.V., Sharp, J.M., Stevenson, K. and Henderson, D.C. (2001). Assessment of surveillance and control of Johne's disease in farm animals in GB. SAC, DEFRA: 67-82. http://www.defra.gov.uk/animalh/diseases/zoonoses/zoonoses_reports/sac2.pdf

Carberry, P.S., Hochman, Z., McCown, R.L., Dalgliesh, N.P., Foale, M.A., Poulton, J.N.G.H., Hargreaves, D.M.G., Cawthray, S. and Hillcoat, N. (2002). The FARMSCAPE approach to decision support: farmers', advisers, researchers' monitoring, simulation, communication and performance evaluation. Agricultural Systems. 74, 141–177

Castaneda, A.J., Munoz-Leiva, F. and Luque, T. (2007). Web acceptance model (WAM): Moderating effects of user experience. Information and Management. 44, 384-396

Chiodini, R.J., van Kruiningen, H.J. and Merkal, R.S. (1984). Ruminant paratuberculosis (Johne's disease): the current status and future prospects. Cornell Vet. 74, 218-262

Collins, M. T., Lisby, G., Moser, C., Chicks, D., Christensen, S., Reichelderfer, M., Hoilby, N., Harms, B., Thomsen, O.O., Skibsted, U. and Binder, V. (2000). Results of multiple diagnostic tests for *Mycobacterium avium* subsp. *paratuberculosis* in patients with inflammatory bowel disease and control. Journal of Clinical Microbiology. 38, 4373- 4381

Collins, M.T., and Morgan, I.R. (1992) Simulation model of paratuberculosis control in a dairy herd. Preventive Veterinary Medicine. 14, 21-32

Food Standards Agency (2001). http://www.johnes.org/handouts/files/Review%20of%20evidence.pdf

Groenendaal, H., Nielen, M., Jalvingh, A. W., Horst, S.H., Galligan, D.T., Hesselink, J.W. (2002). A simulation of Johne's disease control. Preventive Veterinary Medicine. 54, 225-245

Humphrey, R.W., Stott, A.W., Adams, C. and Gunn, G.J. (2006). A model of the relationship between the epidemiology of Johne's disease and the environment in the suckler-beef herds. The Veterinary Journal. 172, 432-445

Kennedy, D., Holstrom, A., Plym Forshell, K., Vindel. E. and Suarez Fernandez, G. (2001). On farm management of Paratuberculosis (Johne's disease) TB in dairy herds. Bull. Int. Dairy Federation. 362, 18-31

Kudahl, A., Ostergaard, S., Sorensen, J.T. and Nielsen, S.S. (2007). Stochastic model simulating paratuberculosis in a dairy herd. Preventive Veterinary Medicine. 78, 97 - 111.

Matthews, K., B., Schwarz, G., Buchan, K., Rivington, M. and Miller., D. (2008). Wither agricultural DSS? Computers and Electronics in Agriculture. 61, 149-159

McCown, R., L. (2002). Locating agricultural decision support systems in the troubled past and socio-technical complexity of 'models for management', Agric. Systems.74, 11–25.

McInerney, J. (1996). Old economics for new problems - livestock disease: Presidentialaddress. Journal of Agricultural Economics. 47, 295-314

Parker, C. (1999). PhD Thesis: Bridging the Gap: User-Centred Design and Support Methods for Decision Support Systems in Crop Production. Loughborough University

Pennsylvania State University, (2007). Pennsylvania State University Vet Extension Service http://vetextension.psu.edu/biosecurity/

Whitlock, R.H. and Buergelt, (1996) Preclinical and clinical manifestation of paratuberculosis (including pathology). Vet. Clin. N. Am. Food Animal Practice. 12, 245-356

DECISION SUPPORT

META-ANALYSIS ON THE EFFICACY OF DRY COW THERAPY INTERVENTIONS

T. HALASA*, M. NIELEN, A.C. WHIST, T. VAN WERVEN, H. HOGEVEEN AND O. ØSTERÅS

SUMMARY

The aim of this study was to perform two meta-analyses on dry period interventions. The first investigated the efficacy on prevention of new intra-mammary infections (IMI), while the second meta-analysis quantified the efficacy of dry cow therapy (DCT) to cure existing IMI at dry off. Studies that had a treatment and control group were selected. Publication bias was assessed. Blanket DCT provided significant protection against quarter new IMI caused by *Streptococcus* spp., but not against new IMI caused by coliforms and *Staphylococcus* spp., after correcting for publication bias. Selective DCT protected quarters from new IMI, but depending on the selection unit for treatment. Teat sealant provided significant protection against quarter new IMI caused by *Staphylococcus* spp., but not against quarter new IMI caused by *Streptococcus* and coliform pathogens. Blanket DCT provided a higher cure rate from quarter IMI caused by *Staphylococcus* spp. and *Streptococcus* spp. than untreated IMI quarters.

INTRODUCTION

The dry period (DP) is an important risk period for new intra-mammary infections (IMI). Several interventions are used to limit new IMI during the dry period. Dry cow therapy (DCT) became one of the 5 points plan and was widely used in North America and several European countries (Dodd et al., 1969; Robert et al., 2006). Raising concerns about bacterial resistance and economic incentives led to the use of selective DCT (SDCT), which was adopted frequently in different countries (Morris et al., 1978; Østerås et al. 1994). The purpose of DCT is not only to prevent new IMI, but also to cure existing IMI at drying off, which might help to prevent new IMI in the healthy quarters of the treated cow during the DP (Østerås et al. 1994).

Another alternative to DCT to prevent bacterial access to the mammary gland was the use of teat sealant (TS) (Meaney, 1976). Internal and external TS were tested in several studies showing a great potential to prevent new IMI at post-calving (Berry et al., 2007; Parker et al., 2008).

Several studies have investigated the effect of DCT with or without TS on the risk of new IMI during the DP and on the cure of existing IMI at dry off (Cummins and McCaskey, 1987; Pankey et al., 1982a,b; Schukken, 1993). The magnitudes of these effects vary noticeably between the studies, which makes it difficult to advise these treatments for controlling IMI during the DP. A meta-analysis summary would be helpful to quantify the preventive and curative effect of DCT on IMI during the DP. Besides, it will also assess the preventive effect of

* Tariq Halasa, Department of Farm Animal Health, Utrecht University, PO Box 80151, 3508 TD Utrecht, the Netherlands. Email: T.H.Halasa@uu.nl

TS against new IMI during the DP. This would ease the economic assessment of DP interventions.

Since studies presenting large and interesting results are more likely to be published, a potential publication bias might arise leading to a biased research body. Using several techniques in the meta-analysis, this potential bias can be investigated to properly draw conclusions on the preventive and curative effect of DCT. The objectives of this research were to provide a summary quantification of: 1) the prevention effects of DCT against new IMI during the DP up to 21 days post-calving; 2) the prevention effects of TS against new IMI during the DP up to 21 days post-calving; 3) the curative effects of DCT of existing IMI at dry off throughout the DP up to 21 days post-calving.

MATERIALS AND METHODS

Paper selection

A search was conducted on literature related to the DP intervention published between 1930 and the beginning of 2008. The search was carried out using two methods: 1) search by using the following key words in Pubmed (the National Library of Medicine, Bethesda, USA) in different combinations: *DP, transitional period, prepartum, peripartum, post partum, lactation, new IMI, cure IMI, mastitis, pathogen, cattle, cow, dairy, management, control, intervention, udder health, dry off, therapy, treatment, teat sealant*, and 2) reference citation procedure in the SIS web of knowledge (The Thompson Cooperation, Philadelphia, USA) where a search was conducted for studies that cited older studies.

Papers to be included in the meta-analysis had to: 1) be original research papers published in peer reviewed journals; 2) report the number or the rate of new IMI at quarter level in at least 2 groups (treated and control group) and the total number of quarters in each group; 3) report the number or the rate of IMI cure at quarter level in at least 2 groups (treatment and control group) and the total number of infected quarters in each group;4) be published in or have a summary in English; 5) report the outcome of a new data set or new protocol. When several studies were published based on the same data, the most detailed study was used. When more than one protocol existed per study roman numbers were used to discriminate between protocols. A total of 31 studies fitted the above criteria for inclusion in the meta-analyses and are listed within the references.

Intervention groups involved in the meta-analyses

Groups in the meta-analysis on the risk of new IMI

Blanket DCT (BDCT) was compared to no DCT, based on studies that reported the number of new quarter IMI during DP up to 21 days post-calving as a cumulative incidence.

The SDCT comparison was based on studies that measured the number of new quarter IMI in the SDCT compared to no DCT during DP up to 21 days post-calving as a cumulative incidence. The analysis was carried out separately for quarter or cow level treatment and reported as a combined overall effect. A separate meta-analysis was carried out for studies that compared SDCT to BDCT as a positive control group.

Studies that investigated the protective effect of TS using negative or positive control groups were analysed together. The studies reported the number or incidence of new quarter IMI during DP up to 21 days post-calving as a cumulative incidence in the treatment and control group.

Groups in the meta-analysis on the cure of IMI

Studies that reported the number or rate of quarter IMI cure during the DP up to 21 days post-calving using BDCT were included in the analysis. In these studies the treatment group was treated IMI quarters at dry off, while the control group was untreated IMI quarters at dry off.

Studies that measured the number or rate of quarter IMI cure using SDCT during the DP up to 21 days post-calving were included in the analysis. Selection of treatment unit was either at quarter or cow level.

Definition and incidence of new quarter IMI

A quarter was considered a new IMI when a pathogen was isolated in the calving or post-calving samples whereas the pathogen was absent in the quarter at previous samplings. The incidence rate of new quarter IMI was re-calculated from all studies as the number of new IMI quarters during the DP up to 21 days post-calving divided by the number of healthy quarters at dry off, to be the number of quarters at risk of new IMI.

Definition and cure of quarter IMI

A quarter was considered cured when a pathogen was no longer isolated at calving or post-calving whereas it was present at drying off. The incidence of cure (cure rate) was re-calculated from all studies to be the number of cured quarters during the DP up to 21 days post-calving divided by the number of IMI quarters at dry off.

Meta-analysis Procedure

Outcome Parameters

The relative risk (RR) of new IMI was calculated as the incidence of new quarter IMI in the treatment group divided by the incidence of new quarter IMI in the control group per study and intervention. The RR of cure was calculated as the cure rate in the treatment group divided by the cure rate in the control group per study and intervention. The calculated RRs were pooled in separate meta-analyses using Comprehensive Meta Analysis (CMA, 2008).

The pooled RRs to prevent new IMI and to cure IMI were calculated per intervention as an overall effect (all pathogens together), and per pathogen group (*Staphylococcus* spp., *Streptococcus* spp., and coliform pathogens); separately. In studies that included more than one protocol, a combined effect was calculated per study (CMA, 2008).

Meta-Regression

The homogeneity of the studies per intervention and pathogen group was checked to examine whether all studies originated from the same meta-population to properly draw conclusions about the estimated pooled RR. The procedure by which the pooled RR and homogeneity parameter (Q) were calculated is explained elsewhere (Borenstein et al., 2007; Duffield et al., 2008). In case of homogeneity, a fixed effect model was used to obtain the pooled RR. In case of heterogeneity, a weighted meta-regression was conducted in an attempt to explain the variation between studies. On the basis of current knowledge, factors involved in the meta-regression were believed to be able to cause variability between studies. These factors were regressed against the results of each study and weighted by the inverse variance (Dohoo et al., 2003). A meta-analysis was carried out only when at least 4 studies were available (Robert et al., 2006).

Publication Bias

The publication bias was assessed using funnel plots. Tests included Duval and Tweedie's fill and trim method (Duval and Tweedie, 2000), Begg and Mazumdar's rank correlation test (Begg and Mazumdar, 1994), and Egger's regression test (Egger et al., 1997). When significant publication bias and change on the estimated pooled RR were detected, the number of studies necessary to reverse the overall pooled effect was calculated using Orwin's fail-safe N method (Orwin, 1983). The study influence was also examined using the one study removed method (Dohoo et al., 2003). When significant publication bias was deemed to exist, the pooled RR was presented based on the Duval and Tweedie's fill and trim method estimation after correcting for the bias. The interpretation of these tests is available in the results section.

RESULTS

Prevention of quarter new IMI

All studies were found to be heterogeneous, but none of the potential explanatory variables in the meta-regression significantly explained the heterogeneity.

When BDCT was compared to no DCT, BDCT provided significantly higher protection against new IMI during the DP up to 21 days post-calving (Table 1). Based on a random effect model, DCT quarters had 0.62 (0.47-0.83) times less risk of new IMI than untreated quarters when *Staphylococcus* spp. were involved. Applying the one study removed method showed that none of the studies altered the random pooled RR significantly. The Begg and Mazumdar rank correlation test suggested no correlation between the study size and effect (P-value = 0.33). However, the regression test of Egger contradicted Begg and Mazumdar's rank correlation test, suggesting a significant association between study size and effect size (p = 0.01). The fill and trim method by Duval and Tweedie indicated no missing studies on the left-hand side of the funnel plot, but 7 studies (black spots) were missing on the right-hand side to reach complete symmetry (Figure 1). This figure indicates that if publication bias did not exist and complete symmetry was reached by including the missing studies, the preventive effect would shift to the null effect (Table 3). Since significant publication bias was indicated, the number of studies necessary to move the pooled RR above 1 was calculated using Orwin's fail-safe N method. According to Orwin's fail-safe N method and when the mean RR in the missing studies was assumed to be 1.10, the number of necessary studies was 17, but when the mean RR in the missing studies was assumed to be 1.20, the number of necessary studies was only 8. This low number of studies supports the insignificant protective effect of DCT against *Staphylococcus* spp. new IMI during the DP up to 21 days post-calving.

BDCT provided high protection against *Streptococcus* spp. (Table 3) and no significant publication bias was indicated by any of the tests. The protection of DCT against coliform was insignificant (Table 1). All publication bias tests indicated an absence of potential bias.

When SDCT was compared to no DCT, the studies were heterogeneous. SDCT provided significant protection against new quarter IMI (Table 3), and protection was slightly higher when selection and treatment were carried out at cow level.

When SDCT was compared to BDCT, the studies were homogeneous. BDCT showed higher protection than SDCT (Figure 2). Nonetheless, there was no significant difference in protection from new quarter IMI between SDCT and BDCT when the selection unit was the cow, with the whole udder treated (Figure 2). When the SDCT selection unit was the quarter, BDCT provided better protection from new quarter IMI than SDCT (Figure 2).

Table 1. Pooled relative risk (RR) of prevention of new quarter IMI during the DP, and RR of cure of existing IMI using the different interventions; overall and per pathogen group, together with the number of studies (n) per group and meta-analysis

Intervention and pathogen group	n	Pooled RR (95% confidence interval) of prevention of new IMI during the DP	n	Pooled RR (95% confidence interval) of cure of IMI during the DP
BDCT vs. no DCT				
Overall	18	0.61 (0.53-0.71)	14	1.78 (1.51-2.10)
Staphylococci	18	0.76 (0.54-1.07)	14	1.65 (1.38-1.96)
Streptococci	14	0.39 (0.30-0.51)	10	1.86 (1.48-2.35)
Coliform	6	0.95 (0.81-1.10)	-	-
SDCT vs. no DCT	5	0.51 (0.30-0.86)	4	1.73 (1.20-2.50)
SDCT vs. BDCT	5	1.83 (1.24-2.71)	-	-
TS vs. no TS				
Overall	6	0.45 (0.27-0.74)	-	-
Staphylococci	4	0.66 (0.51-0.85)	-	-
Streptococci	4	0.50 (0.21-1.19)	-	-
Coliform	4	0.84 (0.63-1.12)	-	-

In general, TS injected quarters have 0.45 (0.27-0.74) times less risk of new IMI than non TS injected quarters (Table 1). TS protected quarters from new *Staphylococcus* spp. IMI, but not from coliform nor from *Streptococcus* spp. IMI (Table 1). All publication bias tests indicated an absence of significant bias.

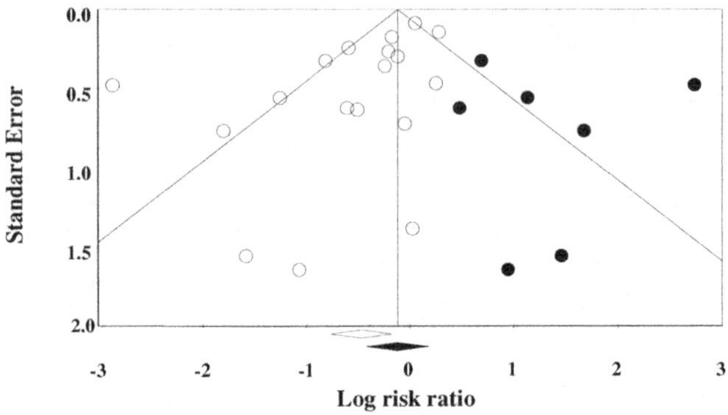

Figure 1. Funnel plot of the pooled relative risk (RR) of studies (empty circles) involved in the protective effect of dry cow therapy against new *Staphylococcus* spp. quarter intra-mammary infections (IMI) during the dry period up to 21 days post-calving (RR = incidence of new *Staphylococcus* spp. quarter IMI in the blanket dry cow therapy group divided by the incidence in the untreated control group). The dark spots are the potential missing studies according to Duval and Tweedie's fill and trim method (if they had existed, the pooled relative risk would have changed toward the null effect; the black diamond under the null effect). The light circles are the 18 studies involved.

Selection unit for treatment	Study	RR	Lower limit	Upper limit
Cow	Browning-I (1994)	1.505	1.048	2.161
Cow	Rindsig (1978)	0.217	0.119	0.394
Cow	Williamson-I (1995)	0.386	0.092	1.612
Pooled RR		**0.519**	**0.117**	**2.308**
Quarter	Hassan (1999)	0.331	0.094	1.161
Quarter	Browning-II (1994)	2.445	1.753	3.410
Quarter	Williamson-II (1995)	2.465	1.328	4.573
Quarter	Robinson (1988)	2.259	1.766	2.888
Pooled RR		**2.010**	**1.339**	**3.017**
Overall pooled RR		**1.831**	**1.238**	**2.710**

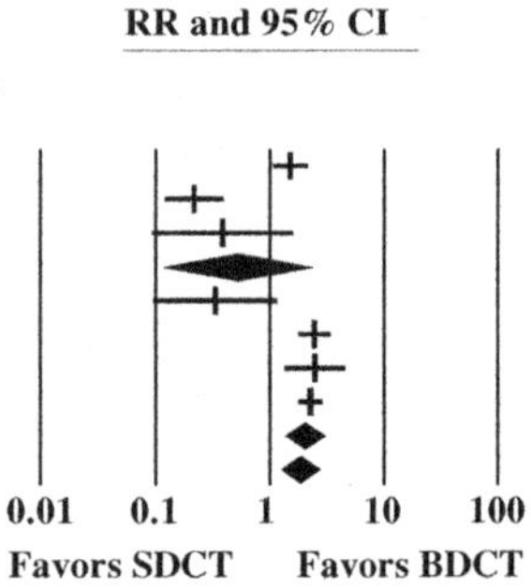

Figure 2. Forest plot of the relative risk (RR) of new quarter intra-mammary infections (IMI) during the dry period up to 21 days post-calving (RR = incidence of new quarter IMI in the selective dry cow therapy group divided by the incidence in the blanket dry cow therapy group) per study, and the pooled RR per selection unit and as an overall pooled RR with the 95% confidence interval (CI).

Cure of quarter IMI

The studies were heterogeneous for all pathogens and none of the potential explanatory variables in the meta-regression explained the heterogeneity significantly. Based on a random model, IMI quarters that had had BDCT had 1.78 (1.51-2.10) times higher cure rate during the DP and early lactation than untreated IMI quarters (Table 1). The RR was not altered by removing any of the studies, and none of the publication bias tests indicated presence of significant bias.

Using a random effect model, DCT would lead to a 1.65 (1.38-1.96) times higher calculated cure rate from *Staphylococcus* spp. IMI compared to no DCT (Table 1). All publication bias tests indicated an absence of significant bias. DCT showed higher cure rate from *Streptococcus* spp. IMI than the spontaneous cure in all studies (Table 1). No significant publication bias was identified by any of the publication bias tests. There were only 3 studies in which the cure rate from coliform IMI was estimated and therefore meta-analysis was not carried out for coliform pathogens.

Studies that challenged the cure rate based on SDCT compared to no DCT were heterogeneous. Meta-regression was not carried out, owing to the small number of studies, and a random effect model was used to present the pooled RR. SDCT provides a higher cure rate of IMI compared to no DCT. Treated IMI quarters at dry off had a 1.73 (1.20-2.50) times higher cure rate during the DP and early lactation than untreated quarters (Table 1)

DISCUSSION

DCT provided high protection against *Streptococcus* spp. new IMI (Table 1). Publication bias tests detected a potential bias, but this was not significant and thus the meta-analysis was deemed correct. DCT did not significantly protect from new coliform IMI during the DP. This was explained by the fact that coliform new IMI occurs late in the DP when DCT might not provide protection against new IMI any longer owing to low concentration (Robert et al., 2006).

On the basis of a random effect model, initially BDCT provided significant protection against *Staphylococcus* spp. new quarter IMI. However, publication bias tests indicated a significant bias. Adding 7 studies to the right-hand side of the funnel plot (Figure 2), led to nullifying the effect and suggested that DCT does not protect significantly against *Staphylococcus* spp. new IMI. Although large and small studies are present on both sides of the plot, 3 large studies including the largest study suggested that DCT does not protect against *Staphylococcus* spp. new IMI (Figure 1). The 7 missing studies might have been conducted, but not published in peer reviewed journals because they showed no protective effect. The fact that 2 of these studies would be small and another 2 studies relatively small (Figure 1), would support the speculation that they were not published (Dohoo et al., 2003). The reason for not publishing the data could be that those studies were sponsored by commercial companies and it would not be commercially beneficial to publish such data. Another reason could be that the results might not have been interesting enough for publication. Many peer reviewed journals do not publish results if they are not striking or interesting enough or show significant differences between treatment effects (Ferguson, 2007). Several studies found that many *Staphylococcus* spp. new IMI occur late in the DP and in early lactation (Soback et al., 1990; Hassan et al., 1999). Soback et al. (1990) indicated that the failure of DCT to prevent new *Staphylococcus aureus* IMI during the DP could have occurred owing to the failure of the DCT to cure existing infections at dry off. Hogan et al. (1994) showed that DCT was not successful in preventing new *Staphylococcus aureus* IMI during the DP. They suggested that since *Staphylococcus aureus* is part of a normal flora of the teat skin and in late DP the teat canal would open and the bacteria would have access causing new IMI. Rindsig et al. (1978) observed that the longer the DP, the higher the chance of new *Staphylococcus* spp. IMI, and reasoned that the decreased DCT concentration provided less prophylactic effect. For all the reasons mentioned above, it was deemed that publication bias existed in the peer reviewed literature and there was no significant protective effect of BDCT against *Staphylococcus* spp. new quarter IMI during the DP up to 21 d post-calving. Although statistically insignificant, the estimated protection effect against new *Staphylococcus* spp. quarter IMI using DCT may be important. Hence an economic analysis is necessary to reveal the importance of the estimated protective effect of DCT against new *Staphylococcus* spp. quarter IMI.

When SDCT was compared to BDCT, and when selection was carried out at cow level for SDCT, there was no significant difference in protection between SDCT and BDCT. However, BDCT showed higher protection when SDCT selection was carried out at quarter level. This might be explained by the fact that an infected quarter in a cow could have a higher chance of infecting other healthy quarters in the same cow during the DP than infecting healthy quarters in other cows (Buddle et al., 1987). Treatment at cow level could or could not cure this infected quarter, but at least would help prevent the infection of other healthy quarters.

Since DCT aims to cure existing IMI and prevent new IMI during the DP and around calving, the current study summarized these two important aspects based on peer reviewed research published in English. The current study found that DCT cured existing *Staphylococcus* spp. and *Streptococcus* spp. IMI at dry off significantly. Significant publication bias was not detected. It also shows that DCT provided significant protection only against new *Streptococcus* spp. quarter IMI. No significant protection was found against new *Staphylococcus* spp. quarter IMI after correcting for publication bias. Using DCT the cure rate against *Staphylococcus* spp. IMI was high in most studies, which made it easy to achieve publication for them because they reached significant levels even in small studies (Dohoo et al., 2003). However, again using DCT, since the rate of prevention of new *Staphylococcus* spp. IMI is not as high as the cure rate, we expected studies that measured new *Staphylococcus* spp. IMI, not to show significant effects and consequently not to succeed in being published. These studies appeared to be missing in the meta-analysis. This could explain the absence of certain studies for *Staphylococcus* spp.

This study provided an important observation in relation to SDCT, i.e. when the cow was the selection unit for treatment SDCT provided equal protection against new IMI as BDCT with a similar efficacy of curing of existing IMI. This might make SDCT based at cow level a good choice to optimize milk production and limit the use of antibiotics. However, the data were limited and more studies on SDCT at cow and quarter level might be helpful to confirm or reject this important observation.

ACKNOWLEDGEMENTS

Authors acknowledge the help of Scott McDougall for providing some hard-to-find papers. This project was financially supported by the Dutch Udder Health Centre (UGCN) and Norwegian School of Veterinary Science.

REFERENCES

Begg, C., and M. Mazumdar. 1994. Operating characteristics of a rank correlation test for publication bias. Biometrics 50:1088-1101.

Berry, E. A., and J. E. Hillerton. 2002a. The effect of selective dry cow treatment on new intramammary infections. J. Dairy Sci. 85:112-121.

Berry, E. A., and J. E. Hillerton. 2002b. The effect of an intramammary teat seal on new intramammary infections. J. Dairy Sci. 85:2512–2520.

Berry, E. A., and J. E. Hillerton. 2007. Effect of an Intramammary Teat Seal and Dry Cow Antibiotic in Relation to Dry Period Length on Postpartum Mastitis. J. Dairy Sci. 90:760–765.

Borenstein, M., L. Hedges, and H. Rothstein. 2007. Meta-Analysis: Fixed effect vs. random effects. Comprehensive meta-analysis, Biostat institute Inc., Englewood, New Jersey, USA.

Bratlie, O. 1973. Dry cow therapy. Vet. Rec. 93:430–431.

Browning, J. W., G. A. Mein, P. Brightling, T. J. Nicholls, and M. Barton. 1994. Strategies for mastitis control: dry cow therapy and culling. Aust. Vet. J. 71:179–183.

Buddle, B. M., M. Herceg, M. J. Ralston, and H. D. Pulford. 1987. Reinfection of bovine mammary glands following dry cow antibiotic therapy. Vet. Microbiol. 15:191-199.

Comprehensive Meta Analysis. 2008. Meta-analysis manual. Biostat institute Inc., Englewood, New Jersey, USA.

Cummins, K. A., and T. A. McCaskey. 1987. Multiple infusions of cloxacillin for treatment of mastitis during the dry period. J. Dairy Sci. 70:2658–2665.

Dingwell, R. T., T. F. Duffield, K. E. Leslie, G. P. Keefe, L. DesCoteaux, D. F. Kelton, K. D. Lissemore, Y. H. Schukken, P. Dick, and R. Bagg. 2002. The efficacy of intramammary tilmicosin at drying off, and other risk factors for the prevention of new intramammary infections during the dry period. J. Dairy Sci. 85:3250–3259.

Dodd, F. H., D. R. Westgarth, F. K. Neave, and R. G. Kingwell. 1969. Mastitis - The strategy of control, J. Dairy Sci. 52:689–695.

Dohoo, I. R., S. W. Martin, and H. Stryhn. 2003. Veterinary Epidemiological Research, Atlantic Veterinary College Inc., Charlottetown, Prince Edward Island, Canada.

Duffield, T. F., A. R. Rabiee, and I. J. Lean. 2008. A meta-analysis of the impact of monensin in lactating dairy cattle. Part 2. production effects. J. Dairy Sci. 91:1334-1346.

Duval, S., and R. Tweedie. 2000. A non-parametric “trim and fill” method of accounting for publication bias in meta-analysis. J. Amer. Stat. Associ. 95:89-98.

Eberhart, R. J., and J. M. Buckalew. 1972. Evaluation of a hygiene and dry period therapy program for mastitis control. J. Dairy Sci. 55:1683–1691.

Egger, M., G. Davey Smith, M. Schneider, and C. Minder. 1997. Bias in meta-analysis detected by a simple graphical test. Br. Med. J. 315:629-634.

Erskine, R., S. Wagner, and F. De Graves. 2003. Mastitis therapy and pharmacology. Vet. Clin. Food Anim. 19:109–138.

Gehring, R., and G. Smith. 2006. An overview of factors affecting the disposition of intramammary preparations used to treat bovine mastitis. J. Vet. Pharmacol. Therap. 29:237–241.

Ferguson, C. J. 2007. Evidence of publication bias in video game violence literature: A meta-analytic review, Agg. Viol. Beh. 12:470-482.

Funk, D. A., A. E. Freeman, and P. J. Berger. 1982. Environmental and physiological factors affecting mastitis at drying off and postcalving. J. Dairy Sci. 65:1258–1268.

Godden, S., P. Rapnicki, S. Stewart, J. Fetrow, A. Johnson, R. Bey, and R. Farnsworth. 2003. Effectiveness of an internal teat seal in the prevention of new intramammary infections during the dry and early-lactation periods in dairy cows when used with a dry cow intramammary antibiotic. J. Dairy Sci. 86:3899–3911.

Harmon, R. J., W. L. Crist, R. W. Hemken, and B. E. Langlois. 1986. Prevalence of minor udder pathogens after intramammary dry treatment. J. Dairy Sci. 69:843–849.

Hassan, Z., R. C. W. Daniel, D. O'Boyle, and A. J. Frost. 1999. Effects of dry cow intramammary therapy on quarter infections in the dry period. Vet. Rec. 27:635-639.

Heald, C. W., G. M. Jones, S. Nickerson, and T. L. Bibb. 1977. Mastitis control by penicillin and novobiocin at drying-off, Can. Vet. J. 18:171–180.

Hogan, J. S., K. L. Smith, D. A. Todhunter, and P. S. Schoenberger. 1994. Efficacy of dry cow therapy and a *Propionibacterum acnes* product in herds with low somatic cell count. J. Dairy Sci. 77: 3331–3337.

Langley, O. H., J. Meaney, N. P. Cullen, and F. Cunningham. 1971. The control of mastitis, Vet. Rec. 89:315-316.

Meaney, W. J. 1976. Dry period teat seal, Vet. Rec. 99:30.

Morris, R. S., D. C. Blood, N. B. Williamson, C. M. Cannon, and R. M. Cannon. 1978. A healthy program for commercial dairy herds. 4. Changes in mastitis prevalence. Aust. Vet. J. 54:247-251.

Natzke, R. P., R. W. Everett, and D. R. Bray. 1975. Effect of Drying Off Practices on Mastitis Infection. J. Dairy Sci. 58:1828:1835.

Orwin, R. 1983. A fail-safe N for effect size in meta-analysis. J. Educ. Stat. 8:157-159.

Østerås, O., J. Aursjo, G. Gronningsaeter Gjul, and A. Jorstad. 1994. Effect of dry-cow therapy on subclinical mastitis - an evaluation of long acting and short acting intramammaria. J. Vet. Med. B 41:529-540.

Pankey, J. W., R. M. Barker, A. Twomey , and G.Duirs. 1982a. A note on effectiveness of dry cow therapy in New Zealand dairy herds, N. Z. Vet. J. 30:50–52.

Pankey, J. W., R. M. Barker, A. Twomey, and G. Duirs. 1982b. Comparative efficacy of dry-cow treatment regimens against *Staphylococcus aureus*. N. Z. Vet. J. 30:13–15.

Parker, K. I., C. Compton, F. M. Anniss, A. Weir, C. Heuer, and S. McDougall. 2007. Subclinical and Clinical Mastitis in Heifers Following the Use of a Teat Sealant Precalving. J. Dairy Sci. 90:207–218.

Parker, K. I., C. Compton, F. M. Anniss, C. Heuer, and S. McDougall. 2008. Quarter-Level Analysis of Subclinical and Clinical Mastitis in Primiparous Heifers Following the Use of a Teat Sealant or an Injectable Antibiotic, or Both, Precalving. J. Dairy Sci. 91:169–181.

Pearson, J. K. L., and C.L. Wright. 1969. Dry cow therapy as a means of controlling bovine mastitis. Vet. Rec. 84:294–298.

Postle, D. S., and R. P. Natzke. 1974. Efficacy of antibiotic treatment in bovine udder. Vet. Med. Small Anim. Clin. 1535-1940.

Rindsig, R. B., R. G. Rodewald, A. R. Smith, and S. L. Spahr. 1978. Complete versus selective dry cow therapy for mastitis control, J. Dairy Sci. 61:1483–1497.

Robert, A., H. Seegers., and N. Bareille. 2006. Incidence of intramammary infections during the dry period without or with antibiotic treatment in dairy cows – a quantitative analysis of published data. Vet. Res. 37:25–48.

Robinson, T. C., E. R. Jackson, and A. Marr. 1988. Mastitis incidence in quarters with different infection status at drying off and calving in two treatment groups. Br. Vet. J. 144:166– 173.

Schukken, Y. H., J. van Vliet, D. van de Geer, and F. J. Grommer. 1993. A randomized blind trial on dry cow antibiotic infusion in a low somatic cell count herd. J. Dairy Sci. 76:2925–2930.

Smith, A., D. R. Westgarth, M. R. Jones, F. K. Neave, F. H. Dodd, and G.C. Brander. 1967. Methods of reducing the incidence of udder infection in dry cows. Vet. Rec. 81:504–510.

Soback, S., G. Ziv, M. Winkler, and A. Saran. 1990. Systemic dry cow therapy – a preliminary report. J. Dairy Sci. 73:661–666.

Swanson, G. H. 1979. Posology and field efficacy study with novobiocin for intramammary infusion in nonlactating dairy cows. Can. J. Comp. Med. 43:440–447.

Tarabla, H., and V. Canavesio. 2003. Prevalence of intramammary infections by major pathogens at parturition in dairy cows after intramuscular antibiotic therapy at drying-off: a preliminary report. J. Dairy Res. 70:233–235.

Williamson, J.H., M. W. Woolford, and A. M. Day. 1995. The prophylactic effect of a dry-cow antibiotic against *Streptococcus uberis*. N. Z. Vet. J. 43:228–234.

ESTIMATING THE PROBABILITY OF FREEDOM FROM PRRS IN SWEDEN: THE QUICK AND DIRTY METHOD OR A MORE THOROUGH APPROACH – DOES IT MATTER?

J. FRÖSSLING*, S. STERNBERG LEWERIN, E. ÅGREN, H. WAHLSTRÖM AND A. LINDBERG

SUMMARY

After the first outbreak and eradication of porcine reproductive and respiratory syndrome (PRRS) in Swedish pigs in 2007, several surveillance activities were performed and almost 25,000 samples were analysed with a negative outcome. Considering the efforts made and resources spent to control this disease, there was a further need to evaluate the surveillance system and to substantiate disease freedom. In this study, four different approaches were used to estimate the surveillance system sensitivity and probability of freedom from disease: 1. Evaluating the total number of test results using Win Episcope, 2. Evaluating results from structured surveys using FreeCalc, 3. Scenario-tree model of the complete surveillance system, assuming independence of observations, 4. Scenario-tree model of the complete surveillance system, adjusting for clustering and overlapping of observations. The approaches were chosen to represent different levels of complexity of calculations and required quality and detail of input data.

The comparison showed that, in this case, the methods gave very similar estimates of surveillance sensitivities and probability of disease freedom. In fact, the estimated probability of disease freedom only varied between 99.8% and 100.0%. However, the different approaches required different degrees of information. In conclusion, although the choice of approach did not make any major difference to the final estimates, the more advanced approach was considered preferable since it produced a more reliable estimate.

INTRODUCTION

In July 2007, porcine reproductive and respiratory syndrome (PRRS) was detected for the first time in Sweden. Within ten days, a total of eight positive herds were identified in the south of Sweden and various measures, including movement restrictions and slaughter of infected herds, were implemented to eradicate the disease (Carlsson et al. 2008). In addition to the continuously ongoing passive surveillance, several active surveillance activities were undertaken.

* Jenny Frössling, Department of Disease Control and Epidemiology, National Veterinary Institute (SVA), SE-751 89 Uppsala, Sweden. Email: jenny.frossling@sva.se

The first case was detected through routine sampling within the Swedish PRRS surveillance programme, which had been in place since 1998. This programme includes all herds affiliated to the Swedish Animal Health Service and has focussed mainly on pedigree herds and sow pool centrals. After detection of the first positive case, an investigation including serological examination of all contact herds and all breeding herds, as well as sampling in regional slaughterhouses. In addition to this, a national slaughterhouse survey was conducted during the last half of 2007. The national survey included >70% of Swedish pig herds and all results were negative.

PPRS has been included in the Swedish Epizootic Act (SFS 1999:657) since 1999. According to this legislation, any suspicion of infection with PRRS virus has to be notified by animal owners, veterinarians or other professionals with animal contact. Moreover, the Swedish Board of Agriculture (the responsible authority under the Department of Agriculture) must investigate all suspect cases and take all necessary measures to eradicate and prevent the spread of the infection, when confirmed.

After six months of intense surveillance activities and in total about 25,000 negative test results, there was a need to substantiate whether the eradication had been successful. A thorough evaluation was considered essential and good quality information related to the outbreak was therefore secured and gathered by the authorities, in collaboration with the Swedish Animal Health Service. The probability of freedom from PRRS was first estimated by scenario-tree modelling (Frössling et al., 2008), which was both a complex and time consuming exercise. Therefore, the aim of this study was to compare the results of the scenario-tree model with results from three less advanced approaches for surveillance sensitivity and the probability of freedom estimation.

MATERIALS AND METHODS

Population and surveillance components

The overall target population of this study is domestic pigs in Sweden. During the study period there were approximately 2400 herds and 1.7 million pigs in the country (Anonymous, 2007b). The surveillance activities performed after the outbreak from 6 July until 31 December 2007 can be categorized into four surveillance system components (*SSCs*): 1) outbreak investigations, 2) a national slaughterhouse survey, 3) the on-going surveillance programme and 4) clinical surveillance. The *SSCs* are described in brief below and a list of activities is included in Table 1, where the target and study populations (number of herds and animals) for each part of the surveillance are given. Note that the figures are of different origin and they can therefore not be directly summarized.

Table 1. Surveillance activities regarding porcine reproductive and respiratory syndrome (PRRS) in Swedish pigs. The table includes activities performed after the outbreak in July 2007 until the 31st of December the same year.

SURVEILLANCE ACTIVITY	TARGET POPULATION OF THE SURVEILLANCE ACTIVITY			STUDY SAMPLE	
	Description	Size		Size	
		Herds	Animals	Herds	Animals
A. Outbreak investigations:					
Trace back and/or forward investigations[a]	Herds considered to be at risk due to the outbreak	199	142000[b]	199	4804
Regional slaughterhouse survey	Herds in the region where the outbreak was detected	1146	506082	67	944
B. National slaughterhouse survey	All pig herds that send animal for slaughter	2400[b]	1700000[b]	876	17077
C. Surveillance programme	Herds affiliated to the Swedish Animal Health Service	1801	1530000[c]	75	2205
D. Clinical surveillance	All pig herds	2400[b]	1700000[b]	1761	1682938[d]

[a] This included sampling of identified contact herds and various outbreak-related sampling in herds.
[b] Exact number not available.
[c] The exact number was not available but as the affiliated herds cover >90% of the total number of pigs in Sweden, this number was set to 90% of the approximate total number of pigs.
[d] The number of pigs present on each of these farms was calculated based on the registered number of sows, the estimated number of weaners and growers, and the reported number of slaughtered individuals.

The outbreak investigations comprised tracings of contacts that may have spread the infection to or from the infected herds. Moreover, initial screenings in herds and slaughterhouses in the affected region were performed. In total, 5,748 samples from 266 herds were included in this surveillance component.

After the first surveillance activities had been initiated, a national slaughterhouse survey comprising 17,077 samples from 876 herds was performed: From all herds sending ≥300 pigs to slaughter each year, 20 pigs were sampled at slaughter. From herds slaughtering <300 pigs annually, 5-13 samples were taken. If less than 5 pigs were slaughtered, the herd was excluded from sampling.

Beside the surveillance activities specifically performed due to the outbreak, pigs were also tested as part of the ongoing surveillance programme for PRRS (Anonymous, 2008a). In this programme, all nucleus or multiplying herds and sow pool centrals, as well as an annual sample of 50 piglet producing herds in southern Sweden, were sampled on a yearly basis. Twenty gilts or sows were sampled in each herd. All boars at artificial insemination centres were also sampled. In all, 2,205 samples from 75 herds were collected within the surveillance programme and evaluated in the calculations.

Finally, clinical surveillance covers all pig herds in Sweden. Herd sizes and information relevant to PRRS clinical surveillance were retrieved from the records of the Swedish Animal Health Service, which are estimated to cover >90% of all pigs in Sweden. For 2007, the records included 1,801 herds and the number of herds with complete information relating to this model and included in the calculations was 1,761. The estimated total number of individuals covered by this *SSC* was 1,682,938 pigs.

Calculations of the probability of disease freedom

Four different approaches were used to estimate the surveillance system sensitivity and probability of freedom from disease. Due to differences in definitions (and assumptions), some were based on data from a subset of *SSCs* while some were based on information from all *SSCs* (Table 2).

Table 2. Surveillance system components considered in four different approaches used to calculate the surveillance system sensitivity and probability of freedom from porcine reproductive and respiratory syndrome (PRRS) in Swedish pigs (2007).

SURVEILLANCE SYSTEM COMPONENT	APPROACH		
	1.[a]	2.[b]	3. and 4.[c]
A. Outbreak investigations:			
Trace back and or forward investigations	x		x
Regional slaughterhouse survey	x	x	x
B. National slaughterhouse survey	x	x	x
C. Surveillance programme	x	x	x
D. Clinical surveillance			x

[a] The total number of test results evaluated using Win Episcope.
[b] Surveys evaluated using FreeCalc.
[c] Scenario-tree models.

In order to get an overall estimate of surveillance sensitivity, i.e. the total surveillance sensitivity (*TotalSSe*), and the probability of freedom based on each approach, the surveillance sensitivities (SSe_j, where j=1...k and k is the number of activities or components included) were summarized as:

$$TotalSSe = 1 - \prod_{j=1}^{k}(1 - SSe_j) \quad (1)$$

The posterior probability of freedom was based on this *TotalSSe* and the prior probability of infection:

$$PostPFree = \frac{(1 - PriorPInf)}{(1 - PriorPInf \times TotalSSe)} \quad (2)$$

The prior probability was set to 0.5, which is a conservative estimate considering PRRS has not been detected in Sweden despite >10 years of active surveillance. However, in the process of temporal discounting (see below, approaches 3 and 4) this was just the starting value for the first month while the prior probability for the following months was a combination of the posterior probability from the previous month and the monthly risk of introduction.

The within-herd design prevalence was set to 20% and the design herd prevalence was set to 0.2%. Note that the number of infected herds at this prevalence would be equal to 5 Swedish pig herds, which is a very low figure. In the most basic approaches (1 and 2), a combination of these prevalences were combined to set the design prevalence for infected individuals in the population, i.e. the between-herd design prevalence was multiplied by the within-herd prevalence (=0.04%). For all methods, the diagnostic specificity was assumed to be 100%. The study time period was 6 months (1st of July to 31st of December 2007). However, the scenario-tree model calculations were made in one-month intervals with temporal discounting between months and a monthly risk of introduction corresponding to 1 introduction in 10 years.

Approach 1: the total number of test results evaluated using Win Episcope

In the most basic approach, all test results were summarized and evaluated by applying traditional statistical methods. The software used was Win Episcope 2.0 (Thrusfield et al., 2001). The probability of detecting disease (i.e. the confidence level or system sensitivity, *SSe*) at the design prevalence (P^*) was based on the number of negative test results (n) related to the total number pigs in Sweden (N) according to the following formula:

$$SSe = 1 - \left(\frac{1-P^*}{N \quad \frac{n-1}{2}} \right)^n \quad (3)$$

Approach 2: surveys evaluated using FreeCalc

In the second approach, test results were evaluated while adjusting for imperfect diagnostic test sensitivity using Survey Toolbox version 1.0 beta, i.e. FreeCalc, described by Cameron & Baldock (1998). These calculations were performed by applying the binomial formula (sampling with replacement) modified to take account of test sensitivity (*Se*) and specificity (*Sp*)

$$SSe = 1 - \left(\left(\frac{n!}{x!\,(n-x)!} \right) \left(P^* \times Se + (1-P^*)(1-Sp)\right)^x \left(P^*\,(1-Se) + (1-P^*)\,Sp\right)^{n-x} \right) \quad (4)$$

where x is the number of test positives in a sample. This approach evaluated surveillance activities that were considered to meet the definition of structured surveys, i.e. the regional slaughterhouse survey in the outbreak investigations, the national slaughterhouse survey and the herds sampled within the surveillance programme. The exact numbers of sample and population sizes are given in Table 1.

The calculations were similar to the basic structure used in the scenario-tree model described below. However, estimation was deterministic and the effect of difference in risk in different groups of the population was not included. In order to enable comparison to the more advanced approaches, the estimated confidence levels of the surveys were combined into a single estimate as described above in Eq. (1) and Eq. (2).

Approach 3: scenario-tree model assuming independence

In the third and fourth approach, stochastic scenario-tree models were built as described by Martin et al. (2007a and 2007b). In this type of model, factors relating to the structure of the study population and to the probability of detection, or infection, are included as nodes for which input proportions or probabilities are given. In our models, system sensitivities and probabilities of freedom were estimated based on all four major *SSCs*: outbreak investigations, the national slaughterhouse survey, the surveillance programme and clinical surveillance.

In the third approach a simplified model was applied, as if information about herd identities and herd sizes was unavailable. In this, model calculations were performed assuming independence of observations. The sensitivity of each surveillance system component was thus calculated as:

$$SSCSe = 1 - (1 - SSCSeU)^{n} \tag{5}$$

where *SSCSeU* is the sum of the probabilities of getting a truly positive test result.

Approach 4: scenario-tree model including adjusting for clustering and overlapping

In the forth and most advanced approach, a full scenario-tree model was built which included adjusting for clustering of individuals within herds and overlapping between surveillance components. This model is fully described in a separate paper (Frössling et al, submitted manuscript). In brief, the probability of a true positive outcome within an infected farm was used to calculate the herd sensitivity, according to an approximation of a hypergeometric distribution (MacDiarmid, 1988) or a binomial distribution, if appropriate. The sensitivity of each surveillance component j ($SSCSe_j$) was based on the product sum of the probabilities of the herds (included in the component) testing negative

$$SSCSe_j - 1 - \prod_{i=1}^{m}\left(1 - SeH \times EPherdInf_r\right) \tag{6}$$

Where $i = 1...m$ and m is the number of tested herds, and $EPherdINF_r$ is each herd's effective probability of infection based on the design prevalence and risk factors as described in Frössling et al. (2008). The risk factors included in the models were herd location (south of Sweden constituting a higher risk relative to north of Sweden) and herd contacts (herds that had had contacts with infected herds where considered as having a higher risk of infection relative to other herds).

The scenario-tree models were run with 10,000 iterations in each simulation, using Microsoft Office Excel® 2007 (Microsoft Co., Redmond, USA) and @RISK 4.5.7 (Palisade Co. Ithaca, USA).

RESULTS

The estimated surveillance system sensitivities (i.e. *TotalSSe*) and probabilities of freedom from disease are presented in Table 3 for the different approaches.

Table 3. Surveillance system sensitivity and probability of freedom from porcine reproductive and respiratory syndrome (PRRS) in Swedish pigs based on surveillance data from July to December 2007 and calculated using four different approaches.

APPROACH	TOTAL SURVEILLANCE SYSTEM SENSITIVITY, %	PROBABILITY OF FREEDOM, %
	Point estimate	Point estimate (CI [b])
1. Win Episcope	100.0	100.0
2. FreeCalc	99.8	99.8
3. Scenario-tree model, assuming independence	96.3 - 100.0[a]	100.0 (99.9, 100.0)
4. Scenario-tree model, adjusting for grouping and overlapping	81.2 - 94.3[a]	99.8 (99.7, 99.9)

[a] Values are minimum and maximum point estimates at the end of each month included in the study period.
[b] Values shown in parenthesis represent the credible interval, i.e. 5th and 95th percentiles of the posterior distribution.

In the second approach, the results from the national slaughterhouse survey alone gave a surveillance sensitivity of 99.4% and were, in other words, adequate to conclude that the population was free from disease at a 99% confidence level. The other two surveys, i.e. the regional slaughterhouse survey in the outbreak investigations and the sampling of herds within the surveillance programme, had surveillance sensitivities of 25.0% and 48.9%, respectively.

Based on the third approach, i.e. a scenario-tree model disregarding lack of independence, the total surveillance system sensitivity varied over time and was highest immediately after the outbreak in July and August and lowest in November

In the fourth and last approach, where estimates were based on a scenario-tree model where grouping of individuals and overlapping between *SSCs* were adjusted for, the estimated total surveillance sensitivity was highest in August. The lowest estimate, on the other hand, was in December. Estimates of surveillance component sensitivity were consistently lower when based on this model compared to the model used in the third approach. For example, the surveillance component sensitivity of the outbreak investigations in August was 87.1% when independence was assumed (approach 3) but only 51.8% when grouping was adjusted for (approach 4).

Based on the results of both approach 3 and 4, it appeared as if the most important *SSC* during the overall study period was clinical surveillance. The outbreak investigations contributed highly to the total surveillance sensitivity in July, whereas the national slaughterhouse survey contributed mainly in August.

DISCUSSION

The estimates of probability of freedom from PRRS based on the methods applied in this study were all close to 100%. In other words, the four different approaches showed a very high probability that the eradication of PRRS in Swedish pigs was successful. Considering the high proportion of herds that was sampled during the study period (approximately >80% of the total population) and the fact that PRRS is a fairly contagious disease, this result seems reasonable. However, although the final estimates of all approaches were similar, there are obvious differences in the information they provide and how convincing the end results are. Substantiating disease freedom based on the total sum of negative samples while ignoring imperfect sensitivity or cluster-effects (as in approaches 1-3) will most likely result in an overestimation of the probability of freedom. Therefore, it will be of limited value when trying to convince e.g. trading partners of the disease status. Moreover, more reliable estimates are necessary for strategic planning and allocating resources for national disease control activities.

In order to document and evaluate freedom from disease there are many aspects to consider besides the actual estimate of probability of freedom. For more advanced approaches, the process of data structuring and search for input valuables in itself gives a great opportunity to scrutinize and document each part of the surveillance system, get an overview and perhaps gain new information about the existing procedures. In addition, this can reveal areas of improvement and help design of future surveillance activities. The scenario-tree models also have the advantage that different weights can be given to test results of different origin thanks to the inclusion of known risk factors. To be able to quantify the sensitivity and define the main steps of the detection chains within the clinical surveillance is also of great value. Based on the results of approaches 3 and 4, clinical surveillance contributed considerably to the total sensitivity of the surveillance system. It makes sense that for newly introduced and highly contagious diseases, clinical surveillance is of main importance. This could not be taken into account in approaches 1 and 2. However, PRRS was detected in Sweden through an active (rather than a passive) surveillance activity and it may be questioned if the sensitivity of the passive clinical surveillance is overestimated.

In the every-day work of surveillance epidemiologists there are often limitations to how advanced we can make our estimations. The selection of approaches used in this study was chosen to represent different degrees of sophistication considering time spent on preparation of data and analysis as well as availability and quality of data.

Because of time-constraint and lack of appropriate data we are often forced to slightly misuse available methods, while trying to be careful when interpreting results and draw conclusions. Summarizing all test results and evaluating these as if they are all part of the same surveillance activity using a traditional statistical method as in approach 1, implies that the limitations of this method are severely ignored. The same is true for parts of the second approach where some, if not all, of the surveys had deficiencies that could be expected to result in e.g. selection bias. By applying the scenario-tree models, the selection procedures and possible non-representative sampling can be incorporated in the model and constitute no threat to assumptions.

By ignoring clustering of individuals within herds, the sensitivities of surveillance components were overestimated. As expected, the third approach rendered higher estimates of sensitivity compared to the fourth approach. However, because the adjusted total sensitivity was relatively high in this study, this made little difference to the estimated probability of freedom. In case the number of negative tests had been fewer, and the estimated sensitivity of clinical surveillance had been lower, the adjusting for grouping could probably have had a larger effect on the final outcome.

Regardless of the approach used to estimate the sensitivity of surveillance and probability of disease freedom, it is important to investigate the coverage of different surveillance activities and define the study population. Non-representative sampling can be captured in the scenario-tree models but even if there are no known risk factors (to be included in the model) it is important to be aware of any systematic exclusion of herd or animal types, e.g. due to geographical distribution, herd size or age and health status of sampled animals. The actual calculations of approaches 1 and 2 did not require much more than the number of negative test results and the size of the target population, while approaches 3 and 4 forced a much more thorough investigation and description of both the background and study populations. Approach 4 also required detailed information about each herd included in the calculations. On the other hand, keeping calculations simple does not necessarily have to exclude that estimates are supplemented by more detailed information about the populations of interest.

It should be noted that in Win Episcope the outcome "Level of Confidence" is the probability of detecting disease, which corresponds to the sensitivity of the surveillance activity. In FreeCalc, the probability of not detecting disease is reported, which can easily be converted to the probability of detecting disease, i.e. the surveillance sensitivity. This facilitates the comparison with estimates of surveillance component sensitivity and total surveillance system sensitivity based on scenario-tree models. For software such as FreeCalc, estimates could be brought even closer to the estimates of scenario-tree models if it was made sure that data was analysed in similar time-steps and including temporal discounting. However, compared to stochastic models, variation and uncertainty of inputs and outputs are not captured and grouping is not easily accounted for. The possibility to include probability distributions in the calculations is of special value when a disease has not been present in the country before, because the epidemiological characteristics in the naïve population are not well documented and several inputs may rely on expert opinion.

Because of the resources spent on the eradication of PRRS and on protecting the Swedish pig population from PRRS, as well as all the efforts made by farmers, veterinarians and others involved in this work, it is our conclusion that quick and dirty just is not good enough when estimating the probability of freedom from this disease. The exact source of the outbreak has not been identified and even though the results from all investigations have been encouraging, the question whether eradication was successful or not did not have an obvious answer. In situations such as this, all information that can improve the estimates of surveillance sensitivity and probability of freedom, as well as our understanding of the surveillance system, matters.

ACKNOWLEDGEMENTS

Dr. Jenny Frössling was funded by a research grant from the Swedish Emergency Management Agency (KBM).

REFERENCES

Anonymous (2008a). Yearbook of Agricultural Statistics, 2007. Swedish Board of Agriculture (SJV) & Statistics Sweden. Available at http://www.sjv.se (accessed 1 April 2008).

Anonymous (2008b). Surveillance and control programmes – Domestic and wild animals in Sweden 2007. National Veterinary Institute (SVA), Sweden. Available at: http://www.sva.se/upload/pdf/Tj%C3%A4nster%20och%20produkter/Trycksaker/surveillance_2007_webb.pdf (accessed 15 December 2008).

Carlsson, U., Wallgren, P., Renström, L.H.M., Lindberg, A., Eriksson, H., Thorén, P., Eliasson-Selling, L., Lundeheim, N., Thörn, C. and Elvander, M. (2008). Emergence of Porcine

Reproductive and Respiratory Syndrome in Sweden; detection – response – eradication. Accepted manuscript.

Cameron, A.R. and Baldock, F.C. (1998). Two-stage sampling in surveys to substantiate freedom from disease. Prev. Vet. Med. 34, 19-30

Frössling, J., Ågren, E., Eliasson-Selling, L. and Sternberg Lewerin, S. (2008). Probability of freedom from disease after the first detection and eradication of PRRS in Sweden: Scenario-tree modelling of the surveillance system. Manuscript submitted for publication.

MacDiarmid, S.C. (1988). Future options for brucellosis surveillance in New Zealand beef herds. N. Z. Vet. J. 36, 39-42

Martin, P.A.J., Cameron, A.R. and Greiner, M. (2007a). Demonstrating freedom from disease using multiple complex data sources 1: A new methodology based on scenario trees. Prev. Vet. Med. 79, 71-97.

Martin, P.A.J., Cameron, A.R., Barfod, K., Sergeant, E.S.G. and Greiner, M. (2007b). Demonstrating freedom from disease using multiple complex data sources 2: Case study – Classical swine fever in Denmark. Prev. Vet. Med. 79, 98-115.

OIE (2007). Terrestrial Animal Health Code. Available at http://www.oie.int/eng/normes/mcode/en_sommaire.htm (accessed May 2008).

Suess, E.A., Gardner, I. A. and Johnson, W.O., (2002). Hierarchical Bayesian model for prevalence inferences and determination of a country's status for an animal pathogen. Prev. Vet. Med. 55, 155-171

Thrusfield, M., Ortega, C., de Blas, I., Noordhuizen and J.P., Frankena, K. (2001). WIN EPISCOPE 2.0: improved epidemiological software for veterinary medicine. Vet. Rec. 148, 567-572

BAYESIAN NETWORKS FOR MASTITIS MANAGEMENT ON DAIRY FARMS

W. STEENEVELD*, L.C. VAN DER GAAG, H.W. BARKEMA AND H. HOGEVEEN

SUMMARY

This manuscript presents the idea of providing dairy farmers with probability distributions to support decisions on mastitis management and illustrates its feasibility by two applications. Naive Bayesian networks were developed for both applications. The networks in the first application were used to compute probability distributions to support decisions on which cows from a mastitis alert list generated by detection sensors in an automatic milking system should be visually inspected for clinical mastitis. The computed probability distribution allows farmers to interpret the uncertainty in an alert. The network in the second application was used to compute probability distributions to support treatment decisions for clinical mastitis cases. The computed probability distribution allows for distinguishing a situation in which a single pathogen has a high probability from the situation where two or more pathogens have almost equal probabilities. The first situation would support choice for a pathogen-specific treatment.

INTRODUCTION

With increasing dairy herd sizes, the need for automated decision support for managing the cows' health is increasing. Fortunately, with increasing automation, more cow data are becoming available that can serve as input for decision support models. Decision support models were developed, for example, to advise on the most appropriate treatment (Jones & Ward, 1990; Kim & Heald, 1999) and to classify cows as either having clinical mastitis (CM) or not (De Mol & Ouweltjes, 2001). Because most of the existing models are not user friendly and have interfaces that are unfamiliar to the end users, most of the developed decision support models are not being used in practice (Groenendaal et al., 2004). Another disadvantage of these models is that they only provide a single qualitative outcome to a farmer, such as the most likely causal pathogen of a CM case (e.g., Jones & Ward, 1990; Kim & Heald, 1999), without any indication of the uncertainty involved.

Providing just a single outcome to a farmer ignores the likelihood of this outcome and of other possible outcomes. Consequently, the risks of misclassification are not visible to the farmer. Providing outcomes with their associated probabilities to a farmer reveals the uncertainty involved and thereby allows more informed decisions. In this manuscript, we illustrate these probabilities for two applications. In the first application, a cow-specific prior probability of CM is used for a better interpretation of mastitis alert lists generated by automatic milking systems. Based on sensor measurements of the milk, these lists mention cows likely to have CM which the herdsman then has to visually inspect. By including a cow-specific prior probability of CM, based on cow factors, the dairy farmer knows which cows on the alert list have the highest probability of CM and can thus make a more informed decision about which cows to inspect. In the second application, the most appropriate treatment for actually detected

*Wilma Steeneveld, Utrecht University, Faculty of Veterinary Medicine, Department of Farm Animal Health, P.O. Box 80151, 3508 TD Utrecht, the Netherlands. Email: w.steeneveld@uu.nl

cases of CM must be decided upon. Based on a combination of cow factors and clinical signs, a probability distribution for the causal pathogen can be established. Providing the farmer with this probability distribution rather than just the most likely pathogen allows more informed decisions regarding treatment. For instance, almost equal probabilities for two or more causal pathogens would support the decision for a broad spectrum antibiotic treatment while a high probability for a single particular pathogen would support the choice for a more specific treatment.

To determine probability distributions for the applications described above, probabilistic models need to be developed. Logistic regression is frequently used for analyzing data and subsequently calculating probabilities (e.g., Steeneveld et al., 2008). This technique, however, has some limitations in view of our applications. First, it cannot handle missing values and, secondly, it is not easy to adapt a once constructed regression model to new insights. In contrast, Bayesian networks are flexible in terms of handling missing values and they allow in essence for computing any prior or posterior probability of interest over the modelled variables. Naive Bayesian networks (NBN) are the simplest type of Bayesian network, well known for their powerful classification performance (Friedman et al., 1997). NBNs have been studied extensively and are being widely applied in human medicine (e.g., Chapman et al., 2005). Although applications are still relatively rare in veterinary medicine, they are gaining in popularity (McKendrick et al., 2000; Geenen et al., 2005). For the two applications described above, NBNs will be used to illustrate the use of probability distributions to support decisions regarding a cow's health.

MATERIALS AND METHODS

Available data and data preparation

The data available for the present study are described elsewhere in detail (Barkema et al., 1998). In short, data on CM were collected from 274 dairy herds during a period of approximately 1.5 years. In the study, farmers were asked to collect milk samples from cows with signs of CM before treatment. From each sample, the causal pathogen was determined by bacteriological culturing. The Dutch national milk recording system (Nederlands Rundvee Syndicaat, Arnhem, The Netherlands) further provided information from the 3- or 4-weekly milk production recording. Only lactations from calving onwards were selected. The dataset for our study consisted of 28,137 lactations from 22,860 cows, which included a total of 5,363 CM cases.

For developing our NBNs, different datasets were derived from the original dataset. To determine cow-specific prior probabilities of CM, two separate datasets were constructed. Dataset1 was constructed to include for each cow the information of the first 30 days in milk (DIM). It was decided to study the data from this period separately, because it was known from previous studies that the incidence of CM can differ considerably within the first 30 DIM (Barkema et al., 1998). The information of the remaining DIM was included in dataset2. To determine a probability distribution for the causal pathogen of a CM case, dataset3 was constructed, containing only the CM cases.

For the purpose of constructing dataset1, the first 30 DIM were subdivided into 6 periods of 5 days each. For each period, it was determined whether or not the cow had CM. The resulting dataset contained 168,822 records with a total 1,617 CM cases. For each period, four additional variables were defined, each representing a risk factor for CM in the first 30 DIM, i.e. 1) the cow's parity, 2) the season of the year, 3) the geometric mean somatic cell count (SCC) of the previous lactation, and 4) whether or not the cow had CM in the previous period of 5 days (Table 1).

Table 1. Description of the study variables with their different levels used for the construction of Bayesian networks for determining cow-specific prior probabilities of having clinical mastitis (CM).

Description	# classes	Levels
Clinical mastitis [a, b]	2	no, yes
Parity [a, b]	4	1, 2, 3, ≥4
First 30 days in milk divided in periods of 5 days [a]	6	1-5, 6-10, 11-15, 16-20, 21-25, 26-30
30-day intervals from 31 days in milk onwards [b]	7	31-60, 61-90, 91-120, 121-150, 151-180, 181-210, ≥211
Season of the year [a, b]	4	January-March, April-June, July-September, October-December
Somatic cell count in the previous 30 days in milk [b]	2	<200,000 cells/ml, ≥200,000 cells/ml
Somatic cell count in the 30 days before the previous 30 days in milk [b]	2	<200,000 cells/ml, ≥200,000 cells/ml
Geometric mean somatic cell count of all test-days in previous lactation [a,b]	2	<200,000 cells/ml, ≥200,000 cells/ml
Having CM in the previous 5-day period [a]	2	no, yes
Accumulated number of CM cases in the previous 30 days in milk [b]	3	0, 1, 2
Accumulated number of CM cases before the previous 30 days in milk [b]	3	0, 1, 2

[a] Included in dataset1, [b] included in dataset2

For dataset2, the DIM from 31 DIM onwards, were divided into 30-day intervals. For every 30 DIM, it was determined for each cow whether it had CM. The resulting dataset contained 195,454 records with a total 3,746 CM cases. For each 30 DIM, moreover, seven additional variables were included, representing risk factors of CM from 31 DIM onwards, i.e. 1) the cow's parity, 2) the season of the year, 3) the SCC in the previous 30 DIM, 4) the SCC in the 30 days before the previous 30 DIM, 5) the geometric mean SCC of the previous lactation, 6) the accumulated number of CM cases in the previous 30 DIM, and 7) the accumulated number of CM cases in the DIM before the previous 30 DIM (Table 1).

To construct dataset3, all CM cases were extracted from dataset1 and dataset2. All cases with contaminated samples, culture-negative samples and cases where no sample was taken were removed. The remaining cases were classified into STREP, containing all *Streptococci* species (*Strep. dysgalactiae*, *Strep. agalactiae*, *Strep. uberis* and other streptococci), STAPH, containing *Staphylococcus aureus,* and COLI, containing *Escherichia coli* and *Klebsiella spp.* Cultures containing two different STREP were classified into this class. All CM cases that could not be classified into STREP, STAPH or COLI were excluded. The resulting dataset contained 962 STREP, 746 STAPH and 979 COLI cases, and hence 2,687 cases in total. In addition to the causal pathogen, the following risk factors were included: the cow's parity, the month in lactation, the location of infected udder quarter, the season of the year, the test-day SCC 1-30 days before CM, the closest test-day SCC > 30 days before CM, the geometric mean SCC of the previous lactation, the causal pathogen 1-30 days and > 30 days before the current CM, the colour and texture of the milk, and whether or not the cow was sick (Table 2). Because continuous variables could not be handled in standard Bayesian networks, the values of all SCC variables in all three datasets were classified as either < or ≥ 200,000 cells/ml (Dohoo and Leslie, 1991).

Table 2. Description of the study variables with their different levels used for construction of a Bayesian network for determining a probability distribution for the causal pathogen of clinical mastitis (CM) cases (dataset 3).

Description	# classes	Levels
Pathogen of current CM case	3	STREP[a], STAPH[b], COLI[c]
Parity	4	1, 2, 3, ≥4
Month in lactation	8	1, 2, 3, 4, 5, 6, 7, ≥8
Season of the year	4	January – March, April – June, July – September, October – December
Infected quarter of the udder	4	right front, left front, right rear, left rear
Somatic cell count 1-30 days before current CM	2	<200,000 cells/ml, ≥200,000 cells/ml
Somatic cell count >30 days before current CM	2	<200,000 cells/ml, ≥200,000 cells/ml
Geometric mean somatic cell count in previous lactation	2	<200,000 cells/ml, ≥200,000 cells/ml
Pathogen history 1-30 days before current CM	4	no previous CM, STREP, STAPH, COLI
Pathogen history > 30 days before current CM	4	no previous CM, STREP, STAPH, COLI
Colour of the milk of cow with CM	5	normal, yellowish, very yellow, watery, blood
Texture of the milk of cow with CM	5	normal, small flakes, big flakes, serous, viscous
Cow sick at the moment of CM	2	not sick, sick

[a] *Streptococcus dysgalactiae, Streptococcus agalactiae, Streptococcus uberis*, other streptococci and mixed cultures of streptococci, [b] *Staphylococcus aureus*, [c] *Escherichia coli* and *Klebsiella spp.*

Model building

An NBN is a probabilistic model consisting of a single class variable which represents the possible classes for the dependent variable of a study, and a set of feature variables modelling the relevant levels of the study's independent variables. In datasets 1 and 2, whether or not a cow had CM was the class variable; in dataset3, the causal pathogen of CM was the class variable. The other variables in the datasets were potential feature variables. Constructing an NBN consists of determining prior probabilities for the class variable and estimating conditional probabilities for the feature variables given the possible classes of the dependent variable. In this study, the prior probabilities for the class variable reflected the incidence of CM per 5 DIM (0.85%) in dataset1, the incidence of CM per 30 DIM (1.76%) in dataset2, and the incidence of the three pathogen groups (STREP: 36.6%, STAPH: 26.0% and COLI: 37.4%) in dataset3, respectively. The conditional probabilities for the feature variables were based on frequency counts in the data. For instance, the conditional probability of a cow being sick, given that it is infected with a STREP, that is, the probability Pr(Sick = yes | causal pathogen = STREP), was computed as the proportion of sick cows among the CM cases reporting a STREP.

In essence, all available feature variables can be included in an NBN. Methods exist, however, for selecting only those feature variables that best serve to discriminate between the different classes of a dependent variable, thereby forestalling over-fitting of the data (Langley & Sage, 1994). For this study, a wrapper method with forward selection was used for selecting appropriate feature variables (e.g., Geenen et al., 2005). With this method, feature variables were selected so as to optimize the accuracy of the NBN under construction. The method started with an NBN including just the class variable and no feature variables. In each subsequent step, it computed the accuracy of the NBN with a single feature variable added, for each such variable separately. It then included the feature variable that increased the accuracy the most, if any. The inclusion of feature variables was continued until the accuracy of the NBN no longer improved.

For the purpose of constructing the NBNs and subsequently studying their performance, all three datasets were split into a construction set and a study set. From each dataset, 2/3rds of the records were selected randomly for construction; the remaining records were included in a study dataset. Constructing the different NBNs, which includes estimating the prior and conditional probabilities required from the available data, was done by using the Bayesian-network editing package Dazzle (Schrage et al., 2005).

Studying model performance

Obtaining posterior probabilities

The three constructed NBNs were used to calculate for each record from the study dataset the posterior probability distributions for their class variables given information on the selected feature variables. For this purpose, an NBN builds upon Bayes' rule, together with the assumption that all feature variables are mutually independent given the class variable. For computing the posterior probability $\Pr(c \mid f_1, \ldots, f_n)$ of the class c given levels $f_1, \ldots, f_n$ for its n feature variables, the model uses Equation (1)

$$\Pr(c \mid f_1, \ldots, f_n) = \frac{\prod_{i=1}^{n} \Pr(f_i \mid c) * \Pr(c)}{\sum_{j=1}^{k} \prod_{i=1}^{n} \Pr(f_i \mid c_j) * \Pr(c_j)} \qquad (1)$$

where $c_1, \ldots, c_k$ are the possible classes for the model's class variable. Using dataset1 as an example, c_1 equals not CM and c_2 equals CM. In the formula, $\Pr(c)$ is the prior probability of the class c of the dependent variable. $\Pr(f_i \mid c_j)$ are the conditional probabilities of the level f_i of the ith selected feature variable given the class c_j. Note that the prior probabilities $\Pr(c)$ and the conditional probabilities $\Pr(f_i \mid c_j)$ for all i and j, have already been estimated from the data upon constructing the NBN and therefore are readily available in the NBN for the computation of posterior probabilities using Eq. (1).

Model accuracy

The main purpose of this study was to illustrate the additional value of providing probability distributions to a farmer to allow more informed decision making. Although constructing the best possible models was not the goal of the study, it is valuable to gain at least some insight in the quality of the constructed NBNs. For this purpose, the accuracy was determined of all three constructed NBNs, where the accuracy was defined as the percentage of correct classifications by the model. From the posterior probability distribution computed for the class variable, the predicted class was established. For the NBN constructed from dataset1, the predicted class was "yes" if the posterior probability of CM was > 0.0085; otherwise, the predicted class was "no". For the NBN constructed from dataset2, the predicted class was "yes" if the posterior probability of CM was > 0.0175; otherwise, the predicted class was "no". The threshold probabilities were chosen to reflect the prevalence of CM in dataset1 and in dataset2, respectively. In the NBN constructed from dataset3, the class variable modelling the causal pathogen had three possible classes. The predicted class was taken to be the one with the highest posterior probability in the computed distribution. The predicted class was compared with the actual class to establish the percentage of correct classifications.

RESULTS

Prior probabilities of clinical mastitis

The NBN constructed from dataset1 included the feature variables DIM and whether or not cow had CM in the previous 5-day period. The accuracy of this NBN was 0.82. With the NBN, for each cow in the first 30 DIM, a prior probability of CM can be calculated based upon the levels of the two selected feature variables. For instance, a cow from 21 to 25 DIM with a previous CM case had a prior probability of CM of 0.007961 (Table 3).

Table 3: A cow-specific prior probability of clinical mastitis (CM) and the corresponding predictive value positive (PV^+) (based on a sensitivity of 43% and a specificity of 97%) of an alert. Illustrations are given for CM alerts for 4 cows before 30 days in milk, differing in prior knowledge.

Days in milk	Having CM in the previous 5-day period	Prior probability of CM	PV^+ (%)
21-25	No	0.002610	3.6
6-10	No	0.004329	5.9
21-25	Yes	0.007961	10.3
1-5	Information not available	0.072573	52.9

The NBN constructed from dataset2 included the feature variables modelling SCC in the 30 days before the previous 30 DIM and the accumulated number of CM cases before the previous 30 DIM. The accuracy of this NBN was 0.65. With the NBN, for each cow after 31 DIM, a prior probability of CM can be calculated based upon the levels of the two selected feature variables. For instance, a cow with an SCC ≥ 200,000 cells/ml and no previous CM case had a prior probability of CM of 0.023238 (Table 4).

Combining the computed cow-specific prior probabilities of CM with the CM detection characteristics of an automatic milking system (sensitivity and specificity), gives the predictive value positive (PV^+) of CM alerts. In our illustrations, assuming a sensitivity of 43% and a specificity of 97%, the PV^+ ranged from 3.6 to 52.9% for alerts in the first 30 DIM (Table 3), and ranged from 13.4 to 46.8% for alerts from 31 DIM onwards (Table 4). A CM alert for a cow with an SCC ≥ 200,000 cells/ml and no CM cases in the 30 days before the previous 30 DIM, had a PV^+ of 25.4%. The alert for this particular cow thus had a probability of 0.254 to be a true positive alert.

Table 4: A cow-specific prior probability of clinical mastitis (CM) and the corresponding predictive value positive (PV^+) (based on a sensitivity of 43% and a specificity of 97%) of an alert. Illustrations are given for CM alerts for 6 cows after 31 days in milk, differing in prior knowledge.

SCC[a] in 30 days before previous 30 DIM[b] (cells/ml)	# CM before the previous 30 DIM[b]	Prior probability of CM	PV^+ (%)
<200,000	0	0.010649	13.4
<200,000	1	0.022290	24.6
≥200,000	0	0.023238	25.4
<200,000	2	0.026536	28.1
≥200,000	1	0.048643	42.3
≥200,000	2	0.057908	46.8

[a] SCC = somatic cell count, [b] DIM = days in milk

<u>Probability distributions for the causal pathogen of clinical mastitis cases</u>

The NBN constructed from dataset3 contained the following eight feature variables: season of the year, whether or not the cow was sick at the moment of CM, colour of the milk, the texture of the milk, SCC 1-30 days before the current CM, SCC >30 days before the current CM, pathogen history 1-30 days before the current CM and pathogen history > 30 days before the current CM. For each CM case from the study dataset, a posterior probability distribution for the causal pathogen was established using the constructed NBN with the eight selected feature variables. For instance, a CM case from a sick cow with watery milk and small flakes in December with an SCC history < 200,000 cells/ml, and without an earlier CM case within this lactation, had a posterior probability for STREP of 0.17, for STAPH of 0.03, and for COLI of 0.80.

Table 5: Predicted and actual numbers of clinical mastitis cases for each group of pathogens using the most likely pathogen as the predicted class.

		Actual			
		STREP[a]	STAPH[b]	COLI[c]	Total
Predicted	STREP[a]	144 (47%)	94 (31%)	67 (22%)	305 (100%)
	STAPH[b]	61 (27%)	126 (55%)	41 (18%)	228 (100%)
	COLI[c]	110 (29%)	67 (17%)	210 (54%)	387 (100%)
	Total	315	287	318	920

[a] *Streptococcus dysgalactiae*, *Streptococcus agalactiae*, *Streptococcus uberis*, other streptococci and mixed cultures of streptococci, [b] *Staphylococcus aureus*, [c] *Escherichia coli* and *Klebsiella spp.*

Table 5 presents the predicted and actual numbers of cases for each pathogen. Of the 920 CM cases in the study dataset, a total of 480 (i.e. 144 + 126 + 210) cases were classified correctly by the NBN, which resulted in an accuracy of 52% (i.e. 480 / 920). Of the 387 CM cases predicted to have been caused by COLI, 210 cases were indeed caused by COLI; 54% of the COLI predicted cases were thus classified correctly.

DISCUSSION

By providing not just a single qualitative outcome of a decision support model to a farmer but also the uncertainties involved, the risks of possible misclassification become visible, which allows the farmer to take a more informed decision. To illustrate this idea, in this study two applications were presented in which probabilities would be provided to a farmer.

Automatic milking systems generate CM alert lists, based on sensor measurements in the milk. These lists mention the cows likely to have CM. Currently, all alerts on the list have the same PV^+ (the probability that a CM alert for a particular cow is a true positive alert) based upon an overall prior probability of CM which is assumed to be the same for all cows. Consequently, it is not possible to rank the CM alerts according to their priority for visual inspection. In the first application, an NBN was constructed to determine a cow-specific prior probability of CM. It was possible to differentiate between CM alerts according to their PV^+ by combining these cow-specific prior probabilities and the test characteristics of a CM detection model of the automatic milking system. The illustrations in Tables 3 and 4 served to support the idea that cow-specific prior probabilities can be used to discriminate between CM alerts. In our illustrations, for alerts from 31 DIM onwards, the PV^+ ranged from 13.4 to 46.8%, indicating that cow-specific prior probabilities can cause a considerable variation in the PV^+. The PV^+ can be used by a farmer to determine which CM alerts have the highest priority for inspection, thereby possibly reducing the workload involved.

In the second application in this study, an NBN was constructed to determine probability distributions for the causal pathogen of CM cases. Based on cow factors, clinical signs and season of the year, a probability distribution of the CM being caused by STREP, STAPH or COLI was established. Simply classifying CM cases according to their causal pathogen, i.e. simply presenting the most likely value, would not provide sufficient information to assist a farmer in deciding upon the most appropriate treatment. Providing a probability distribution for the causal pathogen would reveal the uncertainty involved to the farmer and would thus provide more information for decision making. As an example, consider a CM case with STREP for the most likely class, and assume that the probability distribution for the causal pathogen equals 0.45, 0.15 and 0.40 for STREP, STAPH and COLI, respectively. Providing only the predicted class would ignore the high posterior probability of COLI, which can cause seriously wrong treatment decisions. In practice, only CM cases with a high probability of just a single pathogen will be eligible for more specific treatment. CM cases with almost equal probabilities for two or more pathogens will be eligible for broad spectrum use of antibiotics.

In this study, Bayesian networks were used to compute the probability distributions to be provided to a farmer. Bayesian networks are known as powerful tools for knowledge representation and probabilistic inference (Jensen, 2001). The networks are flexible in terms of handling missing values, capturing complex dependencies among their variables, and allow in essence computing any prior or posterior probability of interest over the modelled variables. These characteristics favour Bayesian networks over other statistical methods such as logistic regression for probabilistic reasoning tasks. In this study, NBNs were used, which are the simplest type of Bayesian network. Although NBNs build upon the assumption that all feature variables are mutually independent given the class variable, they are surprisingly effective (Langley and Sage, 1994), even if the lack of dependencies between the feature variables is somewhat unrealistic. Forward selection was used to select for inclusion in the NBNs only those feature variables that best discriminate between the classes of the class variable. Feature variables were only added if they increase the accuracy of the NBNs under construction. For both NBNs in the first application, just two feature variables were selected. A likely explanation is that the feature variables in the two datasets were, to at least some extent, mutually correlated.

In the presence of an already included variable, adding a mutually correlated feature variable will then not increase the ability to discriminate between the classes of the class variable. Relaxing the independence assumption of an NBN, thus taking correlations between feature variables into account, is likely to lead to more accurate classification models. In our further research, therefore, tree-augmented naive Bayesian networks (Friedman et al., 1997) will be constructed, which allow tree-like dependency structures over their feature variable.

In conclusion, this manuscript presented the idea of providing a farmer with probability distributions in decision support for mastitis management on dairy farms and illustrated its feasibility by means of two applications. The benefits of providing the farmer with a probability distribution instead of just a single qualitative outcome were highlighted in both applications.

ACKNOWLEDGEMENTS

This research was supported by the Dutch Technology Foundation STW, applied science division of NWO, and the Technology Program of the Dutch Ministry of Economic Affairs.

REFERENCES

Barkema, H. W., Schukken, Y. H., Lam, T. J. G. M., Beiboer, M. L., Wilmink, H., Benedictus, G., and Brand, A. (1998). Incidence of clinical mastitis in dairy herds grouped in three categories by bulk milk somatic cell counts. J. Dairy Sci. 81, 411-419.

Chapman, W.W., Dowling, J. N., and Wagner, M. M. (2005). Classification of emergency department chief complaints into 7 syndromes: a retrospective analysis of 527,228 patients. Ann. Emerg. Med. 46, 445-455.

De Mol, R. M. and Ouweltjes, W. (2001). Detection model for mastitis in cows milked in an automatic milking system. Prev. Vet. Med. 49, 71-82.

Dohoo, I. R. and Leslie, K. E. (1991). Evaluation of changes in somatic-cell counts as indicators of new intra-mammary infections. Prev. Vet. Med. 10, 225-237.

Friedman, N., Geiger, D., and Goldszmidt, M. (1997). Bayesian network classifiers. Mach. Learn. 29, 131-163.

Geenen, P.L., Van der Gaag, L. C., Loeffen, W. L. A., and Elbers, A. R. W. (2005). Naive Bayesian classifiers for the clinical diagnosis of Classical Swine Fever. Proceedings of the 2005 meeting of the Society for Veterinary Epidemiology and Preventive Medicine, 169-176. Nairn, Inverness, Scotland.

Groenendaal, H., Galligan, D. T., and Mulder, H. A. (2004). An economic spreadsheet model to determine optimal breeding and replacement decisions for dairy cattle. J. Dairy Sci. 87, 2146-2157.

Jensen, F. V. (2001). Bayesian networks and decision graphs. Springer-Verlag, New York, NY.

Jones, G. F., and Ward, G. E. (1990). Evaluation of a scheme for predicting the Gram-staining reaction of organisms causing bovine mastitis. J. Am. Vet. Med. Assoc. 196, 597-599.

Kim, T., and Heald, C. W. (1999). Inducing inference rules for the classification of bovine mastitis. Computers and Electronics in Agriculture 23, 27-42.

Langley, P., and Sage, S. (1994). Induction of selective Bayesian classifiers. Proceedings of the 10th conference of Uncertainty in Artificial Intelligence, Morgan Kaufmann Publishers, San Francisco, 199-406.

McKendrick, I. J., Gettinby, G., Gu, Y., Reid, S. W. J., and Revie, C. W. (2000). Using a Bayesian belief network to aid differential diagnosis of tropical bovine diseases. Prev. Vet. Med. 47, 141-156.

Schrage, M. M., Van IJzendoorn, A., and Van der Gaag, L. C. (2005). Haskell ready to Dazzle the real world. Proceedings of the 2005 ACM SIGPLAN workshop on Haskell, ACM Press, New York, 17-26.

Steeneveld, W., Hogeveen, H., Barkema, H. W., Van den Broek, J., and Huirne, R. B. M. (2008). The influence of cow factors on the incidence of clinical mastitis. J. Dairy Sci. 91, 1391-1402

EPIDEMIOLOGICAL METHODS

MODELLING HIERARCHICAL AND CROSS-CLASSIFIED DATA STRUCTURES DURING THE INVESTIGATION OF HORSE RACING INJURY

T.D.H. PARKIN*, R. ECOB, L. HILLYER, T. MORRIS, K. ROGERS, A.J. STIRK, P. WEBBON AND J.R. NEWTON

SUMMARY

The majority of previous studies of racecourse fatal or non-fatal injury have ignored the complex data structures that are commonly encountered. These studies assumed that starts made by the same horse in different races; starts made by different horses in the same race; starts made by all horses on the same course and different horses sent out by the same trainer were independent. Wood et al. (2001) and Pinchbeck et al. (2002) have included hierarchical data structures to estimate the variance of random effects at different levels. This study applies this methodology to the investigation of tendon strain injuries during racing and also extends models to include the cross-classified nature of the data to accommodate simultaneous hierarchies. The majority of variability was at the level of the start (level 1) in all models. The largest variance partition coefficients were estimated, in two- and three-level hierarchical models, to be at race, horse and trainer levels. In cross-classified models only the trainer-level variance remained significant. The coefficients and standard errors associated with important risk factors were not significantly affected when different data structures were modelled.

INTRODUCTION

A number of studies have identified risk factors for fatal or non-fatal injury during racing. The majority of these studies have focused on flat racing, without obstacles (Mohammed et al., 1991; Peloso et al., 1994; Estberg et al., 1996 & 1998; Cohen et al., 1997, 1999 & 2000; Hernandez et al., 2001; Boden et al., 2007a). In the UK (Wood et al., 2001; Parkin et al., 2004a & b), Australia (Bailey et al., 1998; Boden et al., 2007b) and the USA (Stephen et al., 2003) risk factors for musculoskeletal injury or fatality in jump racing have been identified. Case definitions that have predominated include fatality, musculoskeletal injury and fracture. Few studies, either on the flat or over jumps, have investigated risk factors for tendon strain injury during racing (Perkins et al., 2005; Parkin et al., 2006; Lam et al., 2007a). Tendon injuries are a major concern to the racing industry worldwide, as although not often life threatening, they often require a long recuperation period and are one of the most common causes of retirement from racing (Perkins et al., 2005; Lam et al., 2007b).

The British Horseracing Authority (BHA) in the UK (formerly the Jockey Club) standardised the system for the collection and recording of racing-related data, from the year 2000. The Equine Welfare database has enabled real-time monitoring of racecourse veterinary-related issues and also formed an important source of data for more complex epidemiological

* Tim Parkin, Boyd Orr Centre for Population and Ecosystem Health, Institute of Comparative Medicine, Faculty of Veterinary Medicine, University of Glasgow, 464 Bearsden Road, Glasgow, G61 1QH. Email:t.parkin@vet.gla.ac.uk

analyses. An investigation of racing-related risk factors for tendon injury was conducted as one of the first welfare concerns to be addressed using the Equine Welfare database (Parkin et al., 2006).

Few of the previous studies of racehorse injury or fatality have attempted to fully account for the complex nature of the data structure. The majority of work has observed outcomes at the level of the individual race start, assuming that all starts are independent. With horses making multiple starts during their career, multiple starts occurring within a single race and many races taking place on the same racecourse this assumption may be difficult to justify. Wood et al. (2001) and Pinchbeck et al. (2002) estimated the proportion of variance residing at different hierarchical levels when investigating risk factors for equine death on racecourses and falls during jump racing, respectively. Wood et al. (2001) identified a significant proportion of variation at the level of trainer in both flat and hurdle races as well as significant race-level variation in hurdle races (but not flat races). Pinchbeck et al. (2002) identified that a significant proportion of the variation in the risk of falling was attributable to both horse and race.

In the current study, the information in the Equine Welfare database relating to all hurdle race starts between 2000 and 2007, inclusive, was used to explore the feasibility of including more complex data structures in the investigation of racing injuries.

The aims of this study were to:

1. determine if inclusion of greater data structure complexity significantly altered the estimates of the coefficients (and the associated standard errors) for important risk factors for tendon strain injury in hurdle racing.
2. identify higher levels that may be important in determining the likelihood of tendon strain injury during racing.
3. model the cross-classified data structure to account for the higher levels with the greatest variance partition coefficient (VPC) on simultaneous hierarchies.

MATERIALS AND METHODS

Case definition and control selection

Case starts were defined as those in which a horse sustained a palpable tendon strain injury, identified by BHA Veterinary Officers after racing in a hurdle race, on any of the 43 UK racecourses that staged hurdle races between January 2000 and December 2007. Tendon injuries recorded as lacerated, severed or bruised were excluded from the case population. Control starts were all other starts in hurdle races made during the study period that did not result in a tendon strain injury.

Data structure

Two slightly different datasets were used during this study. The first dataset included all cases of tendon strain injury. The second excluded the starts associated with the second injury sustained by 24 horses that sustained more than one tendon strain injury during racing. There were a total of 146,545 race starts in the complete dataset and 146,521 starts in the reduced dataset. The complete dataset included 929 starts that resulted in tendon strain injury and the reduced dataset included 905 starts that resulted in tendon strain injury.

The complex nature of the data structure is illustrated in the unit diagram in Fig. 1. The outcome (tendon strain injury) was measured at the level of the individual race start. There were a total of 146,545 race starts made between 2000 and 2007, by 25,674 horses. Horses made a mean of 5.7 starts (median = 4; range 1-96). Within each of 13,143 races there were a mean of 11.1 (median = 11; range 2-30) starts and within each of 43 racecourses there were a mean of 3,407.5 starts (median = 3,486; range 210-6423). Each horse could race for more than one of the 1,299 trainers and be ridden by more than one of the 1,184 jockeys, in different starts, and each of the 2,193 sires could sire multiple horses.

Statistical analysis

Data inconsistencies were identified using SAS (SAS Campus Drive, Cary, USA) and initial single-level models were produced using STATA version 9.1 (Statacorp, College Station, Texas, USA). Two-level models were produced in both STATA version 9.1 and MLwiN version 2.02. Three-level random effects models and cross-classified models were developed in MLwiN version 2.02.

Single-level ordinary multivariable logistic regression models were produced to identify race-, course- and horse-related risk factors for tendon strain injury using standard techniques (Hosmer & Lemeshow, 2000). These results have been reported in detail elsewhere (Parkin et al., 2006). Going (firmness of the racing surface) was included as one of these risk factors in the final model and was classified as heavy or soft, good to soft, good, good to firm, or firm.

The effect of accounting for the hierarchical and cross-classified nature of the data was investigated by developing models of increasing complexity. Initially two-level random intercept models were fitted. Level 1 was defined as the race start in all models. The level 2 random effects that were considered one at a time were race, racecourse, horse, trainer, sire and jockey. Further hierarchical levels (race nested with racecourse and horse nested within trainer, jockey and sire) were then included and finally cross-classified models were developed allowing for the inclusion of more than one simultaneous hierarchy.

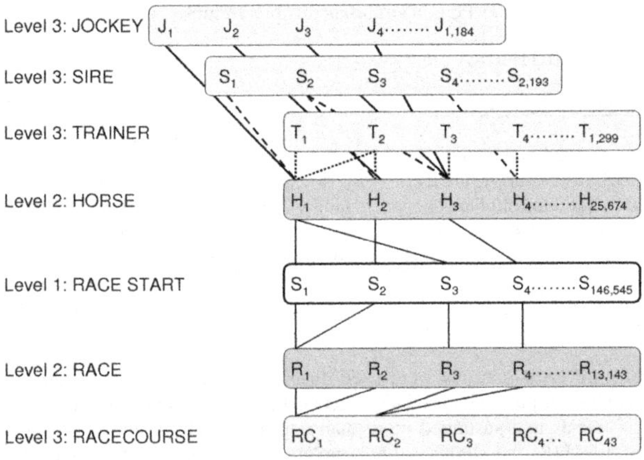

Fig. 1 Unit diagram of the structure of the data associated with tendon strain injuries during hurdle racing in the UK. The number of units at each level in the complete dataset is given as subscripts.

Intercept only models were fitted before fixed effects were added to the models which demonstrated the greatest degree of higher level variance. Initially first-order marginal quasi-likelihood (MQL) models using iterative weighted least squares were produced. As MQL methods have been shown to result in severe under-estimation of variance components, especially where very small cluster sizes exist at one level, 2nd order MQL and 1st and 2nd order penalized quasi-likelihood (PQL) models were also fitted (Rodriguez & Goldman, 1995). It was not possible to fit 2nd order PQL models for all random effect structures. Markov-chain Monte Carlo (MCMC) simulations using Metropolis-Hastings sampling with diffuse priors, a burn in of 10,000 iterations and a run of 500,000 iterations (after an initial assessment of 50,000 iterations) were used to develop cross-classified models (Browne, 2005).

The significance of variance estimates was calculated by using the Wald test for initial hierarchical models and by calculating Bayesian credible intervals for the cross-classified models.

The relative contribution of each random term to the total variance (variance partition coefficient) was estimated using the latent variable approach described by Goldstein et al. (2002). No extra-binomial variation was allowed and the start level was constrained to be 1 on the binomial scale. As described by Goldstein et al. (2002) the total level 1 variance on the logit scale was taken to be fixed and equal to $\pi^2/3 \approx 3.29$. This approach is suitable when it is possible to assume that the binary outcome is a result of an underlying latent process, with a continuous distribution (Snijders & Bosker, 1999; Goldstein et al., 2002). It was assumed in the current investigation that the outcome tendon strain injury would occur once a threshold of tendon pathology or degeneration had been reached (Smith et al. 1999 & 2002). The VPC at different levels is calculated as the ratio of the higher level variance (σ^2_u) to the sum of the level 1 (σ^2_e) and higher level variance [Eq. (1)]. VPC's are reported as percentages.

$$\text{Variance partition coefficient (VPC)} = \sigma^2_u/(\sigma^2_e + \sigma^2_u) \qquad (1)$$

(where $\sigma^2_e = 3.29$)

RESULTS

<u>Single-level multivariable logistic regression (complete dataset)</u>

Between January 2000 and December 2007, 929 hurdle race starts ended in tendon strain injury, from a total of 146,545 hurdle starts (6.3/1,000 starts). Firmer going was associated with an increased likelihood of injury with the odds ratio's (O.R.'s) increasing from 1 for soft or heavy going, to 2.0 (95% confidence interval (CI) = 1.5-2.6) for good-soft going, to 2.8 (95%CI = 2.2-3.6) for good going, to 3.8 (95%CI = 2.9-4.9) for good-firm going and 6.6 (95%CI = 4.2-10.2) for firm going. Starts in races held in the summer months (June, July and August) were 1.2 times (95%CI = 1.0-1.4) more likely to be associated with a tendon strain injury than starts in races held in the spring (March, April, May) or autumn (September, October, November) months. Starts in races held during winter (December, January, February) were 0.72 (95%CI = 0.59-0.87) times as likely to be associated with injury compared to starts in the spring or autumn. For every extra 1000 metres of race distance on the day of the start the likelihood of injury increased by 1.9 times (95%CI = 1.7-2.1). Starts made by older horses were more likely to be associated with injury; for every extra year of age horses were 1.1 (95%CI = 1.0-1.1) times more likely to make a start that resulted in tendon strain injury. Horses that had sustained a tendon strain injury in a previous start were 39 times more likely to be recorded as having sustained a tendon strain injury in a subsequent start (95%CI = 23.4-65.3).

Multilevel modeling

Variance partition coefficient estimates

Two-level intercept only models indicated that the greatest proportion of higher level variance was associated with the race (28.6% – reduced dataset; 31.7% – complete dataset) and horse (20.5% - complete dataset) (Table 1). The VPC for trainer was estimated to be 7.2% (reduced dataset) and 9.3% (complete dataset). In both datasets the VPC for jockey was less than 2%. In the reduced dataset horse-level variance was zero as by definition horses could not sustain more than one tendon injury during racing. Inclusion of all fixed effects, associated with tendon injury, in the two-level models with race included as a random effect resulted in significant reductions in the proportion of variance attributable to race (11.1% - reduced dataset; 12.4% - complete dataset). In the two-level model, developed for the complete dataset, with horse as a random effect the VPC associated with horse was significantly reduced to 7.9% (data not shown).

The VPC's for each of the random effects in the three-level intercept only models for both datasets are presented in Table 2. In these hierarchical models race (33.8% - reduced dataset and 36.4% - complete dataset) and horse (between 14.5% and 16.9% - complete dataset) were associated with the highest VPC's. The VPC associated with trainer was reduced slightly to 6.8% and 6.3% in the reduced and complete datasets, respectively, compared to the equivalent two-level intercept only models.

Table 1. Variance estimates (standard errors) and variance partition coefficients (VPC) for intercept only hierarchical two-level models for the reduced and complete datasets of racecourse tendon injury (level 1 = race start).

2ND LEVEL	REDUCED DATASET (INCIDENT CASES)		COMPLETE DATASET (ALL CASES)	
	Variance (SE)	VPC (%)	Variance (SE)	VPC (%)
Horse	0.0 (0)	0.0	0.850 (0.181)	20.5
Trainer	0.255 (0.053)	7.2	0.337 (0.060)	9.3
Sire	0.180 (0.052)	5.2	0.220 (0.054)	6.3
Jockey	0.054 (0.028)	1.6	0.059 (0.028)	1.8
Race	1.320 (0.188)	28.6	1.529 (0.187)	31.7
Course	0.131 (0.040)	3.8	0.142 (0.043)	4.1

Two cross-classified models were produced for each dataset based on the VPC's observed in the hierarchical models. The VPC's for race cross-classified with trainer and race cross-classified with horse are reported in Table 2.

The VPC associated with race was significantly reduced to 10.9% (from 33.8%) and 12.0% (from 36.4%) for the reduced and complete datasets respectively, when all fixed effects were included in the three-level models including race nested within course (Tables 3 and 4 – model 4). In the complete dataset the horse-level VPC's for the three-level models that included horse at the second level (models 2 and 3) were moderately reduced to between 10.4% and 12.4%, from between 14.5% and 16.9% (Table 4). In the reduced dataset the horse-level VPC increased from 0 to between 5.2% (nested within sire – model 3) and 8.9% (nested within trainer – model 2). The trainer-level VPC was moderately reduced to 4.9% (reduced data set) and 5.1% (complete data set) when all fixed effects were included.

Table 2. Variance estimates (standard errors) and variance partition coefficients (VPC) for intercept only hierarchical three-level (trainer and horse; sire and horse; jockey and horse; course and race) and cross-classified (race and trainer; race and horse) models for incident and all cases of racecourse tendon injury (level 1 = race start).

MODEL TYPE		REDUCED DATASET (INCIDENT CASES)				COMPLETE DATASET (ALL CASES)			
THREE-LEVEL HIERARCHICAL		VARIANCE (SE)		VPC (%)		VARIANCE (SE)		VPC (%)	
3rd Level	2nd Level	3rd level	2nd level	3rd level	2nd level	3rd level	2nd level	3rd level	2nd level
Trainer	Horse	0.239 (0.053)	0 (0)	6.8	0	0.269 (0.057)	0.726 (0.197)	6.3	16.9
Sire	Horse	0.158 (0.049)	0 (0)	4.6	0	0.171 (0.052)	0.589 (0.184)	4.2	14.5
Jockey	Horse	0.054 (0.028)	0 (0)	1.6	0	0.057 (0.028)	0.623 (0.311)	1.4	15.7
Course	Race	0.118 (0.039)	1.738 (0.200)	2.3	33.8	0.133 (0.042)	1.963 (0.199)	2.5	36.4
CROSS-CLASSIFIED									
Race	Trainer	0.799 (0.246)	0.245 (0.077)	18.4	5.7	0.001 (0.001)	0.288 (0.103)	0	8.0
Race	Horse	0.002 (0.001)	0 (0)	0.1	0	0.894 (0.349)	0.001 (0)	21.4	0

In the cross-classified models race-level VPC was significantly reduced from 18.4% (Table 2) to 1.5% with the inclusion of all fixed effects, in the reduced dataset (Table 3). In the same model trainer-level VPC remained effectively unaltered (from 5.7% to 5.9%). When using the complete dataset the highest race-level VPC was significantly reduced from 21.4% to 0.1% (Table 4). Again, trainer-level VPC remained effectively unaltered (from 8.0% to 6.1%).

Effect of accounting for data complexity on estimates for fixed effects

Compared to the single-level model the effect of accounting for different hierarchal structures on the estimates for each of the fixed effects in the model was minimal (Tables 3 and 4). All fixed effects remained significant within all models. The greatest effect was observed in model 2, using the complete dataset, when trainer (level 3) and horse (level 2) were included as random effects. The standard error (SE) of the coefficient associated with previous tendon injury increased by 27% and the coefficient itself reduced by 7% (Table 4).

Table 3. Parameter estimates from the different model data structures with incident racecourse tendon strain injuries as the binary response (i.e. reduced dataset). Model 1 is the single-level model (race start level only); models 2 – 4 are standard three-level hierarchical models with stated third- and second-level random effects; models 5 and 6 are cross-classified models with stated random effects.

	MODEL 1	MODEL 2[a]	MODEL 3[a]	MODEL 4[a]	MODEL 5[b]	MODEL 6[b]

Level 3		Trainer	Sire	Racecourse	Race	Race
Variance	NA	0.189	0.146	0.004	0.053	0.004
(SE)		(0.05)	(0.05)	(0.01)	(0.033)	(0.003)
VPC (%)		4.9	4.0	0.1	1.5	0.1
Level 2		Horse	Horse	Race	Trainer	Horse
Variance	NA	0.341	0.188	0.402	0.209	0.001
(SE)		(0.178)	(0.162)	(0.146)	(0.076)	(0)
VPC (%)		8.9	5.2	10.9	5.9	0
VARIABLE			COEFFICIENT (SE)			
Age	0.076	0.078	0.082	0.076	0.073	0.075
	(0.017)	(0.018)	(0.018)	(0.017)	(0.018)	(0.017)
Season						
Spring/Autumn	Ref	Ref	Ref	Ref	Ref	Ref
Summer	0.165	0.159	0.173	0.155	0.159	0.165
	(0.086)	(0.087)	(0.086)	(0.09)	(0.087)	(0.085)
Winter	-0.353	-0.349	-0.355	-0.349	-0.351	-0.353
	(0.102)	(0.102)	(0.102)	(0.104)	(0.102)	(0.103)
Race distance	0.634	0.639	0.628	0.635	0.641	0.64
(km)	(0.054)	(0.055)	(0.055)	(0.055)	(0.058)	(0.053)
Going						
Heavy/Soft	Ref	Ref	Ref	Ref	Ref	Ref
Good-soft	0.625	0.634	0.629	0.623	0.635	0.625
	(0.141)	(0.142)	(0.141)	(0.143)	(0.139)	(0.140)
Good	1.007	1.019	1.019	1.005	1.021	1.012
	(0.126)	(0.126)	(0.126)	(0.128)	(0.123)	(0.126)
Good-firm	1.3	1.305	1.316	1.292	1.306	1.304
	(0.133)	(0.134)	(0.134)	(0.136)	(0.131)	(0.132)
Firm	1.856	1.864	1.879	1.845	1.849	1.842
	(0.225)	(0.226)	(0.226)	(0.233)	(0.225)	(0.228)
Constant	-8.886	-8.904	-8.927	-8.893	-8.997	-8.910
	(0.246)	(0.252)	(0.251)	(0.253)	(0.252)	(0.246)

[a] 1st order penalized quasi-likelihood; [b] Cross classified model using Markov-chain Monte Carlo methodology (500,000 iterations); SE = standard error; VPC = Variance partition coefficient; Ref = Reference category

Table 4. Parameter estimates from the different model data structures with all racecourse tendon strain injuries as the binary response (i.e. complete dataset). Model 1 is the single-level model (race start level only); models 2 – 4 are standard three-level hierarchical models with stated third- and second-level random effects; models 5 and 6 are cross-classified models with stated random effects.

	MODEL 1	MODEL 2[a]	MODEL 3[a]	MODEL 4[a]	MODEL 5[b]	MODEL 6[b]
Level 3		Trainer	Sire	Racecourse	Race	Race
Variance	NA	0.203	0.144	0.007	0.002	0.001
(SE)		(0.051)	(0.05)	(0.011)	(0.002)	(0)
VPC (%)		5.1	3.8	0.2	0.1	0

Level 2		Horse	Horse	Race	Trainer	Horse
Variance	NA	0.496	0.398	0.450	0.214	0.01
(SE)		(0.175)	(0.162)	(0.143)	(0.053)	(0.004)
VPC (%)		12.4	10.4	12.0	6.1	0
VARIABLE			COEFFICIENT (SE)			
Age	0.072	0.077	0.082	0.073	0.071	0.073
	(0.017)	(0.018)	(0.017)	(0.017)	(0.017)	(0.017)
Season						
Spring/Autumn	Ref	Ref	Ref	Ref	Ref	Ref
Summer	0.195	0.187	0.200	0.176	0.189	0.194
	(0.085)	(0.086)	(0.085)	(0.09)	(0.086)	(0.085)
Winter	-0.332	-0.333	-0.337	-0.326	-0.33	-0.33
	(0.101)	(0.102)	(0.101)	(0.104)	(0.101)	(0.102)
Race distance	0.633	0.641	0.630	0.633	0.639	0.635
(km)	(0.053)	(0.055)	(0.055)	(0.055)	(0.056)	(0.052)
Going						
Heavy/Soft	Ref	Ref	Ref	Ref	Ref	Ref
Good-soft	0.670	0.680	0.676	0.667	0.685	0.681
	(0.140)	(0.141)	(0.141)	(0.142)	(0.142)	(0.140)
Good	1.035	1.046	1.047	1.032	1.052	1.050
	(0.126)	(0.126)	(0.126)	(0.128)	(0.128)	(0.125)
Good-firm	1.33	1.334	1.347	1.319	1.338	1.345
	(0.133)	(0.134)	(0.134)	(0.136)	(0.137)	(0.132)
Firm	1.886	1.893	1.912	1.871	1.883	1.883
	(0.225)	(0.227)	(0.226)	(0.234)	(0.229)	(0.226)
Previous tendon	3.666	3.395	3.490	3.623	3.646	3.658
injury	(0.262)	(0.333)	(0.321)	(0.275)	(0.289)	(0.268)
Constant	-8.891	-8.942	-8.966	-8.898	-8.988	-8.922
	(0.245)	(0.252)	(0.251)	(0.253)	(0.255)	(0.239)

[a] 1st order penalized quasi-likelihood; [b] Cross classified model using Markov-chain Monte Carlo methodology (500,000 iterations); SE = standard error; VPC = Variance partition coefficient; Ref = Reference category

DISCUSSION

Variance at different hierarchical levels

Previous studies by Wood et al. (2001) and Pinchbeck et al. (2002) have identified significant trainer, race and horse level variability associated with death or falling (in jump races). The majority of variance was identified to reside at level 1 (i.e. the start) in both studies. These studies used three-level hierarchical models to produce variance estimates at each level and compared the effect of different techniques (1st and 2nd order MQL/PQL and MCMC methods) in MLwiN. In the current study we extended this approach to include simultaneous hierarchies in the same model by fitting a series of cross-classified models (Rasbash & Browne, 2002).

The VPC's calculated in the two and three-level random effects models indicated that the greatest proportion of variability resides at the start (level 1), as found by both Wood et al. (2001) and Pinchbeck et al. (2002). In the two- and three-level models produced in the current study significant variability at the level of the race (both datasets) and horse (complete dataset), with a small but statistically significant degree of variability at the level of the trainer, was identified. In the three-level models using the complete dataset, where horse was at level 2, the VPC's associated with horse were moderately reduced to between 14.5% and 16.9%. This suggests that some of the variance attributable to horse in the two-level models was actually attributable to the higher 3rd level variance (i.e. trainer, sire or jockey). The trainer-level VPC's were moderately reduced in the three-level models compared to the two-level models. Nevertheless these variance estimates remained statistically significant.

The greatest reductions in race-level variance were estimated when race was cross-classified with trainer or horse. Race-level variance was reduced by up to 50% in cross-classified models compared to three- or two-level hierarchical models. In contrast, trainer-level variance remained essentially unaltered. Horse-level variance was estimated to be zero in these cross-classified models. It may be that the estimates for horse-level variance were unreliable even though models were run for 500,000 iterations as when examining the MCMC diagnostics for this level variance the Raferty-Lewis diagnostic indicated that several million iterations would be required to estimate a 95% confidence interval accurate to within 0.005 with probability 0.95. It may be the case that given the low number of outcomes per horse it is not possible to model the cross-classified nature of the data when including horse as one of the random effects.

The effect of including the relevant fixed effects in the different models was to significantly reduce race-level variance estimates in both the two- and three-level hierarchical models. In the cross-classified models race-level variance was reduced dramatically to non significant levels. But in both datasets the trainer-level variance (in the trainer cross classified with race model) remained unaltered and statistically significant.

These results suggest that further investigation of race- and trainer-level factors associated with tendon injury are appropriate even though significant proportions of both were explained by the inclusion of significant risk factors. Further, given the lack of variance associated with racecourse compared to race, it is important that future studies attempting to identify strategies that racecourses may employ to improve safety should measure race-level variables. Racecourse-level variables such as track circumference, topography and soil structure may be less important whereas race-level variables such as movement of running rails or fences and ground maintenance strategies before individual races may be of greater significance.

<u>Risk factors for racecourse tendon strain injury</u>

Important risk factors for tendon strain injury have been identified and reported in detail elsewhere (Parkin et al., 2006). These risk factors were included as the fixed effects in two slightly different datasets during this study. In the complete dataset, that was used to model any race start resulting in tendon strain injury as the dependent variable, age of horse, season, race distance, going and previous tendon injury were all associated with the outcome. In the reduced dataset, that was used to model race starts that included an incident case of racecourse tendon strain injury as the dependent variable, the same risk factors were identified with the obvious exception of previous tendon injury.

In accordance, with previous studies of tendon injury (Perkins et al., 2005; Lam et al., 2007a) older horses were at greater risk. This most likely reflects the gradual degeneration of tendons that is hypothesised to occur with training and exercise prior to severe tendon injury (Smith et al., 1999 & 2002).

Interestingly summer racing was associated with an increased likelihood of injury even though the confounding effect of going, which is obviously also associated with summer racing (i.e. firmer races during drier/hotter summer months), was accounted for. This indicates that there are further aspects of summer racing which also increase the risk of injury. These may be climatic factors such as temperature and humidity. Alternatively there may be differences in the type or quality of horse that took part in summer jump racing that increased the likelihood of injury, however some measures of ability, such as BHA rating were included in these models. Hurdle starts during the winter were associated with a reduced likelihood of tendon strain injury compared to starts in the autumn or spring months. The reason for this is not immediately obvious, given the fact that going is accounted for, and further investigation of factors associated with winter racing is required.

Race distance has also been identified in previous studies as being associated with fatal or non-fatal injury (Bailey et al., 1998; Wood et al., 2001; Hernandez et al., 2001). We believe that although fatigue may be associated with longer races and an increased likelihood of fatality or injury it is also possible that this association is simply a reflection of time at risk.

Firmer going, identified here as a risk factor, has previously been reported to be associated with many different outcomes including fracture, musculoskeletal injury and fatality (Bailey et al., 1998; Williams et al., 2001; Parkin et al., 2004b; Boden et al., 2007a & b). The size of the effects identified in the current and previous studies suggest that greater efforts to reduce the firmness of turf racecourses would be very likely to have substantial welfare benefits.

The final risk factor identified in the analysis of the complete dataset was having sustained a tendon strain injury in a previous start. It is recognised that a horse with a previous tendon injury is more likely to re-injure (Lam et al., 2007a). This variable was included in the final models using this dataset in order to assess its impact on the estimates of horse level variance. It was not included to infer anything about the risk of injury for a horse with a previous tendon injury. There are likely to be many horses in the database that would have sustained a previous tendon injury during training or even during racing that was only identified after the horse left the racecourse, which would not have been recorded on the Equine Welfare database. In order to better quantify this risk, access to the full medical histories of all horses in the database is required.

It was interesting to note that the coefficients and standard errors for all of the fixed effects were very similar for all final models that included all significant risk factors. This would suggest that the effect of these risk factors on the likelihood of tendon injury did not vary greatly across each of the different higher levels of clustering.

This study has demonstrated that hierarchical models for racecourse injury may be useful in identifying future research priorities. The development of cross-classified models was extremely computationally intensive and the results should be treated with some caution as MCMC diagnostics suggest that a very large number of iterations are required. However, given adequate computational resources and suitable data structures, cross-classified models will ultimately enable the unraveling of higher levels on simultaneous hierarchies. This work has demonstrated that there are likely to be further race- and trainer-level variables that require investigation. Further work is also required to accommodate the complexity of these data to include more than one cross-classification at a time.

ACKNOWLEDGEMENTS

The authors would like to thank Gayle Preston at Weatherbys for assistance with data queries. Tim Parkin is currently funded as a Defra/Scottish Funding Council Veterinary Training and Research Initiative (VTRI) Research Fellow.

REFERENCES

Bailey, C.J., Reid, S.W.J., Hodgson, D.R., Bourke, J.M. and Rose, R.J. (1998). Flat, hurdle and steeple racing: risk factors for musculoskeletal injury. Equine Vet J. 30, 498-503.

Boden, L.A., Anderson, G.A., Charles, J.A., Morgan, K.L., Morton, J.M., Parkin, T.D.H., Clarke, A.F. and Slocombe, R.F. (2007a). Risk Factors for Thoroughbred Racehorse Fatality in Flat Starts in Victoria (1989-2004). Equine Vet J. 39, 430-437.

Boden, L.A., Anderson, G.A., Charles, J.A., Morgan, K.L., Morton, J.M., Parkin, T.D.H., Clarke, A.F. and Slocombe, R.F. (2007b). Risk Factors for Fatality in Jump Starts in Victoria (1989-2004). Equine Vet J. 39, 422-428.

Browne, W. (2005). MCMC estimation in MLwiN Version 2.0. Centre for Multilevel modeling, University of Bristol.

Cohen, N.D., Peloso, J.G., Mundy, G.D., Fisher, M., Holland, R.E., Little, T.V., Misheff, M.M., Watkins, J.P., Honnas, C.M. and Moyer, W. (1997). Racing-related factors and results of prerace physical inspection and their association with musculoskeletal injuries incurred in Thoroughbreds during races. J Am Vet Med Assoc. 211, 454-463.

Cohen, N.D., Mundy, G.D., Peloso, J.G., Carey, V.J. and Amend, N.K. (1999). Results of physical inspection before races and race-related characteristics and their association with musculoskeletal injuries in Thoroughbreds during races. J Am Vet Med Assoc. 215, 654-661.

Cohen, N.D., Berry, S.M., Peloso, J.G., Mundy, G.D. and Howard, I.C. (2000). Association of high-speed exercise with racing injury in Thoroughbreds. J Am Vet Med Assoc. 216, 1273-1278.

Estberg, L., Stover, S.M., Gardner, I.A., Drake, C.M., Johnson, B.J. and Ardans, A. (1996). High-speed exercise history and catastrophic racing fracture in Thoroughbreds. Am J Vet Res. 57, 1549-1555.

Estberg, L., Stover, S.M., Gardner, I.A., Johnson, B.J., Jack, R.A., Case, J.T., Ardans, A., Read, D.H., Anderson, M.L., Barr, B.C., Daft, B.M., Kinde, H., Moore, J., Stoltz, J. and Woods, LW. (1998). Relationship between race start characteristics and risk of catastrophic injury in Thoroughbreds: 78 cases (1992). J Am Vet Med Assoc. 212, 544-549.

Goldstein, H., Browne, W. and Rasbash, J. (2002). Partitioning variation in multilevel models. Understanding Statistics, 1, 223-231.

Hernandez, J., Hawkins, D.L. and Scollay, M.C. (2001). Race-start characteristics and risk of catastrophic musculoskeletal injury in Thoroughbred racehorses. J Am Vet Med Assoc. 218, 83-86.

Hosmer, D.W and Lemeshow, S. (2000). Applied Logistic Regression 2nd Ed, John Wiley, New York.

Lam, K.H., Parkin, T.D.H., Riggs, C.M.R. and Morgan, K.L. (2007a). Evaluation of detailed training data to identify risk factors for retirement because of tendon injuries in Thoroughbred racehorses. Am J Vet Res. 68, 1188-1197.

Lam, K.H., Parkin, T.D.H., Riggs, C.M. and Morgan, K.L. (2007b). Content analysis of free-text clinical records: their use in identifying syndromes and analysing health data. Vet Rec. 161, 547-551.

Mohammed, H.O., Hill, T. and Lowe, J. (1991). Risk factors associated with injuries in Thoroughbred horses. Equine Vet J 23, 445-448.

Parkin, T.D.H., Clegg, P.D., French, N.P., Proudman, C.J., Riggs, C.M., Singer, E.R., Webbon, P.M. and Morgan, K.L. (2004a). Horse level risk factors for fatal distal limb fracture in racing Thoroughbreds in the UK. Equine Vet J. 36, 513-519.

Parkin, T.D.H., Clegg, P.D., French, N.P., Proudman, C.J., Riggs, C.M., Singer, E.R., Webbon, P.M. and Morgan, K.L. (2004b). Race and course level risk factors for fatal distal limb fracture in racing Thoroughbreds. Equine Vet J. 36, 521-526.

Parkin, T.D.H., Rogers, K., Stirk, A.J., Webbon, P.M., Newton, J.R. and Hillyer, L.L. (2006). Risk factors for tendon strain injury during racing in Great Britain. Proc. 16th Int. Conf. Racing Analysts Vet., Tokyo, Japan. pp323-324.

Peloso, J.G., Mundy, G.D. and Cohen ND. (1994). Prevalence of and factors associated with musculoskeletal racing injuries of Thoroughbreds. J Am Vet Med Assoc. 204, 620-626.

Perkins, N.R., Reid, S.W.J. and Morris RS. (2005). Risk factors for injury to the superficial digital flexor tendon and suspensory apparatus in Thoroughbred racehorses. N Z Vet J. 53, 184-92.

Pinchbeck, G.L., Clegg, P.D., Proudman, C.J., Morgan, K.L., Wood, J.L.N. and French, N.P. (2002). Risk factors and sources of variation in horse falls in steeplechase racing in the UK. Prev Vet Med 55, 179-192.

Rasbash, J. and Browne, W.J. (2002). Non-hierarchical structures. In: de Jeeuw, J. and Kreft, I. G. G. (Eds). Handbook of quantitative multilevel analysis. Boston: Kluwer Acad.

Rodriguez, G. and Goldman, N. (1995). An assessment of estimation procedures for multilevel models with binary responses. J Royal Stat Soc, Series A. 158, 73-89.

Smith, R.K., Birch, H., Patterson-Kane, J., Firth, E.C., Williams, L., Cherdchutham, W., van Weeren, W.R. and Goodship, A.E. (1999) Should equine athletes commence training during skeletal development?: changes in tendon matrix associated with development, ageing, function and exercise. Equine Vet J Suppl. 30, 201-209.

Smith, R.K., Birch, H.L., Goodman, S., Heinegård, D. and Goodship, A.E. (2002) The influence of ageing and exercise on tendon growth and degeneration—hypotheses for the initiation and prevention of strain-induced tendinopathies. Comp Biochem Physiol A Mol Integr Physiol. 133, 1039-1050.

Snijders, T.A.B. and Bosker, R.J. (1999). Multilevel Analysis. An introduction to basic and advance multilevel modelling. Sage Publications Ltd., London.

Stephen, J.O., White, N.A., McCormick, W.H., Cowles, R.R. and Corley, K.T.T. (2003). Risk factors and prevalence of injuries in horses during various types of steeplechase races. J Am Vet Med Assoc. 223, 1788-1790.

Wood, J.L.N., Eastment, J., Lakhani, K.H., Harkins, L. and Rogers, K. (2001). Modelling a retrospective study of death on racecourses. Proc. Soc. Vet. Epi. Prev. Med, Noordwijkerhout, The Netherlands. pp115-126.

Williams, R.B., Harkins, L.S., Hammond, C.J. and Wood, J.L. (2001). Racehorse injuries, clinical problems and fatalities recorded on British racecourses from flat racing and National Hunt racing during 1996, 1997 and 1998. Equine Vet J. 33, 478-486.

USE AND VALIDATION OF A NOVEL MARKOV CHAIN MONTE CARLO METHOD OF ANALYSIS FOR FAECAL EGG COUNT REDUCTION TEST DATA

M.J. DENWOOD*, S.W.J. REID, S. LOVE, M.K. NIELSEN, L. MATTHEWS, I.J. MCKENDRICK AND G.T. INNOCENT

SUMMARY

Faecal Egg Count Reduction Test (FECRT) data are frequently characterised by high variability, small sample sizes and frequent zero observations. Accurate analysis of the data therefore depends on the use of appropriate statistical techniques. Analyses of simulated FECRT data by methods based on calculation of the empirical mean and variance, non-parametric bootstrapping, and a novel Markov chain Monte Carlo (MCMC) method are compared. The MCMC method consistently outperformed the other methods, independently of the distribution from which the data were generated. Notional 95% confidence intervals produced by non-parametric bootstrapping contained the correct value between only 84% and 90% of the time, compared to between 92% and 97% of the time for the MCMC method. Computationally intensive parametric techniques such as MCMC should therefore be used for analysis of these kinds of data in order to avoid making erroneous inference about the true efficacy of anthelmintics in the field.

INTRODUCTION

The FECRT is the most widely used method of assessing the in vivo efficacy of anthelmintics against parasitic nematodes of horses, sheep and cattle (Coles et al., 2006; Kaplan, 2002), and is an essential tool in the process of monitoring the increasing prevalence of anthelmintic resistance. The method involves quantifying the egg shedding rate of a group of animals before and after treatment, and inferring the reduction in egg shedding rate. The test is known to have several limitations, including the variability of FEC data (Uhlinger, 1993), leading to a relatively variable FECRT result (Miller et al., 2006). This variability necessitates the use of an appropriate statistical test in order to make appropriate inference about the true reduction in egg shedding rate, especially when combined with the small group sizes and the frequent zero FEC observations that are often encountered with equine data (Kaplan, 2002; Nielsen et al., 2006).

The method currently advocated by the World Association for the Advancement of Veterinary Parasitology (WAAVP) involves calculating the empirical mean and variance before and after treatment, and calculating the empirical mean reduction and estimates of the 95% confidence interval for the true reduction using these figures (Coles et al., 1992). This method takes no account of the difference between uncertainty regarding the true mean of a sample,

*Matthew Denwood, Boyd Orr Centre for Population and Ecosystem Health, Institute of Comparative Medicine, Faculty of Veterinary Medicine, University of Glasgow, UK. Email: m.denwood@vet.gla.ac.uk

introduced by the Poisson variability of the counting process, and variability in the true mean of different samples. Calculation of 95% confidence intervals in this manner also assumes that the distribution of error for the mean is symmetrical on the log scale, although parameter likelihoods (and therefore errors) have been reported to be skewed for FEC data (Denwood et al., 2008), potentially justifying this assumption.

A non-parametric bootstrapping approach has recently been suggested as an appropriate method to generate confidence limits from equine FECRT data (Vidyashankar et al., 2007). The technique involves re-sampling and summarising the observed data, and makes no assumptions about the underlying distribution or processes generating the data (Mooney & Duval, 1993), or the parameter error structure. Non-parametric bootstrapping approaches are therefore widely used and extremely useful when the underlying distribution of data is unknown. A fundamental assumption underlying this approach is that the data obtained are fully representative of the population, an assumption which risks being violated when dealing with small sample sizes, giving misleading results.

Alternative options for analysis of FECRT data include computationally intensive parametric methods. These include parametric bootstrapping, or the likelihood profiling method proposed by Torgerson et al. (2005), but here MCMC (Gilks et al., 1998) is used as an example. Each of these methods requires the use of a parametric distribution in order to describe the FEC data. The negative binomial is the most frequently used parametric distribution for FEC data, and is equivalent to the gamma-Poisson compound distribution implemented here (for the derivation see Vose (2004)). Conceptually, this represents a population of Poisson distributions with gamma distributed means, where the Poisson distributions account for counting variability in observed FEC within a sample, and the gamma distribution describes the variability between samples. The latter could arise as a combination of several factors, including the aggregated distribution of eggs in faeces, variations in worm fecundity over time, and variations in faecal consistency, which are impossible to separate using only a single faecal sample per individual. For the MCMC model, pre-treatment data are assumed to follow a single gamma-Poisson (negative binomial) distribution, while post treatment data are distributed as a different gamma-Poisson distribution, with a mean value which has been scaled relative to the pre-treatment mean, and a value for variability which has separately been scaled relative to the pre-treatment variability. This allows inference on the true change in mean egg shedding, with an additional parameter reflecting the true change in variability between egg counts. From this model, estimates of the mean anthelmintic efficacy and the variability in anthelmintic efficacy between animals can be obtained. The advantage of an MCMC based approach is that the different sources of variability can be taken into consideration, leading to more accurate estimates of the uncertainty of parameter estimates. Disadvantages of this approach include the comparatively high computational effort required to implement the method, and the need to make distributional assumptions about the processes generating the data. FEC between animals is well described by a gamma-Poisson (negative binomial) distribution, however alternatives include zero-inflated distributions (Denwood et al., 2008; Nødtvedt et al., 2002), and the use of a lognormal distribution to describe the variability in means (Morrison, 2004).

Given the worldwide importance of anthelmintic resistance, there is an urgent need to improve and standardise the statistical technique used to analyse FECRT data (Coles et al., 2006; Kaplan, 2002). The usefulness of 95% confidence intervals generated using the three methods outlined above were assessed using simulated data, so that the impact of the assumptions being made using each method could be assessed.

MATERIALS AND METHODS

Statistical Analysis

The analysis currently recommended by the WAAVP was performed as described by Coles et al. (1992). The mean estimate of the reduction along with upper/lower 95% confidence intervals are calculated using Eq. (1).

$$\sigma^2_{reduction} = \frac{\sigma_2^2}{N * \bar{\mu}_2^2} + \frac{\sigma_1^2}{N * \bar{\mu}_1^2}$$

$$mean\ estimate = 100 * \left(1 - \frac{\bar{\mu}_2}{\bar{\mu}_1}\right) \quad (1)$$

$$confidence\ interval = 100 * \left(1 - \left(\frac{\bar{\mu}_2}{\bar{\mu}_1} * exp\left(\pm 2.048 * \sqrt{\sigma^2_{reduction}}\right)\right)\right)$$

Where $\bar{\mu}_1$ is the mean pre-treatment FEC, $\bar{\mu}_2$ is the mean post-treatment FEC, σ^2_1 is the variance in FEC pre-treatment, σ^2_2 is the variance in FEC post-treatment, $\sigma^2_{reduction}$ is the variance of the reduction, and N is the number of animals.

Bootstrapping was conducted using a function written by the author in the R statistical programming language (R Development Core Team, 2008). New pre-and post-treatment pseudo-datasets were sampled from each dataset, and the mean reduction calculated 10,000 times. The mean estimate and 95% confidence intervals for each dataset were then calculated and recorded from these 10,000 iterations.

Bayesian MCMC analysis was performed using a bespoke model, implemented using JAGS (Plummer, 2008) for the MCMC simulation. The model fits a gamma-Poisson distribution to the pre and post-treatment data, with parameters for pre- and post-treatment means and shape parameters. The pre-treatment mean and shape parameters are given minimally informative prior distributions spanning all values that are seen in real FECRT data for each parameter. Post-treatment mean and shape parameters are calculated by multiplying the pre-treatment mean and shape parameters by a "change in mean" and "change in shape" parameter, respectively. The "change in mean" is given an uninformative Beta(1,1) prior, and the "change in shape" a diffuse lognormal prior with a mean of one. The true % FEC reduction is derived from *(1 – "change in mean")*100*. Calling JAGS to run each simulation and summarising of MCMC chains was automated using the runjags package (Denwood, 2008) for R, with two chains. Convergence was assessed using the Gelman-Rubin statistic (Gelman & Rubin, 1992), and necessary sample size using Raftery and Lewis's diagnostic (Raftery & Lewis, 1995). The median estimate and 95% credible intervals for the true egg count reduction were calculated in R using the MCMC output. Software to implement the novel MCMC method is freely available in the form of an add-on package to the R statistical programming language from: http://cran.r-project.org/web/packages/bayescount/index.html

Method evaluation

A total of 1000 parameters for a simulated FECRT were generated in the R statistical programming language. The true proportional FEC reduction was simulated from a Uniform(0.75,1) distribution, so that true egg count reductions varied from reduced efficacy to efficacious reductions. The pre-treatment mean number of eggs counted (equal to FEC if the egg counting technique had an egg detection threshold of 1 egg per gram (EPG)) and sample size (number of animals) were chosen to reflect the values seen in real equine FECRT data obtained from 63 typical Danish equine establishments. The 2.5% and 97.5% quantiles for observed pre-treatment mean and sample size were used as the lower and upper bounds of the distributions used to generate the parameters. Pre-treatment mean was taken from a Uniform(1.45,53.1) distribution, and sample size per group was sampled randomly from integers between 4 and 16 inclusive with each integer having an equal probability of selection. The coefficient of variation (cv) between samples before treatment was sampled from a Uniform(1,1.41) distribution (corresponding to a pre-treatment shape parameter of the gamma distribution, k, of between 1 and 0.5), and the proportional increase in cv after treatment was sampled from the same distribution (corresponding to a post-treatment shape parameter of between 1*1=1 and 0.5*0.5=0.25). These values were also chosen to reflect the values most likely to be encountered in real FECRT data; published values of k are usually less than one (Shaw et al., 1998), and differing efficacy of anthelmintic between animals would be expected to result in an increase in variability post-treatment.

In order to test the implications of the distributional assumptions made by the MCMC and WAAVP methods, simulated datasets were generated using the following three different distributions of underlying sample means; gamma-Poisson (negative binomial), multi-modal lognormal-Poisson, and uniform-Poisson. In each case, the pre- and post-treatment meta-population mean and variance was identical between distributions for each dataset. For the multi-modal data, the number of modes was sampled as between two and ten for each dataset, and a lognormal distribution used to describe the distribution of modes within the group. These modes conceptually represent sub-groups within the population. Further lognormal distributions were then used to describe the distribution of samples at each mode, with the number of animals in each mode taken from a multinomial distribution with equal probability of assignment to each mode for each animal. The cv used for each of the two compound lognormal distributions was equal, and calculated so that the total population variance would be equal to the total population variance of a single gamma distribution with the given mean and shape parameter. This approximation does not hold when the number of modes is not equal to the number of animals, since the variability between animals from the same mode is less than that between animals from different modes. This should not affect the comparisons since the ability of the models to correctly identify the true variance is not being tested. The cv used for the lognormal distributions was calculated using an optimisation algorithm, and Eq. (2) to calculate the effective cv of the population given the cv of two compound distributions.

$$cv_{total} = \sqrt{cv_1^2 + cv_2^2 + (cv_1^2 * cv_2^2)} \quad (2)$$

Where cv_{total} is the effective coefficient of variation (cv) of the population, cv_1 is the cv in the first distribution, and cv_2 is the cv in the second distribution.

For the final distribution, the lower (L) and upper (U) limits of the uniform distribution were calculated using Eq. (3) where μ and cv are the population mean and coefficient of variation, respectively. If the calculated value for L was < 0, then a log-uniform distribution (that is, a distribution which is uniform on the log scale) was used in place of the uniform distribution. In this case, an optimisation algorithm was used to find a solution to Eq. (4) that fit the pre/post-treatment values of μ and cv generated.

$$L = \mu - \sqrt{((cv * \mu)^2 * 12)}$$

$$L = \mu + \sqrt{((cv * \mu)^2 * 12)} \quad (3)$$

$$U = 2 * \frac{\mu^2 + (cv * \mu)^2}{\mu - L}$$

$$\mu = \frac{U - L}{(\log U - \log L)} \quad (4)$$

The log-uniform distribution was only used when the uniform distribution would have required L < 0, so that it was possible for pre-treatment data to be of a different distribution to post-treatment data.

Pre- and post-treatment egg count data were generated using each of these 3 distributions with the 1000 parameter values, to simulate a FECRT for a total of 3000 datasets. These datasets were then analysed using each of the three methods, and credible intervals for the true proportion of datasets contained within 95% confidence intervals calculated using a Bayesian approach with an uninformative Beta(1,1) prior. The mean relative size of these confidence intervals was calculated using Eq. (5).

$$confidence\ interval\ size = \frac{\sum \frac{U - L}{T}}{N} \quad (5)$$

Where L denotes the lower confidence interval limit, U the upper confidence interval limit, T the true parameter value, and N the number of datasets.

To assess the accuracy of the median estimates, the relative root-mean-square-error (RMSE) was calculated using the simulated (true) value for each parameter. The RMSE can also be thought of as the standard deviation of the ratio between each median estimate and the simulated values; however it should be noted that this is not equivalent to the accepted meaning of the term "standard deviation". The term "relative RMSE" will be used to avoid confusion.

RESULTS

Of the 3000 datasets, 35 of the gamma-Poisson datasets, 32 of the multi-modal lognormal-Poisson datasets, and 33 of the (log) Uniform-Poisson datasets gave an empirical reduction of 100%. The median (95% confidence interval) simulated true reduction for these empirical 100% reduction datasets was 99.13% (82.23% - 99.97%). As the post-treatment variance for these datasets was 0, the WAAVP method of calculating 95% confidence intervals could not be applied. In practice, these datasets would be assumed to represent a 100% reduction, so 95% confidence limits of 100% to 100% were assigned to these datasets. The non-parametric bootstrapping approach generated the same confidence limits for these datasets, since all possible combinations of datapoints gave a 100% reduction.

In Fig. 1, the proportion of true reductions that were contained within the notional 95% confidence intervals for each method with all datasets are shown (95% credible intervals calculated using a Bayesian method with an uninformative prior). There is no evidence that the MCMC method did not estimate true 95% confidence intervals for both the gamma-Poisson and (log) Uniform data, but the confidence was lower for the multi-modal data. Non-parametric bootstrapping and the WAAVP method both returned notional 95% confidence intervals that contained the true value between 85% and 90% of the time for all data types. Discounting the datasets with an empirical reduction of 100% improved the apparent performance of the bootstrapping and WAAVP methods, although both methods still generated lower estimates of confidence than the MCMC method for all data types (data not shown).

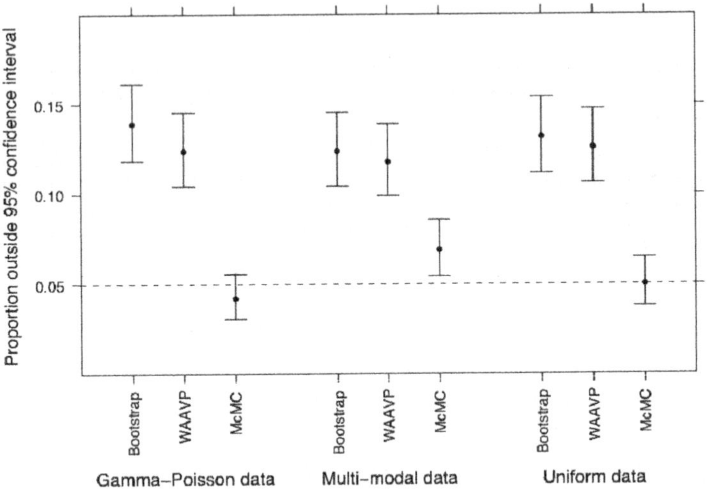

Fig. 1 The proportion of 95% confidence intervals not containing the simulated true mean FEC reduction parameter for each method from the analysis of 1000 datasets simulated using each distribution

In Table 1, the mean relative size of the notional 95% confidence intervals for each method and dataset are shown. The relative RMSE for each combination is shown in Table 2. The MCMC method returned on average slightly larger 95% confidence limits than the other methods for each dataset, although when datasets with 100% apparent reductions are excluded, the 3 methods produce similarly sized 95% confidence intervals (data not shown). The 95% confidence intervals were largest for the (log) Uniform-Poisson data, and most narrow for the multi-modal data. The MCMC median estimates produced a lower relative RMSE than the bootstrapping median and WAAVP mean estimates in every case. The bootstrapping median and WAAVP mean estimates gave similar relative RMSE in all cases, although those produced by the bootstrapping method were lower. As for the relative size of 95% confidence intervals, the relative RMSE was smallest for each method for the multi-modal data and largest for the (log) Uniform-Poisson data.

Table 1. Mean relative size of 95% confidence intervals for the true mean FEC reduction produced by each method from the analysis of 1000 datasets simulated using each distribution

	GAMMA-POISSON	MULTI-MODAL	UNIFORM-POISSON

BOOTSTRAPPING	0.702	0.459	0.803
WAAVP	0.673	0.532	0.786
MCMC	0.746	0.555	0.803

Table 2. Relative root-mean-square-error for median or mean estimate for the true mean FEC reduction produced by each method from the analysis of 1000 datasets simulated using each distribution

	GAMMA-POISSON	MULTI-MODAL	UNIFORM-POISSON
BOOTSTRAPPING	1.69	1.49	2.60
WAAVP	1.70	1.53	2.66
MCMC	1.61	1.46	1.77

DISCUSSION

For all datasets, simulated from each of the distributions tested, the MCMC method provided confidence intervals with the best defined properties, as well as the most precise median estimates for the true FEC reduction. The size of the 95% confidence intervals produced was slightly greater for the MCMC method, but not when datasets with empirical reductions of 100% were removed. This indicates that the MCMC methods were producing more appropriate 95% confidence intervals, rather than merely larger 95% confidence intervals. This was the case not only for data simulated from a gamma-Poisson distribution, where the MCMC method using the same distribution would be expected to perform well, but also using data simulated from different distributions. The performance of the MCMC method was less optimal using the multi-modal data, but even here it out-performed the other two methods. This implies that the distributional assumptions made by the MCMC method have less practical impact on the analysis of these types of FECRT data than the assumption that bootstrapping a limited number of data points can capture all the variability of an inherently very variable system. Vidyashankar et al. (2007) propose dealing with this effect by taking into account inter-farm variability, in effect increasing the sample size of the study. It is likely that this would improve the confidence of the bootstrapping method as long as the total effective sample size is sufficient. The MCMC method is also capable of analysing data from multiple sites, for example by defining a distribution of efficacy that describes the mean FEC reduction at each site and using this extra information to reduce uncertainty in the estimate for the true mean efficacy. Where data from multiple sites is available, and it is reasonable to assume a distribution of efficacy describing the sites, the additional data can be taken into account in order to reduce uncertainty in parameter estimates. However, the intention of this paper was to assess the performance of each method when analysing individual datasets in the absence of any other comparable datasets, so that taking into account inter-farm variability would not have been possible. Based on the results presented, parametric techniques appear to out-perform non-parametric bootstrapping in this regard when sample sizes are small.

Several of the datasets generated with parameters similar to observed equine FECRT data gave an empirical reduction of 100%, even where the true mean reductions were close to 75%. These datasets present difficulties when using both the WAAVP and bootstrap methods, which were unable to generate appropriate 95% confidence limits. Nineteen (19%) of these datasets were simulated using empirical reductions of less than 95%, and so represent a consistent source of false negatives for these methods. The MCMC method was the only method examined in this paper which is capable of analysing datasets with 100% empirical reductions in an appropriate fashion.

The relative RMSE and size of 95% confidence intervals was greater for each method with the Uniform-Poisson data than the other datsets. This was possibly a result of the shape of the Uniform or log-Uniform distribution creating more frequent moderately large values than would be expected with a gamma or lognormal distribution with the same variance. Interestingly, the relative RMSE of the MCMC method seemed to be less affected by the Uniform-Poisson data than with the other methods. The reasons for this were not clear, and it may be a chance observation, or it may be due to the MCMC method accounting for these moderately large values with an increased estimate for the variance. Conversely, the relative RMSE and size of 95% confidence intervals was smallest for each method with the multi-modal data. This is most likely as a result of the population variance being reduced by the clustering effect of the multi-modal distribution, so that the effective variance of the multi-modal distribution was less than the population variance used for the uni-modal distributions.

The question of the true distribution of FECRT data has not been addressed here, although the density distribution of macro-parasites has been extensively studied elsewhere (Barger, 1985; Shaw et al., 1998; Gaba et al., 2005; Morrison, 2004). The use of the gamma-Poisson distribution is widespread, and the equivalence to the negative binomial creates a simple way of calculating the probability mass function without having to integrate the mean value of the Poisson distribution over a further probability distribution. However, the use of the gamma distribution to describe the true distribution of mean faecal egg output rates between animals has not been justified. The lognormal distribution advocated by Morrison (2004) has more theoretical justification, but the variability introduced by the Poisson part of the compound distribution makes the choice difficult to validate with real data. The distribution of egg counts has been found to be bi-modal (zero inflated) in at least one host-parasite system (Denwood et al., 2008), which would suggest that the distribution of egg counts is more complex than a simple lognormal-Poisson.

CONCLUSIONS

Using data simulated with similar values of mean and sample size as observed equine FECRT, both the method currently advocated by the WAAVP and a non-parametric bootstrap method failed to provide true 95% confidence intervals for the FEC reduction. MCMC generated confidence intervals with a true confidence much closer to 95%, independently of the distribution from which data were generated. More computationally intensive parametric methods such as MCMC should therefore be used in preference to nonparametric bootstrapping and more primitive methods, in order to avoid making erroneous inference of the true efficacy of anthelmintics for these kinds of data.

ACKNOWLEDGEMENTS

This research was produced as part of the DEFRA-funded VTRI project 0101. BioSS is partly funded by the Scottish Government. The authors are grateful to Stig Petersen (Equilab Laboratory, Joerlunde Overdrev 7, DK-3500 Slangerup, Denmark) for providing the equine FECRT data discussed.

REFERENCES

Barger, I. A. (1985). The statistical distribution of trichostrongylid nematodes in grazing lambs. Int. J. Parasitol. 15, 645–649

Coles, G. C., Bauer, C., Borgsteede, F. H., Geerts, S., Klei, T. R., Taylor, M. A. and Waller, P. J. (1992). World Association for the Advancement of Veterinary Parasitology (W.A.A.V.P.) methods for the detection of anthelmintic resistance in nematodes of veterinary importance. Vet. Parasitol. 44, 35–44

Coles, G. C., Jackson, F., Pomroy, W. E., Prichard, R. K., von Samson-Himmelstjerna, G., Silvestre, A., Taylor, M. A. and Vercruysse, J. (2006). The detection of anthelmintic resistance in nematodes of veterinary importance. Vet. Parasitol. 136, 167–185

Denwood, M. (2008). runjags: Run Bayesian MCMC Models in the BUGS syntax from Within R. R package version 0.9.2. http://cran.r-project.org/web/packages/runjags/

Denwood, M. J., Stear, M. J., Matthews, L., Reid, S. W. J., Toft, N. and Innocent, G. T. (2008). The distribution of the pathogenic nematode *Nematodirus battus* in lambs is zero-inflated. Parasitology 135, 1225–1235

Gaba, S., Ginot, V. and Cabaret, J. (2005). Modelling macroparasite aggregation using a nematode-sheep system: the Weibull distribution as an alternative to the negative binomial distribution? Parasitology 131 (Pt 3), 393–401

Gelman, A. and Rubin, D. (1992). Inference from Iterative Simulation using Multiple Sequences. Statistical Science 7, 457–511

Gilks, W. R., Richardson, S. and Spiegelhalter, D. J. (1998). Markov chain Monte Carlo in practice. Chapman and Hall, Boca Raton, Fla.

Kaplan, R. M. (2002). Anthelmintic resistance in nematodes of horses. Vet. Res. 33, 491-507

Miller, C. M., Waghorn, T. S., Leathwick, D. M. and Gilmour, M. L. (2006). How repeatable is a faecal egg count reduction test? N. Z. Vet. J. 54, 323–328

Mooney, C. Z. and Duval, R. D. (1993). Bootstrapping: a nonparametric approach to statistical inference. Sage Publications, 2455 Teller Road, Thousand Oaks, CA 91320

Morrison, D. A. (2004). Technical variability and required sample size of helminth egg isolation procedures: revisited. Parasitol. Res. 94, 361–366

Nielsen, M. K., Haaning, N. and Olsen, S. N. (2006). Strongyle egg shedding consistency in horses on farms using selective therapy in Denmark. Vet. Parasitol. 135, 333–335

Nødtvedt, A., Dohoo, I., Sanchez, J., Conboy, G., DesCôteaux, L., Keefe, G., Leslie, K. and Campbell, J. (2002). The use of negative binomial modelling in a longitudinal study of gastrointestinal parasite burdens in Canadian dairy cows. Can. J. Vet. Res. 66, 249–257

Plummer, M., 2008. Just Another Gibbs Sampler (JAGS) http://calvin.iarc.fr/~martyn/software/jags/

R Development Core Team (2008). R: A Language and Environment for Statistical Computing.

R Foundation for Statistical Computing, Vienna, Austria, ISBN 3-900051-07-0

Raftery, A. E. and Lewis, S. M. (1995). The number of iterations, convergence diagnostics and generic Metropolis algorithms. In: Practical Markov Chain Monte Carlo (W.R. Gilks, D.J. Spiegelhalter and S. Richardson, eds.). Chapman and Hall, London, U.K.

Shaw, D. J., Grenfell, B. T. and Dobson, A. P. (1998). Patterns of macroparasite aggregation in wildlife host populations. Parasitology 117 (Pt 6), 597–610

Torgerson, P. R., Schnyder, M. and Hertzberg, H. (2005). Detection of anthelmintic resistance: a comparison of mathematical techniques. Vet. Parasitol. 128, 291–298

Uhlinger, C. A. (1993). Uses of fecal egg count data in equine practice. Compendium On Continuing Education For the Practicing Veterinarian 15, 742–749

Vidyashankar, A. N., Kaplan, R. M. and Chan, S. (2007). Statistical approach to measure the efficacy of anthelmintic treatment on horse farms. Parasitology 134 (Pt14), 2027–2039

Vose, D. (2004). ModelAssist for @Risk. Risk Thinking, Ltd. http://www.vosesoftware.com/modelassist.htm

USE OF A PRE-CLINICAL 'PEN-SIDE' TEST IN THE CONTROL OF SCRAPIE IN A SINGLE UK SHEEP FLOCK

L.A. BODEN, F. HOUSTON, H.R. FRYER AND R.R. KAO*

SUMMARY

A deterministic within-flock model was used to demonstrate that only large flocks with a large proportion of homebred breeding sheep are likely to be a significant risk for onward flock-to-flock transmission of scrapie. For most other flocks it was found that the Compulsory Scrapie Flock Scheme (CSFS) strategy, with its severe consequences for affected farmers, could be replaced by a strategy using a currently available live test without excessive risk to other farmers, even if the proportion of susceptible genotypes was unusually high. Even for flocks that represent a high risk, when scrapie is detected soon after disease introduction (typically less than 5 years), there would be limited risk of onward transmission. However, if detection of disease is delayed, onward transmission remains a concern and the existing CSFS strategy may be the most appropriate control measure in these cases.

INTRODUCTION

Scrapie is an infectious and invariably fatal disease. The first recognised transmissible spongiform encephalopathy (TSE), it has been endemic in the British national sheep flock for over 250 years (Parry, 1983; Radostits et al., 2000). Scrapie occurs naturally and causes progressive neurological degeneration and death. It is associated with an abnormal form of a prion protein (PrP) (Caughey & Chesebro 1997).

The prioritisation of scrapie eradication in Great Britain (GB) occurred after the link between bovine spongiform encephalopathy (BSE) in cattle and variant Creutzfeldt-Jakob Disease (CJD) in humans was discovered (Foster et al., 1993; Hill et al., 1997). The potential for sheep to be a major health risk was based on four concerns: (i) sheep were demonstrated to be susceptible to BSE under experimental conditions (Foster et al., 1993), (ii) they were potentially exposed to the same contaminated feed that had caused the outbreak in cattle (Kao et al., 2002), (iii) the distribution of BSE infected tissue in sheep (Jeffrey et al., 2001; Somerville et al., 1997) has made horizontal transmission a distinct possibility (Kao et al., 2002) and (iv) as BSE and scrapie have very similar clinical signs, scrapie has the potential to mask an incipient BSE epidemic in sheep (Houston & Gravenor 2003). As a result, the National Scrapie Plan (NSP) (Defra, 2007) was implemented in Great Britain in July 2001 (Kao et al., 2001). The NSP's primary objectives were to eradicate scrapie and breed for TSE resistance in the national sheep flock (Baylis et al., 2002), thereby minimising the likelihood that BSE could be present and not detected in the national flock and diminishing the incidence of scrapie in the process.

* Rowland Kao, Institute of Comparative Medicine, Faculty of Veterinary Medicine, University of Glasgow. Email: r.kao@vet.gla.ac.uk

The strategy was adopted due to the exceptionally clear relationship between polymorphisms in a single gene and susceptibility to scrapie and BSE (Goldmann et al., 1994; Foster et al., 2001). At the NSP's inception in 2001, given that BSE incidence in sheep would have been at most low, and masked by the presence of scrapie, any strategy based purely on identifying cases of disease would have been prohibitively risky and expensive and thus a genetically-based breeding strategy targeting susceptibility, rather than disease, provided the most reasonable chance for success.

Participation in the NSP scheme was initially voluntary and remains so for unaffected flocks. Despite evidence that genotypes resistant to scrapie were susceptible to BSE under experimental conditions (Houston et al., 2003), epidemiological evidence remained that this risk was slight (Kao et al., 2003). In 2004, the programme was augmented by a slaughter and replacement scheme. This was initially a voluntary programme aimed at scrapie-affected flocks, but after July 2004 it became compulsory for all flocks with confirmed cases. Upon positive identification of a scrapie case in a flock, the Compulsory Scrapie Flock Scheme (CSFS) (Defra, 2008) requires that either all sheep must be slaughtered, or all susceptible sheep in the flock must be slaughtered and only resistant replacement animals bought in. While this strategy has undoubtedly been effective in reducing scrapie in the British national sheep flock, the economic cost to farmers, industry and government has been high (http://www.defra.gov.uk/animalh/bse/othertses/scrapie/nsp/qanda/q&a.htm#22) and it has also raised issues regarding its impact on performance traits, inbreeding and genetic diversity in flocks (Dawson et al., 2008).

The recent development of a live test for scrapie using lymphoid biopsies obtained from rectal mucosa (González et al., 2008a) suggests that pre-clinical testing may prove a more cost-effective disease-based strategy for scrapie eradication in the UK. Immunohistochemical staining of lymphoid biopsies from tonsil (Schreuder et al., 1998) and third eyelid (O'Rourke et al., 2000), for example, have been recognised as a method for pre-clinical diagnosis of TSEs for some time. The advantages of using rectal biopsies are ease of collection without the need for anaesthesia, the relative abundance of lymphoid follicles in the rectal mucosa, and the ability to adapt the analysis to rapid, high-throughput methods (González et al., 2008b), making this approach more feasible for large-scale application in the field. While there have been several models of scrapie within-flock (Stringer et al., 1998; Hagenaars et al., 2000; Kao et al., 2003; Fryer et al., 2007; Truscott & Ferguson, 2008) and between-flock dynamics in British sheep (Kao et al., 2001; Gubbins, 2005), none have considered the efficacy of a strategy aimed at controlling disease rather than susceptibility. The trade-off between a single or multiple live pre-clinical test(s) and the continuation of the CSFS was explored in this study. Scrapie infectivity has been consistently found in placentae of scrapie-infected ewes (Race et al., 1998) and, more recently, in their milk (Konold et al., 2008), and there is significant circumstantial evidence to suggest that flock-to-flock transmission of scrapie is related to the onward sale of breeding sheep (McLean et al., 1999, Baylis et al., 2002). Thus the number of infected breeding sheep likely to be sold on was used as the basis of comparison between these strategies.

MATERIALS AND METHODS

Within-flock spread of infectivity

A deterministic difference equation model similar to that used in previous analyses (Kao et al., 2003; Fryer et al., 2007) was used to describe the within-flock spread of scrapie. This model incorporates age, infection and breeding structure and the inheritance and impact of the PrP gene. The model takes into account flock size, the number of breeding ewes, proportion of ewes that are home-bred, proportion of ewes sold as replacements, and the genotype distribution of the flock. It also tracks the number of infected sheep that are sold as replacements to other flocks. A full description of the model variables, parameters and equations is presented in Fryer et al. (2007). Model outputs were compared to determine the impact of the different control and eradication strategies on different flock structures.

Flock parameters

In the UK, flock classifications are based on breed and the role they play in the industry and have previously been used in models of BSE and scrapie transmission in sheep (Kao et al., 2002, Truscott & Ferguson, 2008). There is also a recognised flow of animals, genetic material and hence infection based on grazing altitude (hill to lowland) as well as from purebred to cross-breeding flocks (Pollott & Stone, 2006). In this model, flocks are characterised according to the breeding and commercial structure of the UK industry and the role of different flock types in onward transmission of disease.

Flock parameters selected for the model were based on flock type (purebred, commercial or mixed), flock size (25th and 75th percentiles), the proportion of homebred sheep (25th and 75th percentiles), the likelihood of selling sheep on to other flocks and whether scrapie had ever been identified in the flock. All parameters are based on the 2002 anonymous postal survey for scrapie in Great Britain (Sivam et al., 2006). In the survey, flocks are defined as purebred, commercial or mixed. Only purebred and commercial categories were retained in the model; considering the correlation in numbers of sheep sold between flock size and flock type, the numbers of sheep in mixed commercial and purebred scrapie-positive flocks were similar to both commercial and purebred scrapie-positive flock types, and so this flock type was not investigated further.

Further stratification of flock types into small and large commercial, purebred and mixed hill, upland and lowland flocks was also investigated. Farm type (hill, upland and lowland flocks) appears to be correlated with flock type (Pollott & Stone, 2006). Independently, farm type did not appear to play a significant role in the risk of being scrapie positive and did not have an impact on the number of sheep sold on to other flocks (Hoinville et al., 2000). Therefore these sub-classifications were not used.

The analysis was conducted over six different flock structures defined by combinations of the number of sheep in the flock and the proportion of homebred sheep. Specifically, they were classified as: large (>700 sheep) and small (<100 sheep) purebred flocks [with large proportions of homebred sheep (≥89%)] and large (>500 sheep) and small (<200 sheep) commercial flocks [with large (≥89%) and small (≤10%) proportions of homebred sheep]. In the postal survey data, of flocks which have ever had scrapie, commercial flocks represented the majority (77% scrapie negative, 68% scrapie positive). Purebred flocks (12.9% scrapie negative, 14.1% scrapie positive) and mixed flocks (10% scrapie negative, 17.5% scrapie positive) formed smaller proportions of the GB flock demographics.

Ninety eight percent of each of the flocks was assumed to be breeding ewes and the remaining 2% breeding rams. All flocks were assumed to sell ewes as replacements.

Genotype distribution

An average genotype distribution (equal to the national distribution) was used to determine the impact of different control strategies on the different flock types with respect to the number of sheep culled and infected sheep sold on to other farms. This was based on the prevalence of genotypes described in abattoir active surveillance data (VLA 2003a and b). There were six genotypes described: ARR/ARR, ARR/AXX, AXX/AXX, ARR/VRQ, AXX/VRQ and

VRQ/VRQ. The AXX genotype refers to ARQ, AHQ and ARH genotypes. Properties of the 6 genotypes are described in Table 1 (and are reproduced in part from Fryer et al., 2007).

Table 1. Average sheep genotypes: prevalence, susceptibility and mean age at onset of scrapie (reproduced from Fryer et al., 2007)

GENOTYPE	PREVALENCE IN ABATTOIR SCREENING -NATIONAL GENOTYPE (%)	ESTIMATED SUSCEPTIBILITY TO SCRAPIE	MEAN AGE OF ONSET OF SCRAPIE SYMPTOMS (YEARS)
ARR/ARR	19.5	0	NA
ARR/AXX	41.9	0.001	5.9
AXX/AXX	26.5	0.026	3.8
ARR/VRQ	5.5	0.119	5.9
AXX/VRQ	6.2	0.359	3.8
VRQ/VRQ	0.4	1.000	3.2

The number of infected sheep sold on to other farms was also compared for different flock types with different genotype distributions (50%, 75%, 80%, 90% and 95% sensitive genotypes in the flock) to consider the impact of flocks with unusually high proportions of sensitive genotypes. The relative proportions of each of the six genotypes were based on the ratios of each genotype in the abattoir screening data (Table 1).

Control and eradication strategies

The model was adapted to consider the impact of three proposed control and eradication strategies for scrapie. Each strategy was also compared to a strategy where no intervention occurs for up to 15 years (i.e. scrapie positive sheep were allowed to remain in the flock for this period), on the basis that the average large scrapie epidemic has been estimated to last 15 years (Gravenor et al., 2001). In the model, it was assumed that the flock had been identified as having an ongoing scrapie epidemic (through the identification of a sheep with clinical scrapie). Consistent with previous analyses, an ongoing scrapie epidemic was defined as a holding that has at least one case of homebred scrapie in the last year or at least two cases of scrapie in the last five years, of which at least one was homebred (Fryer et al., 2007). The model assumes that most sheep get infected within the first few months of life but that no sheep under the age of 12 months die from scrapie (Fryer et al., 2007). The model runs for a period of 5 years after the year of strategy implementation to consider the short-term impact of the differing strategies. Implementation of each strategy was considered at different time points (detection years) in the model epidemic to determine the effect of within-flock scrapie prevalence on the efficacy of each strategy. This was done to take into account pre-clinical infection which may otherwise go undetected due to the long incubation period of the disease.

Strategy 1: In this strategy, no intervention is implemented. In these flocks, no scrapie positive sheep are culled or removed from the flock at any time during the epidemic.

Strategy 2: This strategy is modelled on the current CSFS (http://www.defra.gov.uk/animalh/bse/othertses/scrapie/nsp/index.html). All sheep are tested for genotype. This is a reactive policy enforced in response to detected disease in the flock.

Genotypes that are considered sensitive to scrapie are culled and resistant genotypes are retained (ARR/ARR ewes and rams and ARR/AXX ewes) (Defra, 2007). For two years after the first year of implementation of this strategy, the model restricts the genotype of bought-in sheep to those genotypes resistant to scrapie (ARR/ARR genotype). After two years of restrictions, replacement sheep are bought in proportion to the distribution of the genotype of the national flock.

Strategy 3: A pre-clinical diagnostic pen-side test is conducted each year over three consecutive years. Like the CSFS, for two years after the first year of implementation of this strategy, the model restricts the genotype of bought-in sheep to those genotypes resistant to scrapie (genotype 1). After two years of restrictions, replacement sheep are bought in proportion to the distribution of the genotype of the national flock. In flocks that are subsequently defined as high-risk flocks with respect to onward transmission of disease, multiple testing over 6 years was also investigated.

Strategy 4: A pre-clinical diagnostic pen-side test is conducted once (over a single year with subsequent restrictions enforced on sale, purchase and breeding on the holding for a period of three years). Like the CSFS, for two years after the first year of implementation, the model restricts the genotype of bought-in sheep to those genotypes resistant to scrapie (genotype 1). After two years of restrictions, replacement sheep are bought in proportion to the distribution of the genotype of the national flock.

Live test parameters

The live pre-clinical pen-side test implemented in strategies 2 and 3 is based on the experimental support for rectal biopsies of lymphoid tissue and was described in detail by González et al. (2008a). They found that the risk of a false negative result in a pre-clinical rectal biopsy sample was 9.3% if the sample contained 10 follicles and that the probability of obtaining a sample containing at least 10 follicles was 87%. The risk of a false positive is believed to be negligible (González, personal communication). Frequency of detection of PrP^d was only slightly higher in samples of palatine tonsil and retropharyngeal lymph node of infected sheep, but these tissues are much less accessible than the rectal mucosa and therefore considered unsuitable for large scale application of a live animal test (González et al., 2006). For this model, it was assumed that at least 10 follicles are retrieved in a single biopsy sample and accordingly, initial test sensitivity of 90% and specificity of 100% was chosen for the model. Test sensitivities of 70% and 35% were also investigated.

In the model, the live pre-clinical testing strategies are applied to sheep at different time points: over 20, 12 and 6 months of age of the sheep tested. González et al. (2008a) suggested that the first positive tests in the rectal mucosa appeared at statistically similar average proportions of the incubation period of experimentally infected sheep (0.5 in AXX/AXX sheep, 0.49 in AXX/VRQ and 0.43 in VRQ/VRQ sheep). The expected age (in months) for a positive rectal biopsy (AXX/AXX 22.8 months; AXX/VRQ 22.3 months; VRQ/VRQ 16.5 months) was calculated from the average incubation periods for natural scrapie (Fryer et al., 2007) (Table 1). There were no data available for ARR/VRQ sheep.

Model outputs

In each flock, after each intervention, in each time period during the course of the epidemic (detection and implementation years 1-15), the average number of breeding sheep removed from the flock and the average prevalence of scrapie per year were calculated. In addition, data from the scrapie postal survey on all flocks were used to estimate the potential number of infected breeding sheep sold to other farms after each intervention for each flock type investigated. A qualitative comparison of the number of sheep sold by each flock type indicated that there was little difference between scrapie positive flocks and scrapie negative flocks so data from all flocks were used. The number of sheep sold was recorded categorically in the scrapie postal survey (0, 1-5, 6-20, 21-50, 50-100 and greater than 100 sheep sold). In order to obtain the maximum number of breeding sheep sold on from an infected flock, categorical data were converted to integers, assuming that the number of sheep sold in each category was equivalent to the upper bounds of each category (i.e. 0, 5, 20, 50, 100 and >100 sheep). An estimate of the upper bounds of the final category (>100 sheep) was based on the size of the breeding ewe flock in each flock type, assuming that each breeding ewe produces at least one ewe lamb per year. The average prevalence of scrapie in the flock, after each strategy was implemented, was used to calculate the number of infected sheep sold on subsequently to other flocks each year for each flock type. For each flock type, the mean number of infected breeding sheep sold onwards per flock per year was calculated for years 1, 5, 10 and 15 and over all years of the epidemic. Model outputs were compared to determine the impact of the different control and eradication strategies on different flock structures.

RESULTS

No intervention

Assuming an average genotypic distribution (38% susceptible genotypes in the flock), over a 15-year period the prevalence of scrapie decreases in smaller flocks (i.e. flocks with ≤132 sheep) due to the depletion of the susceptible population. In these flocks, the smaller the proportion of homebred sheep, the lower the prevalence of scrapie in the flock. In large flocks (≥500 sheep), the prevalence of scrapie remains constant over a 15-year period if the proportion of homebred sheep is small (≤10%). However, if the proportion of homebred sheep is high (≥89%), the prevalence of scrapie in large flocks increases over time.

When the proportions of susceptible genotypes in the flock are low (<38%), only a few small purebred or small commercial flocks sell on greater than one infected sheep to other flocks per year (small purebred and commercial flocks sell a range of 0 to 1 infected breeding sheep per year, with means of 0.35 and 0.15 infected sheep sold respectively on in the worst year) and are thus considered a low risk for onward transmission of the disease (Fig. 1). A small percentage of large commercial flocks (10%) with low proportions of homebred sheep sell on a small number of infected sheep (Fig. 2, range 0 to 2 infected breeding sheep per year, mean of 0.32 in the worst year). These flocks are defined as moderate-risk flocks.

A majority of large purebred flocks pose a high risk of onward transmission, where this is defined as ≥1 infected sheep sold on per year (range 0 to 168 infected breeding sheep sold per year) and this increases from the first year of the epidemic (83% of flocks) until the last year of the epidemic (93% flocks) when there is a mean of just over 100 infected sheep potentially sold on as breeding stock. A smaller proportion of large commercial flocks pose similar risks (range 0 to 65 infected breeding sheep sold) from the first year (28%) to the last year of the epidemic (42% of flocks, mean of 10 infected sheep sold on). Both of these flock types are considered to be high-risk flocks (Fig. 3).

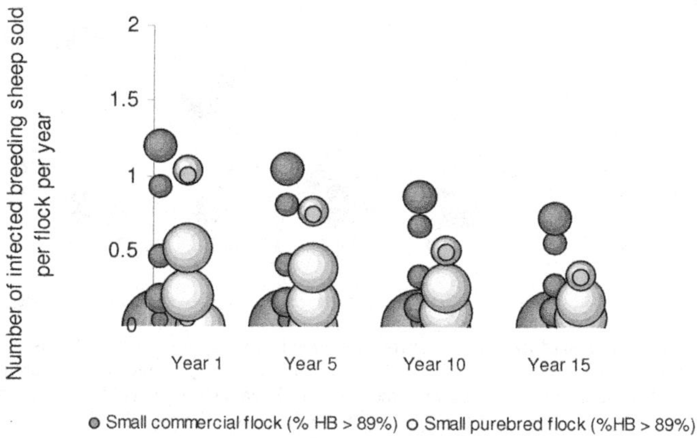

Fig. 1 Comparison of the number of infected breeding sheep sold each year to other farms by different low-risk flock types, where scrapie was identified in years 1, 5, 10 and 15 of an epidemic (size of bubble indicates number of flocks), showing the decline in epidemic size as years to detection increases (x-axis). Small flocks with less than 10% homebred (HB) sheep are not shown as these have insignificant epidemic sizes.

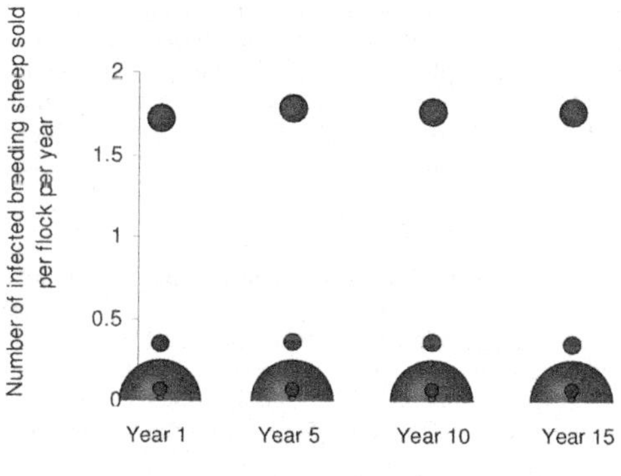

Fig. 2 Comparison of the number of infected breeding sheep sold each year to other farms by large commercial flocks with less than 10% homebred breeding stock in years 1, 5, 10 and 15 of an epidemic (size of bubble indicates number of flocks), showing that epidemics only persist in relatively few flocks, though these maintain infection over a considerable timeframe (x-axis refers to the number of years since the epidemic started).

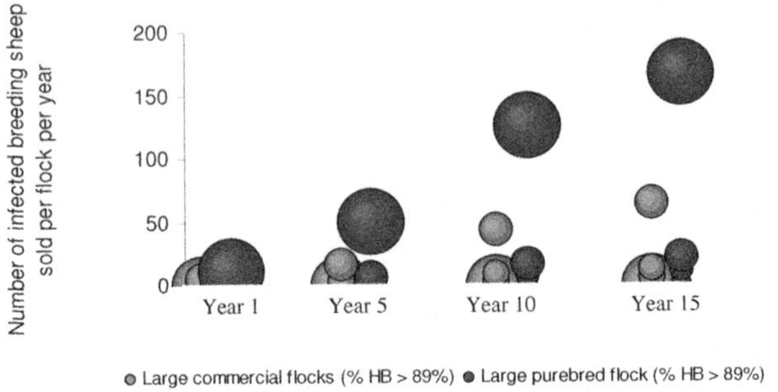

Fig. 3 Comparison of the number of infected breeding sheep sold to other farms each year by different high-risk flock types in years 1, 5, 10 and 15 of an epidemic (size of bubble indicates number of flocks). The x-axis refers to the number of years since the epidemic started. HB refers to the percentage of homebred sheep in the population.

As expected, as the proportion of susceptible genotypes in each flock type increases (≥50%), large and small purebred flocks and large commercial flocks pose a greater risk of onward transmission particularly if scrapie is left undetected in the flock until late in the epidemic. Conversely, small commercial flocks pose little risk of onward transmission even when the proportion of susceptible sheep in the flock is very high (≥95%).

CSFS Strategy (Strategy 2)

While the CSFS strategy is always successful in eradicating disease from all infected flocks and preventing onward transmission of disease to other farms, this invariably results in higher numbers of sheep removed and culled than the two alternative pre-clinical testing strategies (strategies 3 and 4) because it relies on removal of susceptibility, rather than removal of infection. As expected, the proportion of sheep culled by this strategy reflects the proportion of sheep with susceptible genotypes in the flock.

Pre-clinical testing strategies (Strategies 3 and 4)

There is no difference in the results between either of the testing strategies when the tests are applied to sheep at 20 or 12 months of age in any of the flock types. However, as test sensitivity decreases, the average number of sheep removed from the flock decreases and the risk of onward transmission increases. Both multiple and single testing strategies are more effective at reducing prevalence and onward transmission of infection when tests are applied and assumed to be effective in sheep at 6 months of age than when testing and detection is left until 12 and 20 months.

In all flock types, multiple-testing strategies result in increased numbers of sheep culled compared to a single-test strategy. However, multiple-testing strategies still result in a smaller proportion of the flock culled (percentage of flock culled in years 1-15: 0.2-19% in large purebred flocks, 0.2-0.3% in large commercial flocks with small proportions of homebred sheep and 0.3-11% in large commercial flocks with large proportions of homebred sheep) compared with the CSFS (36% of all flocks culled).

Both live testing strategies reduce the risk of onward transmission of disease (Figs. 5 & 6). The effectiveness of each strategy is dependent on when disease is detected during the course of a within-flock epidemic. At high test sensitivities (>90%), in large purebred flocks, if scrapie is detected early in the epidemic (<5 years), multiple testing reduces the risk of onward transmission to zero. However, if scrapie is detected later in the epidemic (≥5 years), 67% (in year 5) to 83% (in year 15) of flocks would still sell on one or more infected sheep depending on the year of implementation. A single test strategy in these flocks would result in a larger percentage of flocks (67% in year 1 to 93% in year 15) selling on one or more infected sheep earlier in the epidemic. In large commercial flocks with a small percentage of homebred sheep (≤10%) multiple and single testing strategies are equally effective in reducing the risk of onward transmission to other flocks (number of sheep sold <1) at any time during the epidemic. When similar testing strategies are applied to large commercial flocks with a high percentage of homebred sheep (>89%), a multiple testing strategy removes the risk of onward transmission of infected sheep if the epidemic is detected early in the epidemic (<10 years). If multiple testing is implemented later in the epidemic, a larger percentage of flocks (17%) sell on infected sheep. A single test strategy is less successful. Early in the epidemic (<5 years), a single test strategy reduces the risk of onward transmission. However if the test is implemented later than this, the percentage of the flock that sell on infected sheep increases from 17% to 40%. The mean number of infected breeding sheep sold per flock per year after implementation of each strategy is illustrated in Fig. 6.

When the number of years over which the live-test is implemented is increased (once a year for 6 years compared to 3 years), the number of infected sheep sold on to other flocks decreases by half, but the proportion of flocks selling on more than one infected sheep is still high in both high-risk purebred and commercial flocks.

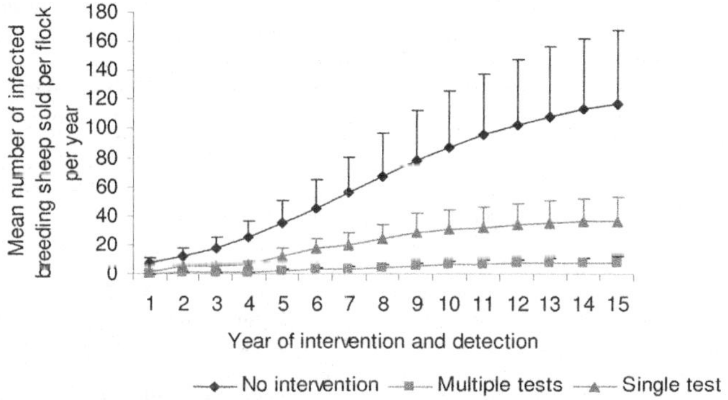

Fig. 5 Mean number of infected breeding sheep sold by large purebred flocks (size ≥700 sheep, proportion of homebred sheep ≥89%) per year (in each year of an epidemic) after implementation of live-test strategies (90% sensitivity). This assumes the national genotypic distribution (38% sensitive genotypes in flock). The upper bars indicate the potential maximum number of infected breeding sheep sold. The minimum number of infected sheep sold is 0 in all years.

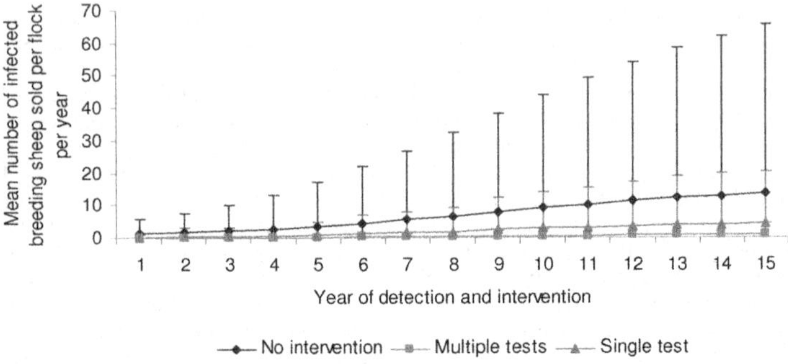

Fig. 6 Mean number of infected breeding sheep sold by large commercial flocks (size ≥500 sheep, proportion of homebred sheep ≥89%) per year (in each year of an epidemic) after implementation of live-test strategies (90% sensitivity). This assumes the national genotypic distribution (38% sensitive genotypes in flock). The upper bars indicate the potential maximum number of infected breeding sheep sold. The minimum number of infected sheep sold is 0 in all years.

DISCUSSION

The British CSFS requires that upon positive identification of scrapie case in a flock, either all sheep must be slaughtered or all susceptible sheep in the flock must be slaughtered and only resistant replacement animals bought in. While this strategy is effective, the cost to farmers, industry and government is high. The recent development of a live-test for scrapie (González et al., 2008a) suggests that preclinical testing may prove a more cost-effective strategy for scrapie control and eradication in the UK. A deterministic model of within-flock scrapie transmission was used in this study to investigate the impact and trade-offs of potential pre-clinical live-test strategies compared to the existing CSFS in the control of scrapie. This study illustrates important differences in the trading patterns and ability of different flock types to sustain or perpetuate scrapie epidemics that are important for understanding the epidemic dynamics at a national level, and which will improve the application and efficiency of targeted control strategies.

While the CSFS is very successful at eliminating a within-flock epidemic of classical scrapie irrespective of flock size or proportion of homebred sheep, this strategy is costly as it relies on the removal of the entire susceptible population in the flock. Additionally, depending on the proportion of susceptible animals and the relatively small incidence of scrapie in the flock, a large number of otherwise healthy sheep are routinely culled in this strategy. A recent study (Truscott & Ferguson, 2008) has demonstrated that not all of the components of the CSFS are equally effective. Trading restrictions alone have little power to limit transmission (Truscott & Ferguson, 2008) and a more efficient implementation may consider either culling or breeding restrictions alone (Truscott & Ferguson, 2008).

Small low-risk flocks (<200 sheep) are less likely to sustain an epidemic or sell on infected breeding sheep which suggests that large-scale control measures such as the CSFS may be unnecessary in preventing the onward spread of disease. The smaller the flock size, the less likely that scrapie is sustained in the population over longer periods of time due to the number of susceptible animals diminishing as a result of loss due to infection and replacement with resistant stock. In closed flocks, susceptible genotypes are not necessarily eliminated but are reduced to a threshold frequency where the density of susceptible sheep is too low to support endemic infection (Woolhouse et al., 1998).

Conversely, large flocks (>500 sheep), especially those with high proportions of homebred sheep, pose the greatest risk for onward transmission of scrapie to other farms due to the increased opportunity for an epidemic to take hold. In these flocks, while live testing dramatically reduces the number of sheep culled compared to the CSFS, it is unlikely to eradicate scrapie completely within a scrapie-positive flock and thus the reduction in cost to the farmer must be balanced against the risk posed to other flocks, in particular if the test sensitivity is low in pre-clinical animals or if the test is too costly or difficult to implement or interpret. The onward risk is likely due to a combination of (i) having a large within-flock epidemic due to there being a large numbers of animals at risk (Healy et al., 2004; Hopp et al., 2001); (ii) large numbers of replacement animals to provide a steady supply of new susceptibles to sustain an epidemic; (iii) large numbers of breeding stock on the premises, due to the risk of sheep-to-sheep transmission at lambing; and (iv) greater risk of onward transmission due to the large numbers of sheep sold on. These factors therefore identify likely scenarios under which stringent control measures may be necessary.

Use of a single test strategy will be cheaper and easier to implement for the farmer, however, may result in the unacceptable exposure of additional flocks via the sale of breeding sheep, unless scrapie is detected relatively early (<5 years) in an epidemic. Extending the number of years in which the live test is applied does not significantly affect the number of sheep culled in the flock and reduces the number of infected sheep sold on to other flocks. However, this reduction is not substantial enough to eliminate the risk of onward transmission altogether and the existing CSFS strategy may remain the most appropriate method of control and eradication in these high risk flocks.

This model assumes that all sheep above a certain age were tested. Future work will investigate different live testing strategies such as testing specific genotypes only or random sampling of sheep within a flock to determine if this has an impact on the efficiency and cost effectiveness of the diagnostic test. Further information to refine flock parameters (such as different genotypic distributions for different flock types) would also assist in the identification of high risk flocks and improve the economic assessment of testing efficacy at a national level. Additional information is still required to determine the cost and ease of test implementation, the cost of culling, restrictions in breeding and trading to the farmer at an individual and national level, before further economic evaluation and comparison with the CSFS can be made.

This study has shown that only large flocks with many homebred breeding sheep are likely to be a risk for onward transmission. In order to determine the role that these flocks might play in the persistence and spread of scrapie in the British national flock, existing datasets characterising the detailed flock-to-flock movement of sheep in GB (Kao et al., 2006; Green et al., 2007) will have to be refined to consider only those movements that are important for scrapie transmission, most likely those movements involving breeding ewes. This will be the subject of future work.

ACKNOWLEDGEMENTS

The authors acknowledge Defra for funding this study. RRK is funded by the Wellcome

Trust, FH by the Royal Society.

REFERENCES

Baylis, M., Houston, F., Kao, R.R., McLean, A., Hunter, N. and Gravenor, M.B. (2002). BSE - a wolf in sheep's clothing? Trends Microbiol. 12, 563-570

Caughey, B. and Chesebro, B. (1997). Prion protein and the transmissible spongiform

encephalopathies. Trends Cell Biol. 7, 56-62

Dawson, M., Moore, R.C. and Bishop, S.C. (2008). Progress and limits of PrP gene selection policy. Vet. Res. 39, 25

Defra (2007). NSP update. Technical Report 9 (Spring/Summer)

Defra (2008). Compulsory scrapie flocks scheme booklet, 2006. (http://www.defra.gov.uk/corporate/regulat/forms/Ahealth/nsp/nsp39.pdf). Accessed August 2008

Foster, J.D., Hope, J. and Fraser, H. (1993). Transmission of Bovine Spongiform Encephalopathy to sheep and goats. Vet. Rec. 14, 339-341

Foster, J.D., Parnham, D.W., Hunter, N. and Bruce, M. (2001). Distribution of prion protein in sheep terminally affected with BSE following experimental oral transmission. J. Gen. Virol. 82, 2319-2326

Fryer, H.R., Baylis, M., Sivam, K. and McLean, A.R. (2007). Quantifying the risk from ovine BSE and the impact of control strategies. Proc. Biol. Sci. 274, 1497-1503

Goldmann, W., Hunter, N., Smith, G., Foster, J. and Hope, J. (1994). PrP genotype and agent effects in scrapie: change in allelic interaction with different isolates of agent in sheep, a natural host of scrapie. J. Gen. Virol. 75 (Pt 5), 989-995

González, L., Dagleish, M.P., Bellworthy, S.J., Sisó, S., Stack, M.J., Chaplin, M.J., Davis, L.A., Hawkins, S.A., Hughes, J., Jeffrey, M. (2006). Postmortem diagnosis of preclinical and clinical scrapie in sheep by the detection of disease-associated PrP in their rectal mucosa. Vet. Rec. 158, 325-331

González, L., Dalgleish, M.P., Martin, S., Dexter, G., Steele, P., Finalyson, J. and Jeffrey, M. (2008a). Diagnosis of preclinical scrapie in live sheep by the immunohistochemical examination of rectal biopsies. Vet. Rec. 162, 397-403

González, L., Horton, R., Ramsay, D., Toomik, R., Leathers, V., Tonelli, Q., Dagleish, M.P., Jeffrey, M. and Terry, L. (2008b). Adaptation and evaluation of a rapid test for the diagnosis of sheep scrapie in samples of rectal mucosa. J. Vet. Diagn. Invest. 20, 203-208

Gravenor, M.B., Cox, D.R., Hoinville, L.J., Hoek, A. and Mclean, A.R. (2001). The flock-to-flock force of infection for scrapie in Britain. Proc. Biol. Sci. 268, 587-592

Green, D.M., Vilas, V.J. del Rio, Birch, C.P.D., Johnson, J., Kiss, I.Z., McCarthy, N.D. and Kao, R.R. (2007). Demographic risk factors for classical and atypical scrapie in Great

Britain. J. Gen. Virol. 88, 3486-3492

Gubbins, S. (2005). A modelling framework to describe the spread of scrapie between sheep flocks in Great Britain. Prev. Vet. Med. 67, 143-156

Hagenaars, T.J., Donnelly, C.A., Ferguson, N.M. and Anderson, R.M. (2000). The transmission dynamics of the aetiological agent of scrapie in a sheep flock. Math. Biosci. 168, 117-135

Healy, A.M., Hannon, D., Morgan, K.L., Weavers, E., Collins, J.D. and Doherty, M.L. (2004). A paired case-control study of risk factors for scrapie in Irish sheep flocks. Prev. Vet. Med. 64, 73-83

Hill, A.F., Zeidler, M., Ironside, J. and Collinge, J. (1997). Diagnosis of a new variant Creutzfeld-Jakob disease by tonsil biopsy. Lancet 349, 99-100

Hoinville, L.J., Hoek, A., Gravenor, M.B. and McLean, A.R. (2000). Descriptive epidemiology of scrapie in Great Britain: results of a postal survey. Vet. Rec. 146, 455-461

Hopp, P., Ulvund, M.J. and Jarp, J. (2001). A case-control study on scrapie in Norwegian sheep flocks. Prev. Vet. Med. 51, 183-198

Houston, F., Goldmann, W., Chong, A., Jeffrey, M., González, L., Foster, J., Parnham, D. and Hunter, N. (2003). Prion diseases: BSE in sheep bred for resistance to infection. Nature 42, 498

Houston, F. and Gravenor, M.B. (2003). Clinical signs in sheep experimentally infected with scrapie and BSE. Vet. Rec. 152, 333

Jeffrey, M., Ryder, S., Martin, S., Hawkins, S.A., Terry, L., Berthelin-Baker, C. and Bellworthy, S.J. (2001). Oral inoculation of sheep with the agent of bovine spongiform encephalopathy (BSE). 1. Onset and distribution of disease-specific PrP accumulation in brain and viscera. J. Comp. Pathol. 124, 280-289

Kao, R.R., Gravenor, M.B. and McLean, A.R. (2001). Modelling the national scrapie eradication programme in the UK. Math. Biosci. 174, 61-76

Kao, R.R., Gravenor, M.B., Baylis, M., Bostock, C.J., Chihota, C.M., Evans, J.C., Goldmann, W., Smith, A.J. and McLean, A.R. (2002). The potential size and duration of an epidemic of bovine spongiform encephalopathy in British sheep. Science 295, 332-335

Kao, R.R., Houston, F.F., Baylis, M., Chihota, C.M., Goldmann, W., Gravenor, M.B., Hunter, N. and McLean, A.R. (2003). Epidemiological implications of the susceptibility to BSE of putatively resistant sheep. J. Gen. Virol. 84, 3503-3512

Kao, R.R., Danon, L., Green, D.M. and Kiss, I.Z. (2006). Pathogen Dynamics on the Network of Livestock Movements in the UK. Proc. Biol. Sci. 273, 1999-2007

Konold, T., Moore, S.J., Bellworthy, S.J. and Simmons, H.A. (2008). Evidence of scrapie transmission via milk. BMC Vet. Res. 4, 14

McLean, A.R., Hoek, A., Hoinville, L.J. and Gravenor, M.B. (1999). Scrapie transmission in Britain: a recipe for a mathematical model. Proc. Biol. Sci. 266, 2531-2538

O'Rourke, K.I., Baszler, T.V., Besser, T.E., Miller, J.M., Cutlip, R.C., Wells, G.A., Ryder, S.J., Parish, S.M., Hamir, A.N., Cockett, N.E., Jenny, A. and Knowles, D.P. (2000). Preclinical diagnosis of scrapie by immunohistochemistry of third eyelid lymphoid tissue. J. Clin. Microbiol. 38, 3254-3259

Parry, H.B. (1983). Scrapie Disease in Sheep: Historical, Clinical, Epidemiological, Pathological and Practical Aspects of the Natural Disease. Academic Press, London, 146p

Pollott, G.E. and Stone, D.G. (2006). The breeding structure of the British sheep industry 2003. Defra, London (http://www.defra.gov.uk/animalh/bse/othertses/scrapie/nsp/publicatsrpts/pollott2003.pdf). Accessed January 2009

Race, R., Jenny, A. and Sutton, D. (1998). Scrapie infectivity and proteinase K-resistant prion protein in sheep placenta, brain, spleen, and lymph node: implications for transmission and antemortem diagnosis. J. Infect. Dis. 178, 949-953

Radostitis, O.M., Gay, C.C., Blood, D.C. and Hinchcliff, K.W. (2000). Diseases caused by viruses and Chlamydia-II. In Veterinary Medicine: a Textbook of the Disease of Cattle, Sheep, Pigs, Goats and Horses (9th Edition). Saunders (W.B.), London, 115-1260p

Schreuder, B.E., van Keulen, L.J., Vromans, M.E., Langeveld, J.P. and Smits, M.A. (1998). Tonsillar biopsy and PrPSc detection in the preclinical diagnosis of scrapie. Vet. Rec. 142, 564-568

Sivam, S.K., Baylis, M., Gravenor, M.B. and Gubbins, S. (2006). Descriptive analysis of an anonymous postal survey of the occurrence of scrapie in Great Britain in 2002. Vet. Rec. 158, 501-506

Somerville, R.A., Birkett, C.R., Farquhar, C.F., Hunter, N., Goldmann, W., Dornan, J., Grover, D., Hennion, R.M., Percy, C., Foster, J. and Jeffrey, M. (1997). Immunodetection of PrPSc in spleens of some scrapie-infected sheep but not BSE-infected cows. J. Gen. Virol. 78, 2389-2396

Stringer, S.M., Hunter, N. and Woolhouse, M.E.J. (1998). A mathematical model of the dynamics of scrapie in a sheep flock. Math. Biosci. 153, 79-98

Truscott, J.E. and Ferguson, N.M. (2008). Control of scrapie in the UK sheep population. Epidemiol. Infect. doi: 10.1017/50950268808001064

VLA (2003a). Summary of the results of the scrapie surveillance in sheep in Great Britain. January 2002 –March 2003: Veterinary Laboratories Agency

VLA (2003b). Summary of the results of the scrapie surveillance in sheep in Great Britain. April –December 2003: Veterinary Laboratories Agency

Woolhouse, M.E.J., Stringer, S.M., Matthews, L., Hunter, N. and Anderson, R.M. (1998). Epidemiology and control of scrapie within a sheep flock. Proc. Biol. Sci. 265, 1205-1210

SCIENCE / POLICY INTERFACE

BARRIERS AND MOTIVATORS FOR ZOONOTIC CONTROL ON CATTLE FARMS

J. ELLIS-IVERSEN* AND H. HOGEVEEN

SUMMARY

The implementation of disease control programs on farms requires an act of behavioral change. This study combined behavioral science with epidemiological principles to investigate and explain the control of zoonotic agents on cattle farms. A socio-ecological model was developed from behavioral science used in human medicine. Field data was used to demonstrate the validity of this model to identify and explain motivational factors for implementation of disease control programs among English and Welsh cattle farmers. The field data originated from interviews of 42 cattle farmers and was used to identify intrinsic and extrinsic barriers. The implementation model was used to illustrate where the barriers affected the implementation process and to classify the farmers according to the current degree of zoonotic control within the model. Statistical analyses were used to identify motivators associated with different levels of implementation. In general, attitudes towards zoonotic control were positive, but 'intent to adopt control measures' was inhibited in approximately half the farmers by non-supportive social norms and/or a lack of belief in self-efficacy. The remaining farmers showed a gradual intent to control, but had not implemented any structured control due lack of knowledge and cultural and economic pressure from society and industry. Farmers with no intent to adopt control measures identified their private veterinarian as the preferred motivator, whereas consumer-demand and financial incentives were significantly associated with farmers who intended to control.

INTRODUCTION

The success of any disease control programme depends on adoption and implementation of disease control practices by individual farmers. In many situations, these practices require changes to established farmer behaviour. In the case of infectious diseases, success is also influenced by the level of coverage of the programme in the broader target population. Behaviour changes are notoriously difficult to induce and sustain, even when interventions are feasible, affordable and acceptable (Grol and Grimshaw, 2003; Panter-Brick et al., 2006). Farm disease control is dependent on the individual farmer's decision whether or not to implement the programme. Behavioural science offers an insight into decision-making and provides tools to classify and map those motivators and barriers that encourage or inhibits behavioural changes. A combination of natural and social sciences, occasionally referred to as social epidemiology, is widely used in human medicine and policy-making. As yet, however, these methods have rarely been applied in veterinary medicine (Prochaska and DiClemente, 1983; WHO, 1989; Grol and Grimshaw, 2003; Panter-Brick et al., 2006; Gunn et al., 2008; Heffernan et al., 2008). Behavioural models mimic basic principles of human behaviour and can provide a framework to classify barriers and motivators that affect the decision to change behaviour at different stages in the process.

---

* Johanne Ellis-Iversen, Centre for Epidemiology and Risk Analysis, VLA, Addlestone, Surrey, KT15 3NB, UK. Email: J.Ellis-Iversen@vla.defra.gsi.gov.uk

The Theory of Planned Behaviour divides behavioural changes by individuals into two distinct steps, 'intent' and 'action', and describes how beliefs and attitudes influence the intent to change (Azjen, 1985). Using a social-ecological model, Panter-Brick et al. (2006) expanded this theory from the individual to the population, to describe factors influencing behavioural change in the context of mosquito net repair in a human population in The Gambia. Social-ecological models can enrich individual models of decision making in behaviour change, thereby allowing interpretation at the level of the population. These models incorporate a schematic overview of external circumstances that are likely to influence action, once intent has been obtained. Population-based behavioural models can provide tools for policy-makers, facilitating resource prioritisation towards motivators, and away from barriers, that are likely to have the greatest impact on both intent and action.

Control of zoonoses, such as salmonella or VTEC O157 on farms initially depends on the farmers' intent to implement and adopt disease control measures. Intent is strongly influenced by intrinsic circumstances, which can be divided into three main groups: 1) Behavioural beliefs, which determine the attitude towards any issue. These are often based on personal experiences and personal core values, including perception of right and wrong or good and bad behaviour. Attitudes can be influenced or changed by increasing focus on successful experiences and demonstrating how core values agree with the recommended change. 2) Normative beliefs, which are determined by perception of social norms. Social norms are derived from the perceived expectations of close social networks such as family, local community, faming/veterinary collaborators and maybe industry partners. Peer pressure will in particular influence a person's normative belief. 3) Belief in self-efficacy is the perception of, and confidence in, one's ability to carry out the behaviour change and sustain the new behaviour. It is more complex than whether or not something can be done or is effective. Factual information does influence this belief, but advice from trusted sources or people who are perceived as "equal" are much more likely to change belief in self-efficacy (Kelly and Thibaut, 1978). However, intent does not necessarily progress into action, noting that this step is mainly dependent on extrinsic circumstances that are generally outside the individual's control. For livestock farmers, three main extrinsic areas influence progress from intent to implementation of a disease control programme: 1) Community and industry influences through financial pressures, traditional reactions and unwritten rules. The opinions and decisions of livestock industries and the rural community influences whether a farmer acts on his/her intent. It requires a great effort to go against tradition or stand outside a communal decision. 2) Cultural and societal circumstances include laws and regulations, economic viability, ethical and moral values of consumers and society. Livestock farmers might be able to change initiating over the long-term changes, but (inter)national campaigns and centralised interventions are often needed for major alterations. 3) Knowledge, skill and ability include availability of knowledge and specialist skills or even the ability to finance the control programme, while keeping a viable enterprise. A farmer may improve this by factual knowledge and skill enhancement, but external intervention might be needed to provide innovation and research to meet the requirements.

This study investigated English and Welsh (E&W) cattle farmers' attitudes and perceptions of barriers and motivators to control for zoonotic pathogens on their farm. A population-based, social-ecological framework was used to: 1) identify intrinsic or extrinsic constraining circumstances, which influence the implementation of a control programme and 2) establish motivators associated with different stages in the implementation model.

MATERIALS AND METHODS

Study Population

A total of 57 cattle farmers were previously enrolled in an intervention trial to investigate the effect of control measures on VTEC O157 in young stock. The relevant selection method and eligibility criteria have been described and discussed in more detail elsewhere (Ellis-Iversen et al., 2007; Ellis-Iversen et al., 2008). Briefly, a stepwise selection process was used to identify study farms. During the trial, all farms were positive for VTEC O157 and all farmers were informed of the risks to humans. The study ended in April 2005 with a visit from the local veterinary investigation officer (VIO), who had been the contact throughout the study, to explain results and discuss experiences of participation. In January 2006, each farmer was again contacted by the VIO via letter and telephone to assess whether they would agree to another visit on the farm to be interviewed about their perceptions, attitudes and opinions about control of zoonoses in cattle. The farmer was offered no incentive to participate apart from a 'chat' with the VIO and an opportunity for the farmer's opinions and ideas to be presented to the policy makers.

Interview Design

A discussion group, which included veterinarians, epidemiologists and risk analysts, was formed to identify topics, methods and potential problems of the planned interviews. These issues were then further discussed with the Veterinary Laboratories Agency's expert cattle veterinary group and with other VIOs. All contributions were collated in the design of the interview.

The interview was conducted using a standardised open-ended questionnaire interview, followed by an informal conversation technique (Berry, 1999). The standardised open-ended interview approach was used for the main topics to ensure responses from every farmer for the analysis, and to minimise the variation in questions asked when using multiple interviewers. A standardised interview 'check-list' was used (available on request) and designed as a multileveled outline with main open questions in the first level and more in-depth questions in the second. The third level consisted of prompting words, which could be used in case the farmer did not understand the question or simply to get the farmer back on track. The informal conversational technique was used to allow farmers to tell the interviewer what was of importance to him/her within each topic without issues being limited by presumptions made by the research team. Furthermore, it also allowed talking patterns to remain as 'normal as possible' during the interview to encourage openness and information flow. Attributes of the farmers were collected at the end of each interview using closed questions with tick boxes.

The interview technique and 'check-list' were piloted on one farm by a team comprising the project leader (observer) and a participating VIO (interviewer). After the trial, the 'check-list' was revised and instructions were included and sent to the ten regional VIOs, who were commissioned to do the interviews. The interview procedures were discussed by phone with each VIO to allow for questions or uncertain issues to be clarified and discussed before the interviews.

If the farmer agreed, the interviews were recorded on a dictaphone and the tapes along with attribute details were sent to the Centre for Epidemiology and Risk Analysis. For confidentiality reasons, the analyst was blinded to the identity of both the farmer and the interviewer, when analysing the data.

The interview outline consisted of various topics. Intent to control zoonoses was assessed by asking the farmer whether any control programme or measures were implemented at present. The farmer was prompted to talk about a zoonotic pathogen of his/her choice and elaborate on what s/he did on a daily basis to control the spread to humans.

The farmers were asked what would influence their decision to implement disease control, where they would seek advice, whom they would listen to, and finally who could convince them to implement control measures. The questions of motivators were initially posed as open questions, but if the farmer did not reply, the interviewer asked whether this or that motivator (from the 'check-list') would influence the decision. Motivators that were not mentioned by the farmer or were described as non-influential after being mentioned by the interviewer were coded equally as negative. The intrinsic motivators listed in the 'check-list' were the private veterinarian, other farmers, proof of effect and cattle/breeding societies. Personal knowledge of someone with a zoonotic disease, having small children, improved health and safety for people on the farm and improved animal welfare were also considered to influence the intrinsic circumstances of beliefs and attitudes. Extrinsic motivators on the 'check-list' included consumer-demand, government recommendation, legislations, financial penalties or gain controlled by any other part of society dependent on implementation of a control programme. Any prompted or unprompted motivators that were mentioned at any time during the interviews were also included.

Data Analysis

All relevant information was deducted from the transcribed interviews or electronic version of non-recorded interviews using MAXQDA software (www.maxqda.com)

Circumstances and barriers

An implementation of disease control model was developed based on the Panter-Brick model (Panter-Brick et al., 2006). The terminology was slightly modified, both in wording and concepts, to improve clarity for animal health professionals. The developed model was used to describe and classify barriers mentioned at anytime throughout the interview (Panter-Brick et al., 2006). Barriers were classified as intrinsic or extrinsic circumstances and entered into the model. The intrinsic barriers were sub-divided into circumstances inhibiting either behavioural beliefs, normative beliefs or the belief in self-efficacy, and the extrinsic circumstances were sub-divided into external and societal barriers, internal and industry barriers or knowledge and ability barriers (Fig. 1).

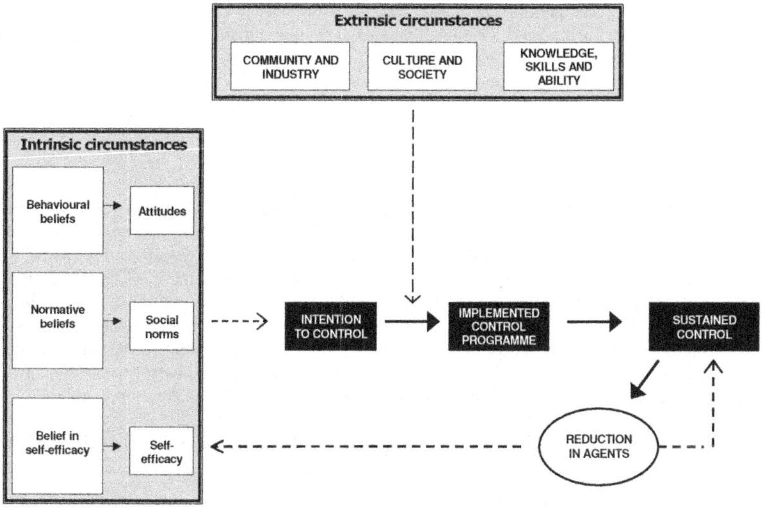

Fig 1. A behavioural model to describe implementation of disease control on farms, modified from Panter-Brick et al., 2006. (Black boxes= stages in process of behaviour change; circle = desired outcome; gray boxes= circumstances that influence behaviour; non-dashed arrows=movements towards desired outcome; dashed arrows= factors affecting movement between stages of behavioural change.)

Classification of farmers at stages in the framework of implementation of disease control

The number of practices, which were mentioned in direct association with reducing spread of zoonotic agents, was interpreted as cognitive actions. Four levels of cognitive actions were identified: no actions, 1 action, 2 actions and >2 actions An action was only considered as cognitive if it was mentioned and applied as a direct intent to protect against zoonoses. Applying individual practices to protect people from zoonotic agents was interpreted as showing intent to control and the more control practices applied, the more intent was shown. The presence of a structured plan to control against one or more zoonotic agents to protect staff and visitors and deliver safe produce was interpreted as an implemented control programme.

Crude associations between the different stages in the model of disease control and farmer attributes were assessed using univariable logistic regression models and only significant results ($p<0.05$) were reported.

Motivators and preferred referents

Associations between farmer attributes and motivators were assessed using univariable logistic regression. A p-value <0.05 was considered significant; non-significant associations were not considered further.

To assess whether preferred motivators differed between farmers at different stages of intent, the ordinal variable for the strength of intent to implement a control programme was fitted as dependent variable in a multivariable ordinal logistic regression model. Initially, all motivators (extrinsic and intrinsic) were included in the model and the final model was derived by stepwise elimination of variables with p-values larger than 0.1, which was considered the significance level. The parallel regression assumption was verified using an approximate likelihood-ratio test. Intercooled STATA 9 was used for all statistical analyses (STATA Corp., College Station, Texas)

RESULTS

Study population

Forty-six farmers out of 57 contacted agreed to an interview resulting in a participation rate of 80.7% and all were visited and interviewed between December 2005 and March 2006. One farmer did not want his/her interview recorded and one interview was conducted in Welsh (and not recorded). The unrecorded interviews were both summarized by the VIO and delivered as written reports. Three interviews were recorded with a lot of background noise, which resulted very few audible whole sentences and they were excluded from the analyses to avoid misinterpretation. Two farmers did not provide attribute details and were, thus, not included in Table 1. However, their interviews were included in the remaining analyses, yielding a total sample size of 43 interviews of which 41 was supported by attribute information (Table 1).

Table 1. Attributes of 41 cattle farmers interviewed about the perception of zoonotic control.

Attribute		Number of farms
Age (years)	25-35	5
	36-45	15
	45-60	16
	>60	5
Gender	Female	5
	Male	35
Role on farm	Manager	15
	Owner	12
	Both	14
Lived on farm	Yes	34
	No	7
Has children < 10 years of age[a]	Yes	12
	No	28
Know someone who suffered from zoonotic illness	Yes	25
	No	16
Member of cattle/farmer society	Yes	31
	No	10
Main production on farm	Dairy	31
	Beef	10
Had side enterprise	Yes	25
	No	16

[a] Missing values are omitted

The average size of the farms was 314 cattle in their main enterprise, ranging from 57-1000. Dairy enterprises (mean=329; median=300) tended to be larger that beef enterprises (mean=272; median=222) and larger enterprises (average herd size of 358 cattle) were more likely to have an additional cattle enterprise than small ones (average herd size of 256 cattle) (p(t)=0.039).

The majority of the interviewees were male, but five women were interviewed. One of these was a manager, one both owned and managed the farm whereas the remaining three categorised themselves as owners only. Children under 10 years of age lived on eight of the farms.

Barriers influencing implementation of zoonotic control

The pathway to implementation of disease control framework shows an overview of the barriers mentioned by farmers, when classified as intrinsic and extrinsic factors (Fig. 2).

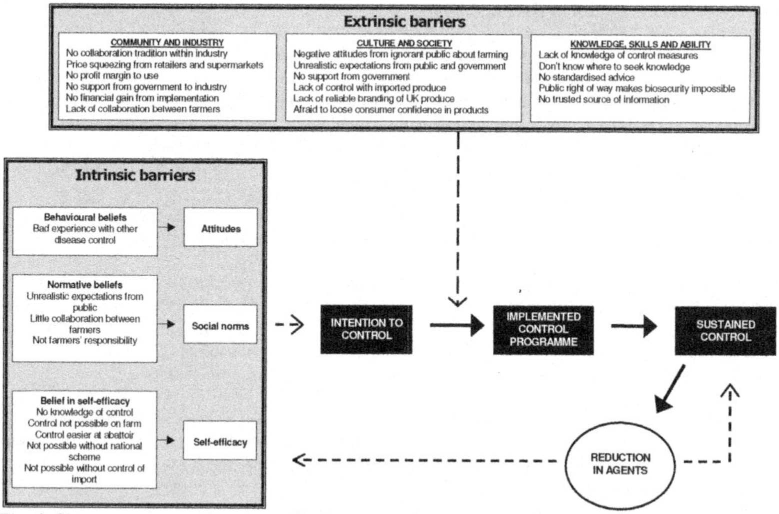

Fig. 2 Circumstances and barriers affecting zoonotic control on English and Welsh cattle farms illustrated in the 'pathway to disease control model' (Black boxes= stages in process of behaviour change; circle = desired outcome; gray boxes= circumstances that influence behaviour; non-dashed arrows=movements towards desired outcome; dashed arrows= factors affecting movement between stages of behavioural change)

Classification of farmers at stages in the framework of the pathway to implementation of disease control

None of the farmers had implemented any structured programme to control zoonotic agents in their herds, but 20 farmers (48.8%) exhibited intent to control by applying at least one measure to avoid spread to humans. Seven farmers mentioned and applied one control action, six farmers two control actions and seven farmers applied several hygiene and management interventions and showed a strong intent to control zoonotic agents. However, none of the farmers applied interventions consistently enough to be considered to have a structured implemented control programme in place. Two farmers were classified as missing values in respect to which stage they were at, because the topic was not pursued by the interviewer.

None of the farmers had a structured control plan and since a haphazard approach is unlikely to result in a reduction in agents, no farmers were classified as having implemented a control programme. However, use of individual measures suggested that barriers in attitudes, social norms and self-efficacy were overcome and that intentions were in some cases transformed into actions, despite external barriers. The group of farmers with strongest intent were more likely to be younger than 45 years of age (p=0.03) and had larger herds (p=0.04) than the farmers, who showed no intent of control.

A total of 21 farmers did not mention any hygiene measures that they applied with the intent to reduce risks for humans. They generally expressed positive attitudes towards zoonotic control on farm, but were inhibited by other intrinsic circumstances such as lack of belief in self-efficacy or normative beliefs. Only two farmers expressed very negative attitudes, which seemed to refer to disease control in general.

The majority of farmers expressed concerns for the health and safety of visitors. The need for interventions with regard to visitors coming on to the farm was motivated mainly by two attitudes: either visitors were perceived as a biosecurity risk for the herd or the animals were considered a safety risk (physical or infectious) to the visitors. The risk of physical harm to visitors appeared to be a stronger driver for precautionary action than the risk of zoonotic transmission, which was more likely to cause concern but did not necessarily result in precautionary action.

Motivators to progress within the implementation of disease control framework

The majority of farmers (65%) would implement a control programme, if recommended by their private veterinarian. In general, the farmers expressed great trust in their veterinarians and felt that the private veterinarians worked for and with them. Only one farmer positively stated s/he would listen to breeding or cattle society recommendations, whereas three farmers stressed that they would not listen to recommendations from breeding or cattle societies.

Improved animal welfare would influence the decision of nine farmers, and people's health and safety (staff and family) would encourage a further six farmers to control zoonotic agents. The farmers motivated by welfare had larger enterprises than the ones, who were not (460 cattle vs. 279 cattle: p=0.01).

Twenty percent of the farmers revealed that recommendations from the government would influence their decision to implement control measures positively. Of the remaining 32 farms, six stressed that governmental recommendations would not have any influence on practices on their farms. Ten farms would implement measures if legislation was passed, whereas one farmer emphasised that legislation would not have any influence on his/her decision. The remaining 29 farmers did not mention legislation as a motivator.

Eight farmers mentioned that consumers influenced their decision to implement controls either through demand for VTEC-free produce or through the fear of losing consumer confidence in the produce, e.g. due to a media-scare. One third of the farmers would listen to their customers if they demanded control measures, especially if rewards or penalties were connected to implementation. Seven farmers said that they would be motivated by financial gains or penalties, independently of where they originated.

Farmers with a strong intent to control zoonotic agents were more likely to be motivated by changes in extrinsic circumstances such as financial incentives or penalties and demand from consumers, than farmers who did not intend to control (table 2). The farmers who did not show any intent were more likely to identify a trusted source (in this case their private veterinarian) as the best motivation to progress towards zoonotic control than their counterparts, who had already overcome intrinsic inhibiting circumstances.

Table 2. Preferred motivators identified by farmers with intent to control zoonotic agents in their cattle compared to farmers with no intent.

Motivators	Coefficient	CI 95%	P-value
Financial incentives or penalties	4.32	2.1; 6.6	<0.001
Consumer demand	1.64	-0.08; 3.4	0.061
Recommendations from veterinarian	-1.75	-3.3; 0.23	0.024

Proportionality of odds likelihood ratio-test p=0.1, N=38

DISCUSSION

Behavioural models are widely used in human health policy and commercial marketing to identify motivators, which might increase the success of a behavioural change. Animal health policy-makers can also benefit from behavioural science models. Because the livestock industry is very dependent on market fluctuations and on the public perception of their industry, there is a need for behavioural models, which acknowledge and incorporate the influences of extrinsic circumstances on a farmer's decision making process (Lloyd et al., 2001). This study applied a model, which enabled schematic classification of barriers influencing decision making at the different steps in the process of behaviour change. Furthermore, the model also enabled classification of farmers into two groups according to stage in the process of behavioural change.

Approximately half of the farmers in the study population showed intent to control zoonotic agents in their herds. This is likely to be an overestimate and should not be extrapolated to the general population of cattle farmers, because all participants were previously enrolled in a trial of zoonotic control on their farms. Despite the skewed study population, it is likely that the differences in motivators and characteristics between the farmers with and without intent are realistic and reasonably unbiased.

Younger farmers and/or larger farms were more likely to intend to implement a control programme than their counterparts. This may reflect the generic human behaviour trait, where younger people are more dynamic and more willing to accept changes (Crabtree et al., 2001; Mathijs, 2003). However, it may present a changing attitude and shift in perception of responsibility among English and Welsh cattle farmers along side the emerge of the responsibility and cost sharing initiative (Defra, 2008).

The Theory of Interdependence explains how extrinsic motivators such as experts, legitimate authority, coercive actions and rewards are considered useful in securing action (compliance), whereas information/marketing approaches and using 'liked' referents are essential for conversion of beliefs (Kelly and Thibaut, 1978). Applied to our study, we observed that farmers, who showed no intent to control, were significantly more likely to mention their veterinarian (a trusted source) as motivator than their counterparts, who had an established intent. The non-intent farmers were less likely to identify barriers such as financial barriers, because extrinsic factors were not relevant to them, when belief in self-efficacy and normative beliefs of responsibility were lacking. The financial motivation was of greater importance to the other group of farmers, who had progressive beliefs, had overcome the intrinsic hurdles and showed intent to control zoonotic agents within their herd.

The differences in motivators within the farming population identify a need for multiple communication tools and motivators to reach all farmers and implement zoonotic control on all cattle farms. The private veterinarian was seen as an impartial advisor working for the farmer, which suggests that the proportion of farmers with intent could be increased by educating private veterinarians to advise on zoonotic control. One of the biggest extrinsic barriers was lack of accessible knowledge on how to reduce zoonotic pathogens and it is likely that farmers with intent would implement a feasible and effective zoonotic control programme if available. Optimal knowledge transfer could be done by a central body such as government, industry or an expert science organisations (e.g.: European College of Veterinary Public Health), which insures that information is consistent and easily available. Acknowledgment of the different needs or motivators among subgroups of farmers enables targeted support and encouragement and ultimately is more likely to result in action and successful implementation.

More research and structured studies in the area of implementation and motivation for improving animal and public health is needed to confirm the trends and observations in our study. The social-ecological model applied in this paper was useful and accurate tool, which can be recommended as investigation tool to aid the adoption of other disease control programmes. The ability of the model to correctly identify motivators according to behavioural science theory, using statistical analyses, could be considered a validation of fit-for-purpose of the model. The model provides a tool for policy-makers to aid prioritisation of resources to remove the barriers that inhibit the largest part of a population.

ACKNOWLEDGEMENTS

We would like to thank all the farmers, who were interviewed and provided us with the data. Thanks to all the VIOs who conducted the interviews, especially Geoff Pritchard for also participating in interview design and trial. We are also grateful for the assistance of CERA staff, especially Richard Smith, who managed the data collection process. We would also like to thank Eamon Watson, Alex Cook, Marion Wooldridge, Mirjam Nielen and Lesley Larkin for their invaluable contributions. The research was funded by Defra under project OZ0145.

REFERENCES

Azjen, I., 1985. From intentions to actions: A theory of planned behaviour. In Kuhl, J. and Beckman, J. (Ed): Action-control: From cognition to behaviour. Springer, Heidelberg.

Berry, R. S. Y., Collecting data by indepth interview, http://www.leeds.ac.uk/educol/documents/00000172.htm. Accessed: 18/09/08.

Crabtree, B., Chalmers, N. and Eiser, D., 2001. Voluntary incentive schemes for farm forestry: Uptake, policy effectiveness and employment impacts. Forestry. 74, 455-65.

Defra, Responsibility and Cost Sharing, http://www.defra.gov.uk/animalh/ahws/sharing/index.htm Accessed: 15/12/08.

Ellis-Iversen, J., Smith, R. P., Snow, L. C., Watson, E., Millar, M. F., Pritchard, G. C., Sayers, A. R., Cook, A. J., Evans, S. J. and Paiba, G. A., 2007. Identification of management risk factors for VTEC O157 in young-stock in England and Wales. Prev. Vet. Med. 82, 29-41.

Ellis-Iversen, J., Smith, R. P., Van Winden, S., Paiba, G. A., Watson, E., Snow, L. C. and Cook, A. J., 2008. Farm practices to control E. coli O157 in young cattle - A randomised controlled trial. Vet. Res. 39, 1-3.

Grol, R. and Grimshaw, J., 2003. From best evidence to best practice: effective implementation of change in patients' care. Lancet. 362, 1225-30.

Gunn, G. J., Heffernan, C., Hall, M., McLeod, A. and Hovi, M., 2008. Measuring and comparing constraints to improved biosecurity amongst GB farmers, veterinarians and the auxiliary industries. Prev. Vet. Med. 84, 310-23.

Heffernan, C., Nielsen, L., Thomson, K. and Gunn, G., 2008. An exploration of the drivers to bio-security collective action among a sample of UK cattle and sheep farmers. Prev. Vet. Med. 87, 358-72.

Kelly, H. H. and Thibaut, J. W., 1978. Interpersonal relations: A theory of interdependence. Wiley, New York.

Lloyd, T., McCorriston, S., Morgan, C. W. and Rayner, A. J., 2001. The impact of food scares on price adjustment in the UK beef market. Agricultural Economics. 25, 347-57.

Mathijs, E., 2003. Social capital and farmers' willingness to adopt countryside stewartship schemes. Outlook on agriculture. 32, 13-6.

Panter-Brick, C., Clarke, S. E., Lomas, H., Pinder, M. and Lindsay, S. W., 2006. Culturally compelling strategies for behaviour change: a social ecology model and case study in malaria prevention. Soc. Sci. Med. 62, 2810-25.

Prochaska, J. O. and DiClemente, C. C., 1983. Stages and processes of self-change of smoking: toward an integrative model of change. J. Consult. Clin. Psychol. 51, 390-5.

WHO, 1989. Knowledge, attitudes, beliefs and practices. Global programme on AIDS. Social and Behavioural Unit.

DEVELOPMENT OF A PARTICIPATORY METHODOLOGY TO PRIORITISE MILK-BORNE DISEASE IN DATA-SCARCE ENVIRONMENTS

D. GRACE* AND T. RANDOLPH

SUMMARY

Most poor people buy and sell food in informal markets which escape safety and quality regulation and where high levels of hazards are present. We developed a methodology to prioritise milk-borne pathogens by combining epidemiological, microbiological and behavioural data and evaluated this in a case study in Debre Zeit, Ethiopia. The methodology comprises: 1-Hazard identification to screen for potential hazards and associated syndromes; 2-Key Informant Interviews and Syndromic Surveillance with stakeholder groups to generate evidence on the presence/prevalence of hazards; 3-Rapid Exposure Assessment to identify risk amplification or reduction on the cow-to-consumer pathway and also assess consumption; 4-Development of a Risk Matrix to support stakeholder prioritisation.

Literature review found that out of nearly 60 important hazards known to be milk-borne, 27 were probably relevant to Ethiopia. Local veterinarians (n=3) considered 17 zoonotic diseases present in cattle but doctors (n=3) considered only 8 were present in the human population. However, all groups reported presence high presence of syndromes compatible with milk-borne disease (doctors: 6 out of 10 human syndromes present; consumers: 16 out of 16 present; veterinarians: 8 out of 8 cattle syndromes; farmers: 11 out of 11 present). Risk mitigating measures included heating and fermenting milk; risk amplifying measures included storing and mixing milk; children were considered to consume more milk, old people less and pregnant women the same amount as adults. Stakeholders developed a matrix in which hazards of concern were assessed against criteria of concern including: disease severity and prevalence, equity and livelihood impacts, and ease of control.

The participatory methodology produced scores that were sufficiently differentiated between pathogens to be useful for ranking them on the basis of risk. It allowed a rapid, low-cost assessment that engaged stakeholders and is a step towards evidence-based prioritisation of food-borne pathogens.

INTRODUCTION

Food-borne disease is the most common illness in both rich and poor countries and a major cause of morbidity and mortality. In less developed countries, food and water-borne disease kill an estimated 2.1 million people annually, most of whom are children (WHO, 2001). Characteristics of poor countries expected to increase risk include: higher proportions of vulnerable people (e.g. young, immuno-suppressed and malnourished); a greater variety and often higher levels of pathogens; less food preservation infrastructure; environmental conditions

* Delia Grace, International Livestock Research Institute, Nairobi. PO Box 30709, d.grace@cgiar.org

that favour pathogen survival and growth; generally inadequate food safety systems; and lack of knowledge about the detection and management of food safety problems. Most poor people buy and sell in informal markets which by definition escape safety and quality regulation and studies on livestock products in these markets typically find high levels of hazards.

In contexts where disease burden has been systematically evaluated, the Pareto Principle or Law of the Vital Few appears to apply. This states that, for many events, the greater part of the effects come from the smaller part of the causes. For example, the Global Burden of Disease study shows 6 infectious diseases (20% of the total classified) are responsible for 75% of the total disability-adjusted life years (DALY's) lost (WHO, 2008) ; similarly 90% of health research is devoted to 10% of the world's health problems (the 10/90 gap) (www.globalforumhealth.org). In countries where good quality attribution data on food-borne disease exists, *Campylobacter* spp., *Yersinia enterocolitica, Salmonella* spp., and *Clostridium perfringens* typically cause more than 80% of the total morbidity burden and the latter two diseases along with *Toxoplasma gondi* and *Listeria monocytogens* account for most mortality (Adek et al., 2005; Hall et al., 2005, CDC, 2005). If the majority of the disease burden is attributable to a minority of pathogens then targeting resources towards the vital few diseases will be much more effective than targeting resources at the trivial many. However, it cannot be assumed that the 'vital few' will be the same in every country; countries which differ in dietary habits and disease ecosystems may also differ in the subset of food-borne pathogens responsible for the majority of disease. As a result, risk-targeting or prioritisation of hazards according to their potential to cause harm must be context specific.

MATERIALS AND METHODS

A methodology was developed to prioritise milk-borne pathogens by combining epidemiological, microbiological and behavioural data and evaluated in a case study in Debre Zeit, Ethiopia. The methodology drew on Risk Analysis, Syndromic Surveillance and Participatory Learning and Action. The first step was Hazard Identification: in this, a systematic literature review was conducted to generate a list of milk-borne diseases (which term we will use to cover disease associated with milk and dairy products), the evidence for their relevance to the context of the case study, and the disease syndromes associated with them. To do this we carried out a PubMed search using the keywords "food-borne disease", "milk", "milk-borne disease", "attribution", separately and in combination, as well as a review of grey literature. The list of syndromes associated with these relevant milk-borne disease in both people and cattle was constructed by consulting standard text-books.

In the second stage, field work started with interviews of medical and veterinary key informants and participatory rural appraisals (PRAs) with farmers and consumers to estimate the presence and prevalence of milk-borne disease, the presence and prevalence of syndromes compatible with milk-borne disease, and the proportion of vulnerable groups in the community. In order to check experts' ability to recognise milk-borne disease and control for affirmative bias, we added pathogens to the list provided to medical informants which are not responsible for food-borne illness, and to the list provided to veterinarians a disease which is not present in cattle. For the PRAs with farmers, we developed a series of picture cards to represent the different syndromes. Interviews were carried out with 9 key informants (3 doctors, 3 veterinarians, 3 managers of large commercial farms). PRAs were carried out with 4 groups of farmers (25 men and 18 women); three of these groups were linked to dairy co-operatives and one were farmers who were not co-operative members.

Next a Rapid Exposure Assessment was developed to identify opportunities for risk amplification or reduction for each pathogen on the cow-to-consumer pathway and assess consumption disaggregated by food product and vulnerable groups. Interviews were carried out with 5 groups of consumers (41 men and 34 women). Four groups of consumers were the end clients of the four groups of farmers consulted and the remaining group worked for a floriculture enterprise. In addition, the 4 groups of farmers provided information about household consumption. The study started in April 2008 and is due to be completed in April 2009.

In the fourth and final step, a risk matrix was constructed with stakeholders to aid in their prioritisation of milk-borne hazards. This added two dimensions to the prioritisation of disease; first a 'concern axis' and secondly a 'manageability axis'. The concern axis reflects people's consistent deviation from reliance on health metrics in order to achieve desired social goals, such as preference to improve the situation of the worst-off or to support survival. The 'manageability axis' reflects the costs and feasibility in mitigating risk and the logic that it may be more cost effective to target a disease of less prevalence and/or impact but which can be easily and cheaply controlled rather than a disease that is of higher burden but also more difficult to control.

RESULTS

Step 1: Hazard Identification

We used evidence from three sources to prepare an initial risk estimate for dairy products (including milk) in Ethiopia. Firstly, studies on the proportion of food-borne disease outbreaks attributable to milk and dairy products, secondly population studies on the role of dairy products in food-borne disease, thirdly reports on presence of pathogens dairy products. Animal-source foods are responsible for the majority of food-borne disease outbreaks. However, milk-borne disease is considered relatively rare in developed countries. Milk was responsible for 2% of all reported outbreaks of food-borne disease in the UK (Gillespie et al., 2003), 1% in the USA (Lynch et al., 2006), 4% of outbreaks in Australia (FSANZ, 2006), 4% in Austria (Much et al., 2007) and from 1 to 5% in France and other industrialised countries (De Buyser et al., 2001). Although raw (unpasteurised) milk constitutes only a small proportion of the total consumed, it made up a large proportion of outbreaks, suggesting milk may be a more important vehicle in places where the majority of milk and milk products is consumed without effective heat treatment or other processing. Furthermore, dairy products were an important cause of disease in the nineteenth century before widespread pasteurisation and disease eradication schemes (especially tuberculosis, brucellosis, typhoid, paratyphoid and food poisoning) gain, this might be more analogous to the situation in developing countries.

Outbreak reports are known to greatly under-estimate disease burden because only a fraction of outbreaks are reported (and fewer still followed through to identification) and also because isolated cases, for many diseases is the most common manifestation, are by definition not reported as outbreaks. Population surveys typically suggest far higher levels of food-borne disease than outbreak data: incidences of acute gastro-intestinal disease vary from 0.2 to 1.3 episodes per person per year, of which a third or more may be due to food-borne illness (Flint et al., 2005). However, attribution of illness to food type is obviously difficult in these surveys as it is rarely possible for respondents to accurately identify the food causing illness.

The isolation of disease-causing bacteria in raw milk is another indicator of potential risk to human health and has been reported most extensively from Canada and the United States; these show around 1-10% of samples are contaminated with important pathogens including *Salmonella* spp., *Y. enterocolitica*, verocytotoxigenic *Escherichia coli* and *C. jejuni* (Jayero and

Henning, 2001). Pathogens frequently detected in raw milk include *Aeromonas* spp., *B. cereus*, *Brucella* spp., *Campylobacter* spp., *Coxiella burnetii*, pathogenic *E. coli*, *L. monocytogenes*, *Mycobacterium spp.*, *Salmonella spp.*, *S. aureus*, *Streptococcus* spp. and *Yersinia* spp. (Oliver et al., 2005). Systematic data from Africa is largely lacking and, with the exception of a few well-studies pathogens such as brucellosis consists mainly of isolated case studies. A recent review by Grace et al. (2007) suggested *B. abortus*, *C. parvum*, *C. burneti*, *C. jejuni*, verocytoxigenic *E. coli*, *L. monocytogenes*, *M. bovis*, *Salmonella* spp., antibiotic residues and mycotoxins were probably important and *Streptococcus equi*, *Str. zooepidemicus*, *S. aureus*, *T. gondii*, *Y. enterocolitica*, *B. cereus* and Rift Valley fever virus were possibly important pathogens.

Using a heuristic to combine the data, we arrived at a list of 27 hazards which were likely to be potential sources of risk to human health in Ethiopia which we later presented to expert informants. This list consisted of 23 pathogens plus 4 chemical hazards. We also included 3 pathogens which are not associated with milk-borne disease in people (*Ehrlichia ruminantium*, *Campylobacter fetus*, and *Pasteurella haemolytica* (now renamed *Mannheimia haemolytica*) as false or check hazards in order to check the accuracy of key informant reporting.

For each of the hazards, we identified associated disease syndromes. Separate lists were generated for syndromes in animals and in people, and for key informant interviews with experts and for PRAs with farmers; in total 4 sets of syndromes. These varied from non-specific syndromes associated with food-borne disease e.g. (vomiting and diarrhoea) to syndromes more closely associated with specific food-borne pathogens (e.g. bloody diarrhoea followed by renal failure in children associated with verocytoxigenic *E. coli* and carpal hygroma associated with brucellosis in cattle).

<u>Step 2: Key informant interviews and Participatory Rural Appraisals</u>

The key medical informants (n=3) considered that 14 of the 27 hazards were present in Debre Zeit. However, there was only consensus (defined for our study as a majority of the informants agreeing on presence) for 8 hazards. None of the 3 non-zoonotic (false) hazards were considered hazards to humans. Among the 6 hazards on which there was consensus, the importance ranking was identical (Table 1). The key veterinary informants (n=3) considered 25 of the 27 hazards were present, and there was consensus on the presence of 19. However, only one informant was able to provide estimates of prevalence (Table 1). None of the respondents indicated that the non-zoonotic (false hazard) pathogen (*Corynebacteria diphtheriae)* was zoonotic).

Table 1. Assessment of the presence and prevalence of potential milk-borne hazards by key informant interviews with doctors (Drs) and veterinarians (Vets) in Debre Zeit, Ethiopia

Hazard	Presence		Prevalence[a]	
	Drs	Vets	Drs	Vets
Aeromonas hydrophila	0	0		
Bacillus cereus	0	1		H
Brucella abortus	0	1		M
Brucella melitensis	0	1		M
Campylobacter fetus	0	1		M
Campylobacter jejuni	1	0	M	
Chlamydia psittaci	0	0		
Clostridium perfringens	0	1		H
Corynebacterium diphtheriae	0	0		
Coxiella burnetti	0	0		
Cryptosporidium parvum	0	1		
Dysentery organisms (e.g. Shigellae)	1	1	H	
Ehrilichia ruminantium	0	1		M
Verocytotoxigenic E. coli	0	0		
Haemolytic streptococci	0	0		
Giardia lamblia	1	0	H	
Leptospira interrogans	0	1		
Listeria monocytogenes	0	1		
Mycobacterium paratuberculosis	0	1		
Multiple drug resistant bacteria	1	1	M	H
Mycobacterium bovis	1	1		M
Salmonella species	1	1	M	H
Staphylococcus aureus	1	1	H	M
Streptococcus zooepidemicus	0	1	M	
Toxoplasma gondii	0	0		
Yersinia enterocolitica	1	0	M	
Antibiotic residues	0	0		
Heavy metals	0	1		H
Mycotoxins	0	1		M
Pesticide residues	0	0		

a. M = medium prevalence (1 to 10%); H = high prevalence (>10%)

Out of 25 syndromes presented to medical experts, 10 were indicative of specific milk-borne disease and there was consensus that 6 of these were present in the community. These syndromes were indicative of campylobacteriosis, salmonellosis and toxigenic infection (believed by medical experts to be present), and with brucellosis, zoonotic tuberculosis and listeriosis (believed by medical experts to be absent). Syndromes consistent with verocytotoxigenic *E. coli* infection and toxoplasmosis were not reported present. Consumers reported presence of all of a simplified list of 16 syndromes including some that were considered absent by medical experts. Interestingly, while all experts considered food-borne disease was present, one considered milk-borne disease was not present. Eight of the 21 sets of syndromes in cattle provided to veterinary experts and managers of large farms were indicative of specific milk-borne disease (brucellosis, listeriosis, tuberculosis and salmonellosis). Veterinarians considered all of these to be present (consensus) but farm managers considered only those consistent with brucellosis to be present. Farmers, however, reported presence of all 11 of the syndromes in the simplified list, including syndromes not reported present by experts.

We added the milk-borne diseases for which syndromic surveillance provided evidence of presence to those identified by either medical or veterinary experts. This generated the list of 19 hazards shown in Table 2 from the initial list of 27 hazards.

Table 2. List of potential hazards in milk in Debre Zeit, Ethiopia derived from key informant interviews and syndromic surveillance

Hazard	
Bacillus cereus	Multiple drug resistant bacteria
Brucella abortus	*Mycobacterium bovis*
Campylobacter jejuni	*Salmonella species*
Clostridium perfringens	*Staphylococcus aureus*
Cryptosporidium parvum	*Streptococcus zooepidemicus*
Dysentery organisms (e.g. Shigellae)	*Toxoplasma gondii*
Verocytotoxigenic *E. coli*	*Yersinia enterocolitica*
Giardia lamblia	Heavy metals
Leptospira interrogans	Mycotoxins
Listeria monocytogenes	

Step 3: Rapid Exposure Assessment

The Rapid Exposure Assessment had two components: firstly an inventory of practices which were likely to amplify or reduce risk on the pathway from cow to consumer and secondly an estimation of the proportion of vulnerable groups and their differential consumption of dairy products. Milk was mainly consumed boiled in tea or coffee (2 out of 5 groups reported daily consumption, typically 250 ml per day). Boiling is a risk mitigating process. The next most common consumption pattern (reported by 2 out of 5 groups) was drinking liquid milk (typically 500 ml per household per day); one group drank pasteurised milk (risk mitigating) while the other drank raw milk. The other consumption pattern was drinking of home-fermented milk or '*ergo*'. Only one group reported this, with a typical consumption of 500 ml per household per day. Groups reported that other dairy products (cottage cheese and butter) were not typically consumed. Milk was bought fresh every day (risk mitigating) from the dairy co-operative (risk mitigating), kiosks selling pasteurised milk (risk mitigating) or neighbours selling raw milk (risk amplifying). Most liquid milk was drunk immediately after bringing to the household (risk mitigating) but some respondents reported storing milk for several hours without refrigeration (risk amplifying) or mixing milk from different sources (risk amplifying). We considered 4 groups of vulnerable people: young (<5 years), old (>60 years), pregnant or lactating women and the immuno-suppressed. Medical key informants estimated their proportions in the population as 15%, 5%, 5% and 3% respectively while consumers estimated their proportions as typically 9%, 3%, 3% and 2%. Relative to adult men and women, consumers considered that children consumed more milk and dairy products, old people less, and pregnant women the same amount. We concluded that a significant minority of respondents consumed substantial quantities of raw, unprocessed milk and so were at risk from milk-borne diseases and that children were at increased risk because of increased exposure.

Step 4: Construction of a risk matrix

Stakeholders identified the following factors as influencing their concern over milk-borne disease: susceptibility of children; ability to cause serious illness or death; ability to cause disease in animals as well as people; high prevalence. They identified two factors affecting the manageability of control: affordability of control and effectiveness of control. The control methods considered were vaccination of animals, testing animals to ensure they were disease free and boiling milk before consumption. The results of this scoring and ranking are shown in Table 3 (this is a preliminary analysis; more detailed results will be available later).

Table 3. Potential hazards in milk in Debre Zeit, Ethiopia ranked according to stakeholder concern and manageability

Hazard	CS	SI/D	AC	HP	AC	EC	Rank
Mycobacterium bovis	1	1	1	0	1	2	6
Brucella abortus	0	1	1	0	1	2	5
Salmonella species	1	1	1	0	1	1	5
Leptospira interrogans	0	1	1	0	1	2	5
Verocytotoxigenic *E. coli*	1	1	0	0	1	1	4
Dysentery organisms	1	0	0	1	1	1	4
Campylobacter jejuni	0	1	0	1	1	1	4
Listeria monocytogenes	0	1	1	0	1	1	4
Clostridium perfringens	0	0	0	1	1	1	3
Cryptosporidium parvum	1	0	0	0	1	1	3
Giardia lamblia	0	0	0	1	1	1	3
Multiple drug resistant bacteria	0	0	0	1	1	1	3
Streptococcus zooepidemicus	0	1	0	0	1	1	3
Toxoplasma gondii	0	0	0	0	1	1	2
Yersinia enterocolitica	0	0	0	0	1	1	2
Mycotoxins	0	1	1	0	0	0	2
Heavy metals	0	0	0	1	0	0	1
Bacillus cereus	0	0	0	1	0	0	1
Staphylococcus aureus	0	0	0	1	0	0	1

CS = Children susceptible, SI/D = Severe illness or death, AC = Affects cattle also, HP = High prevalence, AC=Affordable control, EC=Effective control

DISCUSSION

A fundamental of risk-based approaches to food safety is risk-targeting or prioritisation of hazards according to their potential to cause harm. However, unlike risk assessment there are no standard or consensus methodologies, and currently one of the most active areas of non-laboratory research is Risk Ranking (also known as Hazard Ranking, Risk Attribution, Risk-Based Priority Setting, Comparative Risk Assessment [CRA], or Maintaining a "Risk Register"). While several models have been proposed, their application has been limited in developing countries by cost and complexity.

The method proposed here for Hazard Identification and Exposure Assessment using participatory methods and Syndromic Surveillance was rapid and low cost. We found risk matrices assisted decision-making to help stakeholders systematically address the problem and reach consensus. An advantage of participatory methods is they build on existing knowledge and by triangulating information from different sources improve accuracy and reliability. This was the case in our study. There was reasonable consensus between key informants and none of the key informants failed the check for accuracy and affirmative bias. A disadvantage is that group wisdom fails to detect unknowns, for example verocytotoxigenic *E. coli* is an emerging disease which has not been investigated in the study area and neither medical nor veterinary key informants considered it present. Given its widespread distribution in Africa and its presence in neighbouring countries it is quite likely to be present in Ethiopia and indeed communities recognised the syndrome of renal failure in children after bloody diarrhoea which is strongly associated with this disease. The hazards identified were broadly consistent between stakeholder groups and with literature; in the ongoing phase of the project their presence is being validated through a cross-sectional survey of milk at point of consumption which will provide additional information of the utility of the method.

An interesting finding was the disconnect between veterinary and medical experts in knowledge of zoonotic disease. For example, veterinarians considered brucellosis, leptospirosis and listeriosis to be present in the cattle population but medical respondents were not aware of presence of these contagious zoonotic diseases in people. This finding supports the recent move for better collaboration between the human and medical professions as witnessed by the growing interest in "one medicine" and "one health". Another finding was that disease syndromes were reported present by both farmers and consumers which were consistent with diseases not reported present by professionals. One explanation is that lay people are more sensitive but less specific in their recognition of symptoms; it is also possible the there failure in surveillance and diseases present at community level are not being adequately addressed.

In conclusion, the participatory methodology allowed a rapid, low-cost assessment that engaged stakeholders and is a step towards evidence-based prioritisation of food-borne pathogens.

ACKNOWLEDGEMENTS

This work was supported by the Italian Ministry of Foreign Affairs, Directorate General for Development Cooperation and the Netherlands Development Organisation.

REFERENCES

Adak, G.K., Meakins, S.M., Yip, H., Lopman, B.A., O'Brien, S.J., 2005. Disease risks from foods, England and Wales, 1996-2000. Emerg. Infect. Dis. 11, 365-372.

CDC, 2005. Centers for Disease Control and Prevention. FoodNet, Foodborne Disease Active Surveillance Network, CDC's Emerging Infections Program. Available at: http://www.cdc.gov/FoodNet. Accessed 15 February 2005

DeBuyser, M.L., Dufour, B., Maire, M., Lafarge, V., 2001. Implication of milk and milk products in food-borne diseases in France and in different industrialized countries. Int. J. Food Microbiol. 67, 1–17.

Flint, J., A., Duynhoven, Y.T. Angulo, J., Delong, S.M., Braun, P., Kirk, M., Scallan, E.,

Fitzgerald, M., Adak, G.K., Sockett, P., Ellis, A., Hall, G. Gargouri, N., Walke, H., Braam, P., 2005. Estimating the burden of acute gastroenteritis, foodborne disease, and pathogens commonly transmitted by food: an international review. Clin. Inf. Dis. 41(5), 698-704.

Gillespie, I.A., Adak, G.K., O'Brien, S.J., Bolton, F.J., 2003. Milkborne general outbreaks of infectious intestinal disease, England and Wales, 1992–2000. Epidemiol. Infect. 130, 461–468.

Grace, D., Randolph, T., Omore, A., Schelling E., Bonfoh B., 2007. Place of Food Safety in Evolving Pro-Poor Dairy Policy in East and West Africa. Revue Elev. Med. Vet. Pay Trop. Vol 60, (in process of validation)

FSANZ, 2006. A Risk Profile of Dairy Products in Australia. Food Safety Standards Australia New Zealand, pp. 181.

Hall, G.V., Kirk, M.D., Becker, N., et al., 2005. An estimate of foodborne gastroenteritis in Australia, allowing for uncertainty. Emerg. Infect. Dis. 11, 1257–1264

Jayarao, B.M., Henning, D.R., 2001. Prevalence of Foodborne Pathogens in Bulk Tank Milk. J. Dairy Sci. 84, 2157–2162.

Lynch, M., Painter, J., Woodruff, R., Braden, C., 2006. Surveillance for Foodborne-Disease Outbreaks United States, 1998—2002. Surv. Summ. 55(SS10), 1-34.

Much, P., Pichler, J., Allerberger, F., 2007. Food borne infectious outbreaks, Austria 2005, 1: Wien Klin. Wochenschr. 119(5-6), 150-157.

Oliver S.P., Jayarao, B.M., Almeida, R.A., 2002. Foodborne Pathogens in Milk and the Dairy Farm Environment: Food Safety and Public Health Implications. Foodb. Path. Dis. 2 (2),115-129.

WHO, 2001. The World Health Report 2001. World Health Organisation (WHO), Geneva, Switzerland.

WHO, 2008. The global burden of disease: 2004 update. World Health Organisation (WHO), Geneva, Switzerland.

IMPACT OF THE IMPLEMENTATION OF REST DAYS IN LIVE BIRD MARKETS ON THE DYNAMICS OF H5N1 HIGHLY PATHOGENIC AVIAN INFLUENZA: A MODELLING APPROACH

G. FOURNIE*, F.J. GUITIAN, P. MANGTANI AND A.C. GHANI

SUMMARY

Live bird markets act as a network "hub" and potential reservoir of infection for domestic poultry, thus they may be responsible for sustaining avian influenza virus circulation within the poultry sector. Rest days are periods during which markets are emptied and disinfected. Their potential to modulate the dynamics of highly pathogenic avian influenza (HPAI) within the poultry sector is investigated here using a stochastic meta-population model. A vertical market system with a unidirectional flow of poultry is assumed: from farms, poultry are stored in a unique wholesale market before being transferred to regional markets. Compared to interventions applied in farms, the model shows that frequent rest days are an effective means with which to reduce HPAI transmission. Furthermore, the model predicts that permanent market closure would only be slightly more effective than frequent rest days to reduce transmission. These results are also sensitive to the degree to which indirect transmission occurs directly between farms, and between farms and the regional markets.

INTRODUCTION

Since December 2003 outbreaks of H5N1 Highly Pathogenic Avian Influenza (HPAI) affecting domestic poultry have been reported in 49 countries across the world (OIE, 2008). The virus has also shown potential for cross-species transmission, sporadically infecting humans and other mammals (Peiris et al., 2004). Both the massive economic losses and the putative pandemic threat make H5N1 HPAI one of the greatest current public health concerns. Although interventions have been implemented, the disease is now considered to be endemic in several countries, especially in South-East Asia. Indeed, the drastic measures which allowed developed countries to eradicate past and ongoing HPAI epidemics are not appropriate in all affected areas. Therefore, locally adapted control strategies need to be designed. Some risk factors associated with the local characteristics of poultry production in affected countries have been identified as playing a key role in the sustainability of the virus (Martin et al., 2006; Webster et al., 2006). Among them, live bird trade is considered to be the main pathway for disease transmission (Sims, 2007), making the live bird chain a potential target for implementing control strategies.

From the late 1970s, the abundance and diversity of Avian Influenza (AI) viruses has been recognized in live bird markets (LBMs) (Shortridge et al., 1977): gathering a high density of hosts, live bird markets offer conditions for virus amplification, reassortment and cross-species

---

*Guillaume Fournié, VEPH Group, Royal Veterinary College, Hawkshead Lane, North Mymms, Hatfield, Hertfordshire, AL9 7TA, United Kingdom, email: gfournie@rvc.ac.uk

transmission (Webster, 2004). Therefore, LBMs are thought to play a key role in the epidemiology of avian influenza viruses (Senne et al., 1992). Acting as a network "hub", they may be responsible for sustaining endemic infection within the poultry sector.

Several surveys have highlighted the diversity and abundance of Low Pathogenic Avian Influenza (LPAI) viruses in East Asian LBMs (Guan et al., 2002; Liu et al., 2003; Chen et al., 2006). Moreover H5N1 viruses have been identified in markets where they circulated silently. Whereas no outbreak has been notified in Vietnam before 2003, H5N1 virus had been identified in a LBM around Hanoi in 2001 (Nguyen et al., 2005). During the H5N1 epidemic which affected Hong Kong in 1997, LBMs were found to be highly infected, the prevalence of infection in chickens reaching almost 20% (Guan et al., 2007).

Following multiple outbreaks of H5N1 HPAI in Hong-Kong between 1997 and 2003, control strategies were implemented across the live bird market chain (Sims et al., 2003a; Sims et al., 2003b; Guan et al., 2007). These interventions appear to have been successful as only one outbreak has been notified since 2003 (ProMED-mail, 2008). Among them, rest days, during which markets are emptied and disinfected, have been associated with a significant decrease in the rate of isolation of LPAI viruses in the retail markets (Kung et al., 2003; Lau et al., 2007). Similar observations have been made in the United States: surveys here highlighted that rest days, frequent cleaning and disinfection are factors decreasing the risk that the market is positive for LPAI (Bulaga et al., 2003; Garber et al., 2007; Yee et al., 2008). These observations show on the one hand that rest days may be effective at reducing the prevalence of AI viruses in LBMs, and on the other that the level of infection in markets is not the simple result of multiple introductions of infected birds, but the consequence of virus re-circulation and amplification within them. LBMs could thus sustain the virus. LBMs have also been recognized to be a likely source of infection for domestic poultry flocks: retail marketing of live poultry was implicated as the main source of exposure to infection on chicken farms in Hong Kong during the 2002 H5N1 epidemic (Kung et al., 2007).

The evidence from observational studies therefore suggests that H5N1 HPAI dynamics across the live bird market chain could drive the H5N1 HPAI dynamics in the global poultry sector and that measures implemented in LBMs and further along the market chain could control the spread of the disease. However it remains unclear what the relative contribution of the many other controls implemented simultaneously were in reducing both HPAI and LPAI transmission. Using a modeling approach, we aim to determine the likely impact of strategies implemented within the market chain on the transmission of HPAI H5N1 within poultry sectors and to assess what aspects of the system need to be understood and quantified to determine the success of interventions implemented in LBMs.

MATERIALS AND METHODS

A stochastic meta-population model was constructed to explore the dynamics of HPAI transmission and the impact of various interventions within a poultry production system incorporating LBMs. The model was implemented in Berkeley Madonna version 8.4.14 (Macey and Oster, 2000).

Structure and functioning of the market chain

A vertical market system with a unidirectional flow of poultry comparable to the one in use in Hong-Kong was assumed (Lau et al., 2007): from farms all poultry are stored in a unique wholesale market before being transferred to regional markets (Fig. 1). There are no poultry movements direct from farms to regional markets. Each farm rears 5,000 broiler chickens with a cycle length of 45 days according to all-in-all-out system. When a cycle ends, the infectious reservoir, if present, is then assumed to be removed through disinfection. Mortality due to other causes than HPAI is considered to be negligible.

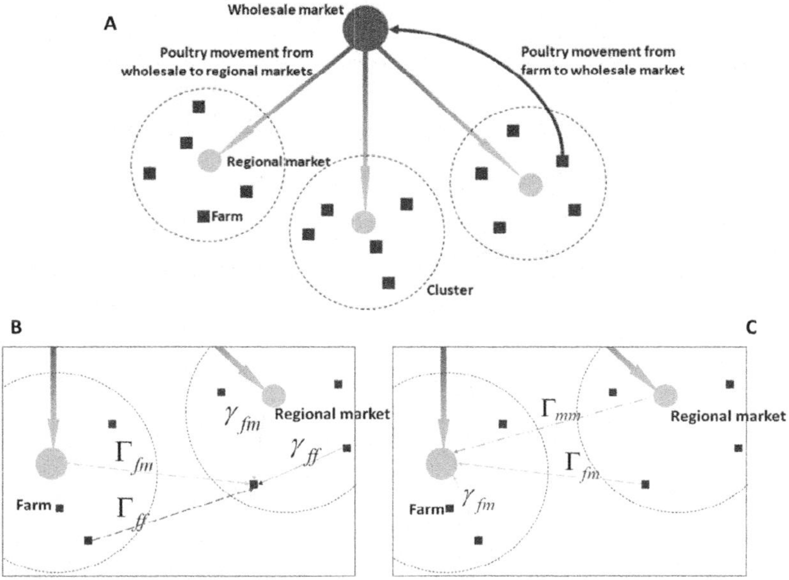

Fig. 1 Diagram of the poultry sector and routes of disease transmission **A** – Diagram of the poultry sector: farms are clustered around regional markets. Poultry movements are from farms to the wholesale market and from the wholesale to regional markets. **B** – A given farm can be infected by farms located in the same cluster (relative strength of mixing: γ_{ff}), by farms in other clusters (Γ_{ff}), by markets in the same cluster (γ_{fm}) and by markets in other clusters (Γ_{fm}). **C** – A given regional market can be infected by introduction of infected birds from the wholesale market, by markets in other clusters (Γ_{mm}), by farms in the same cluster (γ_{fm}) and, by farms in other clusters (Γ_{fm}).

Disease transmission

Within farms, wholesale and regional markets, birds pass through three infection states: susceptible, infected but not infectious and infectious. They die at the end of the infectious period.

Infectious birds contaminate their environment by releasing faeces at each time-step. Faeces infectiousness decreases exponentially with time. Therefore, during the infectious period of a bird, disease is transmitted directly by contact with susceptible birds and indirectly by the contaminated environment. Transmission continues after the death of the infectious bird via the remaining environmental reservoir.

Between flocks, the infection can spread by (i) commercial poultry movements across the market chain from farms to the wholesale market, and from the wholesale market to regional markets, or by (ii) indirect contacts between farms, between farms and regional markets, and between regional markets.

The infection process is stochastic, frequency dependent via direct contact and density dependent via the environment. Homogeneous mixing is assumed. Thus, the force of infection applied to birds within a farm (or a market) depends on the prevalence φ (or ψ) and the environmental load Φ (or Ψ) within this farm (or this market), and the environmental load in other farms and markets. Farms are clustered around each regional market, and the rates of transmission differ within and between clusters (Figure 1): γ_{ff}, γ_{fm} are the relative strength of mixing between farms, and between farms and markets belonging to the same cluster respectively. Γ_{ff}, Γ_{fm}, Γ_{mm} are the relative strength of mixing between farms, between farms and markets, and between markets belonging to different clusters respectively.

In a farm i in a cluster j with $S_{i,j}$ susceptible birds at time t, the number of newly infected birds at $t+dt$ is given by a stochastic binomial variable $B(\lambda_{i,j}(t),S_{i,j}(t))$, with $\lambda_{i,j}(t)$ the force of infection (i.e. the rate at which poultry get infected between t and $t+dt$) defined as follows:

$$\lambda_{i,j}(t) = 1 - exp\left\{-\beta \times \begin{pmatrix} \varphi_{i,j}(t) + \eta \times \Phi_{i,j}(t) \\ +\gamma_{ff} \times \sum_{l \neq j} \Phi_{i,l}(t) \\ +\Gamma_{ff} \times \sum_{k \neq i,l} \Phi_{k,l}(t) \\ +\gamma_{fm} \times \Psi_i(t) \\ +\Gamma_{fm} \times \sum_{k \neq i} \Psi_k(t) \end{pmatrix} \times dt\right\} \quad \begin{matrix} \text{Within farm infection process} \\ \text{Farms in the same cluster} \\ \text{Farms in other clusters} \\ \text{Market in the same cluster} \\ \text{Markets in other clusters} \end{matrix} \tag{1}$$

Similarly in a regional market i:

$$\lambda_i(t) = 1 - exp\left\{-\beta \times \begin{pmatrix} \vartheta \times (\psi_i(t) + \eta \times \Psi_i(t)) \\ +\gamma_{fm} \times \sum_{l = j} \Phi_{i,l}(t) \\ +\Gamma_{fm} \times \sum_{k \neq i,l} \Phi_{k,l}(t) \\ +\Gamma_{mm} \times \sum_{k \neq i} \Psi_k(t) \end{pmatrix} \times dt\right\} \quad \begin{matrix} \text{Within market infection process} \\ \text{Farms in the same cluster} \\ \text{Farms in other clusters} \\ \text{Markets in other clusters} \end{matrix} \tag{2}$$

Here β is the within farm rate of transmission between chickens, η is the relative rate of transmission of environmental load compared to β, and υ is the relative strength of mixing within market.

We assume that $\Gamma_{fm}=\Gamma_{mm}$. f/m is then defined as the ratio between farm-to-farm and farm-to-market rates of transmission:

$$f/m = \frac{\gamma_{ff}}{\gamma_{fm}} = \frac{\Gamma_{ff}}{\Gamma_{fm}} \quad (3)$$

If *f/m* is low, the routes of transmission involving markets are more important than the ones involving only farms (i.e. the main source of infection of farms are markets). In contrast, if *f/m* is high the routes of transmission involving markets are less important than the ones involving only farms (i.e. the main source of infection of farms are other farms).

Outcome

We calculate the flock reproduction number *r*, defined as the expected number of secondary cases (market or farm) per single infected case in a fully susceptible population, using the approach advocated by Diekmann and Heesterbeek (2000). The reproduction number assesses the potential for infection to be sustained: if it is greater than one, the epidemic will almost always spread whereas if it is less than one the infection is more likely to go extinct.

We denote r^f to be the flock reproduction number when the market chain has been removed (i.e. markets are no longer infectious).

r and r^f were calculated using R software 2.7.1 (R Development Core Team, 2008).

Scenarios

The flock reproduction number *r* is assumed initially to be equal to five. Three scenarios corresponding to three different values of *f/m* are considered:

- *f/m*=1 (r^f/r=0.04): almost all farm outbreaks are due to market-to-farm transmission
- *f/m*=10 (r^f/r=0.32): most farm outbreaks are due to market-to-farm transmission
- *f/m*=50 (r^f/r=0.7): most farm outbreaks are due to farm-to-farm transmission

The impact of the following control strategies on *r* is assessed:

Early detection of outbreaks in farms and stamping out: An outbreak is detected if the mortality rate exceeds 0.5% during two successive 24 hours periods, two days after which birds are culled out, the farm is emptied and the infectious reservoir is assumed to be removed through disinfection and/or isolation.

Vaccination in farms: 50% of chickens are vaccinated at the start of each cycle. The vaccine is assumed to be fully protective two weeks after vaccination occurs.

Diagnostic tests in farms: These tests refer to detection of virus by PCR from tracheal and cloacal swabs. At the end of each cycle, some birds are sampled and tested for detection of viral shedding. If at least one test is positive, the flock is culled out, before being sent to the wholesale market.

Rest days in live bird markets: Rest days, times during which LBMs are emptied, remaining birds are culled out and the infectious reservoir is assumed to be removed via disinfection. We assume that these days are synchronized in the wholesale and regional markets.

Live bird market closure: The live bird market chain is permanently closed.

RESULTS

Figure 2 compares the impact of control strategies applied in farms (stamping out and vaccination) with rest days in LBMs on the flock reproduction number r. For f/m=1, the relation between r and the frequency of rest days is non-linear (Figure 2): when the time between two successive rest days is shortened (i.e. the rest days are more frequent), the slope of the curve increases and the additional impact of an increase in the frequency of rest days on r is amplified. However, as f/m is increased (i.e. as farm-to-farm transmission becomes more important), the relationship between r and the frequency of rest day becomes linear and the benefit of more frequent rest days is lost. Furthermore, the impact of rest days on r is smaller as f/m is increased. Whereas rest days applied every ten days in LBMs are enough to reduce r below one when f/m=1, they would need to be implemented in combination with stamping out and vaccination to decrease r below this threshold when f/m=10 or 50.

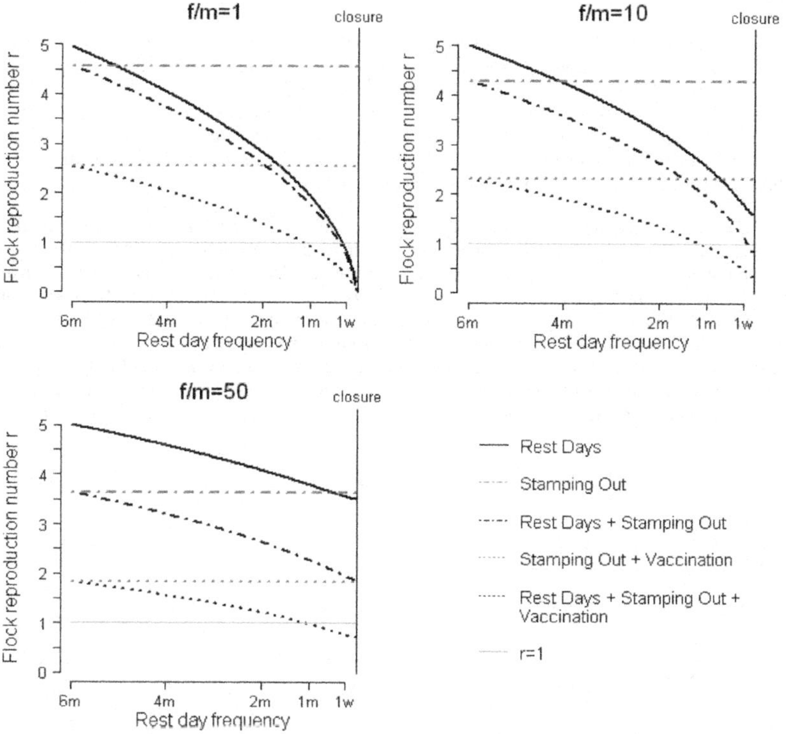

Fig. 2 Comparison of the effects of stamping out, vaccination and rest days on the flock reproduction number *r*. *f/m* refers to the ratio between the rate of transmission from farm to farm and rate of transmission from market to farm – for *f/m*=1 transmission from farm-to-market dominates whereas for *f/m*=50 transmission from farm-to-farm dominates whilst *f/m*=10 is an intermediate scenario. *6m*: rest days every 6 months; *1w*: rest days once a week; *closure*: the market chain is closed

Control strategies applied in farms show an opposite pattern: they have a greater impact on *r* as *f/m* increases (i.e. the extent of farm-to-farm transmission increases). Compared to rest days, stamping out plus vaccination is less effective when *f/m* is low: for *f/m*=1 and 10, an equivalent reduction in the reproduction number *r* to that achieved by stamping out plus vaccination can be achieved with rest days alone implemented every seven and three weeks respectively. In contrast, if farm-to-farm transmission dominates (*f/m*=50), then vaccination plus stamping out is a much more effective policy than frequent rest days or market closure. However, even for a high degree of farm-to-farm transmission (*f/m*=50), stamping out without vaccination is still less effective than rest days implemented twice a month. For all values of *f/m*, monthly rest days implemented in combination with stamping out and vaccination could reduce *r* below its threshold of one.

Permanent market closure appears to be only slightly more effective than weekly rest days. Indeed, in all scenarios in which market closure results in *r* falling below the threshold value of one, weekly rest days also achieve this reduction (e.g. for *f/m*=1). Moreover, as the degree of farm-to-farm transmission (*f/m*) increases and the relation between *r* and rest day frequency becomes linear, the difference between *r* in a system with weekly rest days and *r* in a system without markets becomes smaller: for *f/m*=1, this difference is equal to 0.55, for *f/m*=10 and 50, this difference is then equal to 0.17 and 0.04 respectively.

The impact of diagnostic testing on the proportion of infected flocks sent to the market chain and the flock reproduction number *r* is shown in Figure 3. Sampling and testing 20 birds at the end of each cycle will reduce the number of infected flocks introduced into the market chain by 50%, but its impact on *r* is low, *r* decreasing only by between 22% and 33%, depending on the value of *f/m* and with *r* remaining higher than 2.8. Moreover, as the number of birds tested increases, the slope of the curve decreases. Therefore the benefit of testing a large number of birds is limited. Indeed, increasing the sampling to 100 birds per cycle would only lead to a reduction in infected flock movements by 63% compared to 50% reduction achieved if 20 birds are sampled and *r* would remain higher than 2.6.

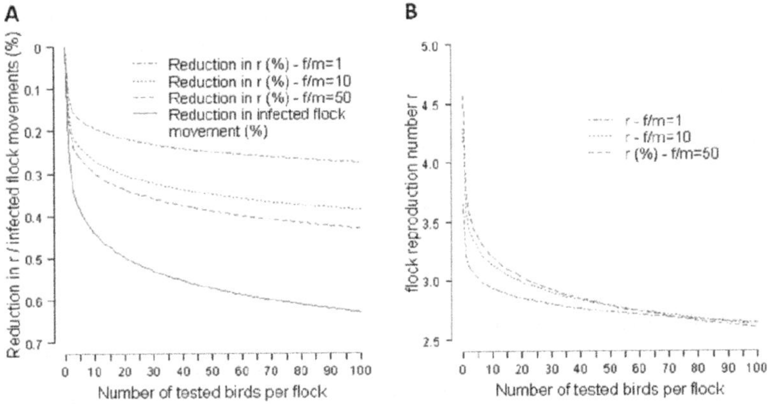

Fig. 3 Effect of diagnostic testing on the movement of infected flocks and the flock reproduction number *r* **A** – Reduction in *r* and infected flock movement (expressed in percentage) as a function of the number of tested birds per flock. **B** – Flock reproduction number *r* as a function of the number of tested birds per flock. All flocks are assumed to be tested. Stamping out is also applied.

DISCUSSION

In this study a meta-population model has been used to assess if LBMs could be an appropriate target for controlling the spread of H5N1 within the poultry sector. The results show that rest days implemented in LBMs can have a strong impact on disease dynamics within the poultry sector. Depending on the characteristics of the system, and especially the relative importance of transmission routes involving markets compared to those only involving farms, rest days can be more effective than control strategies applied in farms to reduce disease transmission. Moreover, as rest days will target other transmission routes, their effect acts in synergy with stamping out and vaccination.

For scenarios in which most transmission occurs from market-to-farm (low values of *f/m*), this study has shown that the impact of rest days on *r* is amplified as the time between two successive rest days decreases. In fact, if rest days are implemented sufficiently frequently, virus amplification would be halted in the market before it reaches endemic levels and as a result, the infectivity from the market to other flocks will be drastically reduced.

In contrast virological tests appear to be less effective than rest days under all considered parameter settings. In relatively large flocks, such as those considered in the model, detection of the disease at the start of the infection course would require a far higher number of tests than is feasible. With the numbers of tests considered here this intervention fails to prevent infected flocks from entering into the market chain. However, the influence of flock size on the effectiveness of virological testing needs to be taken into consideration in generalizing these results.

Compared to weekly rest days, the benefit of permanent market closure seems to be limited. Instead this measure could have some strong unintended effects on the structure of the live bird trade chain. Indeed, in societies where this habit is culturally well entrenched, and where this activity ensures the livelihood of many stakeholders, such a ban may not stop this activity (Meleigy, 2007), but it may change the structure of the market chain, which would then be more difficult to control. The rationale behind the banning of LBMs, as it has been implemented in some countries, should thus be put into question.

In conclusion, frequent rest days in live bird markets are an effective means with which to reduce HPAI transmission. Indeed, if LBMs are a driver of the disease dynamics, they are also focal points where it may be possible to implement effective interventions which may be more cost-effective than the ones applied in farms. However, their impact will depend on the patterns of contacts between farms, regional markets and wholesale markets as well as the risk of transmission between each of these locations. The relative weight of transmission routes involving or not LBMs will be key to determine which interventions are best suited to local circumstances and at which levels they should be applied. Here, the poultry system is assumed to be highly structured and homogeneous, yet most countries where H5N1 is a recurrent problem have a heterogeneous poultry sector and a much more complex market chain. The impact of control strategies implemented in LBMs could thus vary. Moreover, whilst there is some evidence to suggest that markets amplify and sustain the virus cycle, further investigations on their role are required. Therefore, further data on the different market systems in AI-affected countries could help to elucidate the potential impact of rest days as well as to define their optimal frequency in terms of their impact on circulating HPAI virus.

ACKNOWLEDGEMENTS

GF thanks the Bloomsbury consortium for PhD funding. ACG acknowledges support from the MRC as part of the MRC Centre for Outbreak Modelling and Analysis.

REFERENCES

Bulaga, L.L., Garber, L., Senne, D.A., Myers, T.J., Good, R., Wainwright, S., Trock, S., Suarez,

D.L., 2003. Epidemiologic and surveillance studies on avian influenza in live-bird markets in New York and New Jersey, 2001. Avian Dis 47, 996-1001.

Chen, H., Smith, G.J., Li, K.S., Wang, J., Fan, X.H., Rayner, J.M., Vijaykrishna, D., Zhang, J.X., Zhang, L.J., Guo, C.T., Cheung, C.L., Xu, K.M., Duan, L., Huang, K., Qin, K., Leung, Y.H., Wu, W.L., Lu, H.R., Chen, Y., Xia, N.S., Naipospos, T.S., Yuen, K.Y., Hassan, S.S., Bahri, S., Nguyen, T.D., Webster, R.G., Peiris, J.S., Guan, Y., 2006. Establishment of multiple sublineages of H5N1 influenza virus in Asia: implications for pandemic control. Proc Natl Acad Sci U S A 103, 2845-2850.

Diekmann, O. and Heesterbeek, J.A.P., 2000. Mathematical Epidemiology of Infectious Diseases : Model Building, Analysis and Interpretation. Wiley Series, Chichester.

Garber, L., Voelker, L., Hill, G., Rodriguez, J., 2007. Description of live poultry markets in the United States and factors associated with repeated presence of H5/H7 low-pathogenicity avian influenza virus. Avian Dis 51, 417-420.

Guan, Y., Chen, H., Li, K.S., Riley, S., Leung, G.M., Webster, R., Peiris, M., Yuen, K.Y., 2007. A model to control the epidemic of H5N1 influenza at the source. BMC Infect Dis 7, 132.

Guan, Y., Peiris, J.S., Lipatov, A.S., Ellis, T.M., Dyrting, K.C., Krauss, S., Zhang, L.J., Webster, R.G., Shortridge, K.F., 2002. Emergence of multiple genotypes of H5N1 avian influenza viruses in Hong Kong SAR. Proc Natl Acad Sci U S A 99, 8950-8955.

Kung, N.Y., Guan, Y., Perkins, N.R., Bissett, L., Ellis, T., Sims, L., Morris, R.S., Shortridge, K.F., Peiris, J.S., 2003. The impact of a monthly rest day on avian influenza virus isolation rates in retail live poultry markets in Hong Kong. Avian Dis 47, 1037-1041.

Kung, N.Y., Morris, R.S., Perkins, N.R., Sims, L.D., Ellis, T.M., Bissett, L., Chow, M., Shortridge, K.F., Guan, Y., Peiris, M.J., 2007. Risk for infection with highly pathogenic influenza A virus (H5N1) in chickens, Hong Kong, 2002. Emerg Infect Dis 13, 412-418.

Lau, E.H.Y., Leung, Y.H.C., Zhang, L.J., Cowling, B.J., Mak, S.P., Guan, Y., Leung, G.M., Peiris, J.S.M., 2007. Effect of Interventions on Influenza A (H9N2) Isolation in Hong Kong's Live Poultry Markets, 1999–2005. Emerg Infect Dis 13, 1340-1347.

Liu, M., He, S., Walker, D., Zhou, N., Perez, D.R., Mo, B., Li, F., Huang, X., Webster, R.G., Webby, R.J., 2003. The influenza virus gene pool in a poultry market in South central china. Virology 305, 267-275.

Macey, R., Oster, G., 2000. Berkeley Madonna: Modelling and analysis of dynamics systems. Available from: http://www.berkeleymadonna.com

Martin, V., Sims, L., Lubroth, J., Pfeiffer, D., Slingenbergh, J., Domenech, J., 2006. Epidemiology and ecology of highly pathogenic avian influenza with particular emphasis on South East Asia. Dev Biol (Basel) 124, 23-36.

Meleigy, M., 2007. Egypt battles with avian influenza. Lancet 370, 553-554.

Nguyen, D.C., Uyeki, T.M., Jadhao, S., Maines, T., Shaw, M., Matsuoka, Y., Smith, C., Rowe, T., Lu, X.H., Hall, H., Xu, X.Y., Balish, A., Klimov, A., Tumpey, T.M., Swayne, D.E., Huynh, L.P.T., Nghiem, H.K., Nguyen, H.H.T., Hoang, L.T., Cox, N.J., Katz, J.M., 2005. Isolation and characterization of avian influenza viruses, including highly pathogenic H5N1, from poultry in live bird markets in Hanoi, Vietnam, in 2001. J Virol 79, 4201-4212.

OIE, 2008. H5N1 Reported in Domestic Poultry 2003-2008. Paris. Available from http://www.oie.int/eng/info_ev/en_AI_factoids_3.htm

Peiris, J.S., Yu, W.C., Leung, C.W., Cheung, C.Y., Ng, W.F., Nicholls, J.M., Ng, T.K., Chan, K.H., Lai, S.T., Lim, W.L., Yuen, K.Y., Guan, Y., 2004. Re-emergence of fatal human influenza A subtype H5N1 disease. Lancet 363, 617-619.

ProMED-mail, 2008. Avian Influenza (75): China (Hong Kong S.A.R.) Bird flu virus found in market stalls. Available from:

http://www.promedmail.org/pls/otn/f?p=2400:1001:4465822385385527::NO::F2400_P1001_BACK_PAGE,F2400_P1001_PUB_MAIL_ID:10001,72755

R Development Core Team, 2008. A Language and Environment for Statistical Computing and Graphics. Available from: http://www.r-project.org

Senne, D.A., Pearson, J.E., Panigrahy, B., 1992. Live poultry markets: a missing link in the epidemiology of avian influenza. In: Beard, C.W., Easterday, B.C. (Eds.), Proceeding of Third International Symposium on Avian Influenza. United States Animal Health Association, Richmond, VA, pp. 50-58.

Shortridge, K.F., Butterfield, W.K., Webster, R.G., Campbell, C.H., 1977. Isolation and characterization of influenza A viruses from avian species in Hong Kong. Bull World Health Organ 55, 15-20.

Sims, L.D., 2007. Lessons learned from Asian H5N1 outbreak control. Avian Dis 51, 174-181.

Sims, L.D., Ellis, T.M., Liu, K.K., Dyrting, K., Wong, H., Peiris, M., Guan, Y., Shortridge, K.F., 2003a. Avian influenza in Hong Kong 1997-2002. Avian Dis 47, 832-838.

Sims, L.D., Guan, Y., Ellis, T.M., Liu, K.K., Dyrting, K., Wong, H., Kung, N.Y., Shortridge, K.F., Peiris, M., 2003b. An update on avian influenza in Hong Kong 2002. Avian Dis 47, 1083-1086.

Webster, R.G., 2004. Wet markets--a continuing source of severe acute respiratory syndrome and influenza? Lancet 363, 234-236.

Webster, R.G., Peiris, M., Chen, H., Guan, Y., 2006. H5N1 outbreaks and enzootic influenza. Emerg Infect Dis 12, 3-8.

Yee, K.S., Carpenter, T.E., Mize, S., Cardona, C.J., 2008. The live bird market system and low-pathogenic avian influenza prevention in southern California. Avian Dis 52, 348-352.

INFECTIOUS DISEASE MODELING

EPIDEMIOLOGY AND ENVIRONMENTAL RISK FACTORS OF WEST NILE VIRUS INFECTION IN THE SENEGAL RIVER BASIN

V. CHEVALIER*, A. DUPRESSOIR, A.L. TRAN, O.M. DIOP, E. ETTER, A.A. SALL, N. GAIDET, M. DIA , V. SOTI AND M. NIANG

SUMMARY

West Nile virus (WNV) transmission was shown to be endemic in the Ferlo area, a sahelian part of Senegal. A serological study was carried out on horses in the Senegal river basin to assess the epidemiological status of this area for WNV transmission and try to identify environmental risk factors of this transmission. Two Landsat Enhanced Thematic Mapper satellite images from the dry and wet seasons were used to provide a land-cover map of the study area. Using a generalized linear mixed model and a component analysis strategy, the results showed that (i) WNV is endemic in this region; (ii) the transmission differed with landscape despite a global high transmission level. This first landscape approach in an endemic area may provide a method to identify risk areas in non-endemic regions and target surveillance

INTRODUCTION

West Nile fever (WNF) is an emerging arbovirosis caused by West Nile virus (WNV) (*Flavivirus, Flaviviridae*). WNF epidemiology is complex: the virus is transmitted between birds (wild and domestic) by *Culicidae* mosquitoes (mainly *Culex* genus). Horses and man are accidental hosts. WNV circulation has been often recorded in wetlands (Durand et al., 2002) but also in urban (Savage et al., 1999) or in dry areas (Chevalier et al., 2006) The influence of environmental factors on WNV circulation remains poorly understood.

WNV has been isolated several times from *Aedes* and *Culex* mosquitoes in the Senegal River Valley (northern Senegal) (Traore-Lamizana et al. 1994). Known as a major wintering area for European migratory birds, this area is suspected to be a source of WNV for Europe, WNV being transported by migrating birds.

In 2005, an eco-epidemiological study was carried out in the Senegal River valley. The goals were (i) to estimate the serological point prevalence of anti-WNV antibodies in horses thereby assessing the epidemiological situation for WNV infection and (ii) to identify environmental factors potentially linked to WNV infection.

* Veronique Chevalier, International Centre of Agronomy for Development (CIRAD), UR AGIRs, Campus International de Baillarguet, 34398 Montpellier Cedex 5, France, email: chevalier@cirad.fr

MATERIALS AND METHODS

Study area

The study area was located in the north-west part of Senegal, between 15.72° and 16.65° North and -16.64° and -15.55° East. This area presents contrasting landscapes with wet areas (swamps, rice fields) bordering the Senegal River and dry areas (herbaceous savannah, coastal dunes). This region has two seasons, the rainy season from June to October, characterized by heat, humidity and storms, and the dry season from November to May characterized by Harmattan wind. Within this area, 5 study zones were identified to carry out the epidemiological survey on WNV infection. These 10 km radius zones were chosen to be representative of the different land cover found in this zone, based on image interpretation of a Landsat Enhanced Thematic Mapper (ETM+) satellite image (4 March 2003) and field observations (Figure 1). From west to east, the first zone was chosen around Saint Louis town. The heart of St Louis is located on a narrow island (just over 2 km long and about 400 m wide) in the Senegal River, 25 km from its mouth. At this point the river is separated from the Atlantic Ocean to the west by a narrow sand stretch, the Langue de Barbarie (300 m wide), which has also been urbanized. A third part of the city, lies on the eastern mainland and is nearly surrounded by tidal marches. Saint-Louis is situated on the Mauritanian border and the landscape is characterized by occasional acacias and is disturbed by sand storms during the dry season. When the river overflows into the countryside, Saint Louis is surrounded by flood basins. The salt water creates small ponds and stretches of mangroves. Many birds come here to feed, including flamingos and pelicans. The second zone was located in the Djoud'j National Park (PNOD). The PNOD is a 16,000-ha wetland located on the border between Mauritania and Senegal, in the Senegal River delta. It is made of a large lake surrounded by streams, ponds and backwaters. Land cover is mainly composed of acacia swamps, muddy areas, reed bed, and rice fields. PNOD is known as a major African wintering area for palearctic birds. The third study site was centred on Ross-Bethio town. The landscape surrounding Ross-Bethio is typically sahelian, characterized by sand dunes, absence of green vegetation apart from some scattered trees and shrubs during the dry season. During the rainy season the vegetation is composed of a herbaceous layer and a sparse woody plant population. The fourth study zone was centred on Richard-Toll town. Richard-Toll is located near the Senegal River, 80 km far from St Louis. Apart from the city, this study site was mainly composed of small areas of agriculture, such as rice, crops, sugar cane and savannah. The last study site one was centred on Nguith village located on the border of the Lac de Guiers, known for its large population of migrating birds. The West part of this site was mainly composed of dry savannah (Figure 1).

Environmental data

Two ETM+ satellite images from the dry (4 March 2003) and wet (4 November 1999) seasons were used to provide a land-cover map of the study area. This type of sensor was chosen because the resolution (pixel size of 30x30 m) is adapted for the extraction of birds' habitats, hosts of the WNV, and because it allows coverage of the whole study area. An ecological characterisation of bird habitats was first conducted at 230 sites spread over the entire study area during a field survey conducted in March 2006. A supervised classification was then performed on the image from March using these sites as a training dataset (image processing software: ERDAS Imagine). The second image from the wet season was processed to map the flooded areas after the rainfall period. The accuracy of the classification was evaluated from a confusion matrix using a different set of training data (190 ground control points).

From this land-cover map, the surface covered by each land-cover type was calculated for each study zone using Geographic Information System (GIS) functionalities (GIS software:

ESRI ArcGIS™, Spatial Analyst).

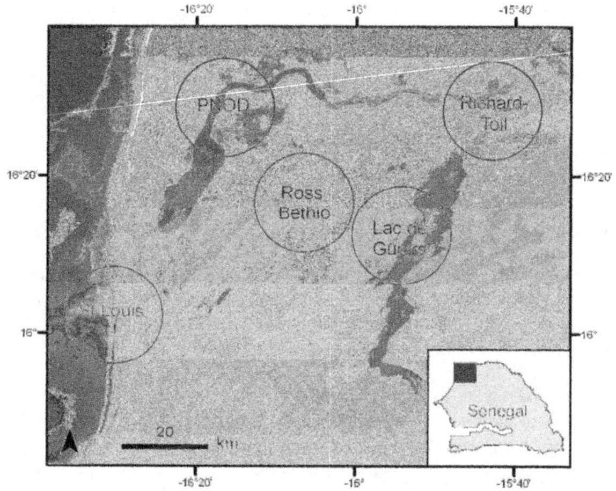

Fig. 1 Study area and location of the field study sites for the serological survey (Background: Landsat ETM+ image, 4 March 2003, © NASA Landsat Program, USGS, Sioux Falls. Data source: Global Land Cover Facility, www.landcover.org)

Epidemiological and serological data

In each study site, a market was purposively identified, this market being the centre of a buffer zone of 10km radius. In each site, 80 horses were randomly selected in the corresponding market and blood sampled. Horse ages as well as the GPS coordinates of the place they were living were recorded. Horses living out from the buffer were discarded from the study. Samples were centrifuged, stored at 4°C before being analysed for anti-WNV antibodies, IgM and IgG, using an ELISA test. Positive sera were confirmed by seroneutralisation test. Horse prevalence data were used to estimate the annual incidence rate in horses, following a method previously used and assuming (a) a constant annual incidence, (b) a lifelong persistence of neutralizing antibodies, and (c) that mortality related to WNV was nil (Chevalier et al., 2006).

Statistical Analysis

Horses were grouped in 3 age classes: 2-7 years (n=102), 8-10 years (n=120) and 10-24 years (n=145). Because of the sampling frame (horses clustered in sites), serological data were firstly analysed using a generalized linear mixed model (GLMM, R software), with age classes as a fixed effect and the site as potentially grouping effect. The individual serological status was the response. To assess the effect of environmental variables on the site prevalence, serological data were secondarily analysed with the serological status of sites as response. As the surfaces occupied by the cover types within a buffer were highly correlated, a principal component analysis (PCA) was carried out to synthesize the initial information on the landscape into independent factors, i.e. principal component (PC). These factors were included in the second statistical model as the explanatory variables.

RESULTS

The landscape map derived from the satellite imagery included 23 classes, that belonged to four main landscape types: human and cultivated areas (urban area, market gardens, rice-fields, sugar-cane plantations, bare soil, other cultures), arid land areas (shrubland, thorn-bush savanna , grassland), wetlands (temporary and permanent ponds, open water, backwater, floating aquatic vegetation, marshes with scirpus and rushes; alluvial grassland) and coastal areas (sea, estuarine and_intertidal mudflats, herbaceous, shrubby and woody coastal sand dune, mangrove, seasonally inundated brackish lagoons, saline flats with vegetation). The overall accuracy of the classification estimated was correct (82.54 %) with 0.79 for the Kappa index.

Four synthetic variables (PC) resulted from the PCA. The main negative contributor of PC1 was sea water, grassy vegetation and inundated during rainy season "tan" (banks of mudflats). PC2 was mainly composed of halophyte vegetation, PC3 of free water, and PC4 positively with sugar cane and negatively with never inundated naked "tan".

A total of 367 horses were included in the study, their ages ranging from 2 to 24 years. The overall IgG seroprevalence rate was 85% [95% CI=0.81-0.89]. The prevalences (P) were significantly different from one study site to the remainder (Chi-square=16.17; df=4; p=0.003), with the highest prevalence rate in the Nguith site (P=95%, n=56), then in Richard Toll (P=92%, n=79), Ross Bethio (P=86%, n=50), PNOD (P=82%, n=71). The lower prevalence rate was observed in Saint Louis site (P=74%, n=80). The IgM seroprevalence was nil. The estimated serological prevalence was 21%.

Results of the generalized linear mixed model showed that the prevalence rate significantly increased with age (Table 1). The estimated random effect's standard deviation was 0.49, suggesting that prevalence site was linked not only with age but also with the site ecological components. PC1 and PC4 were statistically linked to the site serological status ($p=8.10^{-4}$ and p=0.04, respectively) suggesting that the components of PC1, sea water, grassland and inundated during rainy season "tan", were protective factors whereas the main component of PC 4, sugar cane, was a risk factor for WNV transmission.

Table 1. Results of the generalized linear mixed model (horse's serological data, Senegal River Basin, 2005)

Variable	Reference	Coef	z	p-value
Intercept		1.168	3.564	0.00037
Age 8-10 yrs	Age 2-7yrs	0.931	2.519	0.0118
Age 10-24 yrs	Age 2-7yrs	1.329	3.444	0.00057

DISCUSSION

This study confirms that WNV circulation is endemic in the Senegal River basin. Serological results were in accordance with a previous study performed in the Ferlo area where the seroprevalence rate in horses was estimated to be 78% in 2003 (Chevalier et al., 20006).

With respect to IgM seroprevalence being nil, horses were sampled in July which is the beginning of the rainy season. In the Senegal River basin, the *Culex* population is almost nil from November to June (B. Mondet, personal communication) and starts to increase with the first rain events, at the end of July.

The location where horses were living was taken into account for the environmental analysis because *Culex* mosquitoes have a crepuscular or nocturnal activity. Therefore the location where horses live was also the place where they were infected.

Based on expert opinion and previous field knowledge, we assumed that people walked no more than 10 km from their house to join the market. This estimation was used to define the radius of the area from which environmental data were extracted considering that horses located in this buffer were equally exposed to mosquito bites.

Despite an overall prevalence estimated as 21%, we showed that the transmission level varied according to the study site and that the transmission level was linked to the type of landscape. The biology of *Culex pipiens*, one of the main vectors of WNV in Senegal, probably explains the results of the environmental analysis. *Culex* mosquitoes prefer water contaminated with organic matter for the development of the larvae and feed preferentially on mammals. "Tan" are very dry surfaces where nothing but acacias may survive. This land cover type is thus particularly unfavorable to these mosquitoes. *Culex* larvae can not survive in salted water. Moreover, the wind resulting from the proximity with the sea may explain why WNV transmission is lower in St Louis than in the other selected sites. Organic components are highly represented in sugar cane fields, possibly explaining why the presence of sugar cane is a risk factor.

The preliminary results need be confirmed and extended. The identification of risky landscapes in endemic areas should help to understand the key factors of WNV transmission and to target virological and serological surveillance either in these areas or in risky European areas.

ACKNOWLEDGMENTS

This work was granted by GOCE-2003-010284 EDEN grants.(www.edenfp6project. net)

REFERENCES

Chevalier V., Lancelot R., Diaité A., Mondet B., Sall B., de Lamballerie X. (2006) Serological assessment of West Nile fever virus activity in the pastoral system of Ferlo (Senegal). Ann NY Acad Sci. 216-225.

Durand B., Chevalier V., Pouillot R., Labie J., Marendat I., Murgue B., et al. (2002) West Nile Virus outbreak in horses, Southern France, 2000: results of a serosurvey. Emerg Infect Dis. 8, 777-782.

Savage H.M., Ceianu C., Nicolescu G., Karabatsos N., Lanciotti R., Vladimirescu A., et al. (1999) Entomologic and avian investigations of an epidemic of West Nile fever in Romania in 1996, with serologic and molecular characterization of a virus isolate from mosquitoes [published erratum appears in Am J Trop Med Hyg (2000) 62, 162]. Am J Trop Med Hyg. 61, 600-611.

Traore-Lamizana M., Zeller H.G., Mondo M., Hervy J.P., Adam F., Digoutte J.P. (1994) Isolations of West Nile and Bagaza viruses from mosquitoes (*Diptera: Culicidae*) in central Senegal (Ferlo). J Med Entomol. 31, 934-938.

RELEVANCE OF HYPOTHESIS IN EPIDEMIOLOGICAL MODELLING: APPLICATION TO PATHOGEN SPREAD WITHIN PIG HERDS

A. LURETTE*, M. ANDRAUD, N. ROSE AND C. BELLOC

SUMMARY

Due to economic and public health consequences, control of pathogens spread within pig herds is a major concern for the pork food chain. To study the pathogen spread within pig herds, and then, assessing potential control measures, models describing both population dynamics and epidemiology are needed.

The objective of this study was to assess the relevance of the modelling hypotheses concerning both the population and the infection dynamics representation level, and of the implications of these hypotheses on the pathogen spread results.

Two models describing the pigs' and sows' dynamics within farrow-to-finish pig herds were developed. The first model was an individual based model with a time step of one day (IBM/day model). The second one used the batch as the modelling unit and a time step of one week (batch/week model). Firstly, the adequacy of the zootechnical parameters of the two models was checked. Then, the two population dynamics models were coupled, firstly with a PCV2 (Porcine Circovirus type 2) epidemiological model and secondly with a *Salmonella* epidemiological model.

The results of seroprevalence in batches of pigs from birth to slaughterhouse delivery were compared for each pathogen combined with each model of population dynamics. The evolution of PCV2 seroprevalence with time in a batch obtained from both population models was very close. However, the variability of the seroprevalence was lower for the batch/week model than for the IBM/day model. The mean seroprevalence of *Salmonella* was slightly higher for the IBM/day model than for the other one. Gain in terms of simulation time is significant (30 seconds for the batch/week model instead of 3 minutes in the case of the IBM model for a one-year simulation) and can lead to assessment of the effect of a higher number of control measure and combinations of measures.

Simplifying the representation level and increasing the time-step could not perfectly handle the variation in infectious potential according to time since infection. This major issue in the case of PCV2 infection might have led to homogenize the animal health status. However, this representation level is suitable to represent *Salmonella* spread. Depending on the pathogen considered and the objectives targeted, the modelling hypothesis can allow assessment of the effect of control measures on the mean comportment of the model and/or on its extreme cases.

---

*Amandine Lurette, INRA, ENVN, UMR1300 Bio-Agression, Epidémiologie et Analyse de Risque, F-44300 Nantes, France. Now at : Population and Disease Group, Dept of Biological Sciences, The University of Warwick, Coventry CV4 7AL UK. E-mail : A.Lurette@warwick.ac.uk

However, to assess the efficiency of control measures, a large number of scenarios are needed. Simplifying the population dynamics could be then a good trade-off to optimise the use of epidemiological models for scenario assessments.

INTRODUCTION

Control of pathogen spread within pig herds is a major concern for the swine industry. Actually, the related infections can lead to economic and public health consequences. For studying infectious diseases, the modelling approach is a useful tool which complements the experimental or observational data. Epidemiological models can help to improve knowledge about infectious processes by contributing to identify the key factors for pathogen spread. It can also help to improve pathogen control through the *ex-ante* assessment of control measures efficiency. For studying the pathogen spread within pig herds, which are structured and dynamic populations, models describing both population dynamics and epidemiology are needed.

Many different types of epidemiological models can be found in the literature and most of the time, different models can be built for a given issue (Wearing et al., 2005). Modelling hypothesis are needed which are influenced by (i) the pathogen of interest (route of transmission, speed of transmission,...), (ii) the host population and (iii) the interaction between epidemiology and population dynamics (added mortality, growth retardation...). For instance the modelling scale can vary from the very precise individual-based model to aggregate models. The choice of relevant scale is therefore an important issue in a modelling project (Keeling and Rohani, 2008). Conversely, aggregate models take less time for simulation. The modeller usually chooses modelling hypothesis considering factors influencing the pathogen spread within the population. For instance animal individual characteristics (sow parity, passive immunity...) are relevant to represent an individual based model. However, individual-based model (IBM), which permit a fine description of the dynamics of epidemics are costly in computation time and need many simulations to obtain mean comportment of models.

The objective of this study was to assess the relevance of the modelling hypothesis concerning both the population and the infection dynamics representation level, and of the implications of these hypotheses on the pathogen spread results. Two infections with drastically different epidemiological characteristics were chosen: (i) a viral infection with economic consequences and (ii) a bacterial infection with public health consequences.

MATERIALS AND METHODS

General presentation of the models, similarities and differences

Population dynamics models

Two models are developed to describe pig and sow population dynamics within farrow-to-finish pig herds. In the two developed models, the farrowing batch system including a three-week interval between batches is represented. This management system includes both the entire reproduction cycle of sows and the entire growth of pigs from birth to slaughterhouse delivery. The sow herd is divided into groups called batches. The reproduction cycle of sows is represented by the occupancy of three successive rooms: the mating room (4 weeks), the gestating room (12 weeks) and the farrowing room (5 weeks). The duration in each room, the same for one batch, and the transfer between rooms are governed by the animals' physiological stage. The cycle ends in the farrowing room at the weaning of piglets. The growth of pigs corresponds to the occupancy of three successive rooms: the farrowing room (4 weeks), the post-weaning room (8 weeks) and the finishing room (between 12 and 16 weeks). In farrowing, post-weaning and finishing rooms, pigs of a batch, which have the same age, enter and leave the room at once. This all-in/all-out housing system allows a cleaning-disinfecting process and a down period of one week between two batches.

For each model, the time step is chosen according to the infectious process considered. The time step is one day for the first model and is one week for the second. In the same way, the representation level for the population dynamics differs in these models.

Actually, the first model was developed to study the spread of PCV2. Characteristics of this pathogen (transmission from the dam to the offspring, importance of passive immunity intake) led to use an individual based model (IBM). This model, denoted by IBM/day model, was developed with Visual Basic for Access (Copyright© 1997-2001 Microsoft Corporation).

The second model aims at studying the *Salmonella* spread (Lurette et al., 2008). The one-week time step is the basic unit for grouping tasks and moving animals between rooms in a batch management system. It is also well suited to the *Salmonella* infection dynamics, since no process occurs under this weekly time-step. This is a compartmental model; the same process occurs for all pigs in a batch. A batch of pigs is reared in only one room at once. This model, denoted by batch/week model, was implemented with Scilab 4.07 (www.scilab.org).

Epidemiological models

PCV2 epidemiological model

PCV2 infectious statuses and transition probabilities (Figure 1) are based on a classic SEIR (Susceptible, Exposed, Infectious, Recovered) model with 5 supplementary states representing the effect of passive immunity intake on the infectious process and the possibility for piglets to be infected at birth when sows were inseminated with infected semen. The sow's lifespan is long enough for active immunity to be lost, so recovered sows can possibly go back into the susceptible class. Additional states are:

- S_m: Piglets susceptible at birth with passive immunity. These piglets are not fully protected by maternal antibodies and might become infected, then moving to compartment P.
- P: Piglets infected by contact with an infectious individual while having passive immunity.
- E_n: Piglets vertically infected by infected semen.
- I_n: Infectious piglets without passive immunity. These piglets were vertically infected by infected semen but did not receive passive immunity from their dam.
- I_m: Infectious piglets with passive immunity. These piglets were vertically infected by infected semen but received passive immunity from their dam. The effect of passive immunity relies on a decrease in the transmission rate.

C represents an environmental pool of virus from which susceptible individuals can acquire the infection, especially in farrowing crates during the lactation period (Fig. 1). Purchased gilts obtained from multiplier herds are supposed to have contracted PCV2 infection during their growing phase. For this reason, the gilts are either infectious or recovered when entering the herd depending on the time elapsed since their infection. This is randomly fixed, the underlying assumption being that purchased gilts would have acquired infection in the nursery phase, between 1 and 145 days (uniform distribution). All gilts infected for more than 55 days were supposed to be in a state of recovery (Andraud et al., 2009).

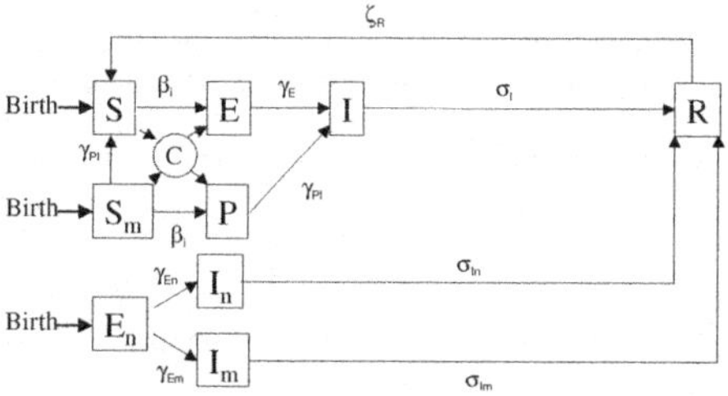

Fig. 1 PCV2 infectious model: states and transitions.

Transmission parameters were derived from three experimental studies and 6 transmission rates were determined. The infectious potentials of the infectious individuals (class I) are defined in terms of the time elapsed since they acquired infection using the time-dependent transmission rates estimated in a previous study (Andraud et al., 2009). Hence, individual transmission rates, corresponding to the route of acquired infection (horizontal or pseudo-vertical) and physical locations (within- and between-pen) of infected pigs, are calculated daily using a lognormal-like function defined by:

$$\beta_l(\tau) = R_{0l} f_{Ln}(\tau - Lat, k, \theta), l = 1,...,6.$$

In this, f_{Ln} is the lognormal probability density function with k and θ being its mean and variance respectively ($k = 2.2$ and $\theta = 0.54$), and τ represents the time since infection. Lat corresponds to the latency period duration. R_{0l} s are the 6 basic reproduction ratios according to location (within- or between-pen) and presence or not of passive immunity (Table1). The other parameters are related to the departure rates from the different compartments which are represented by cumulative probability density functions (Table 1). Because of high resistance in the environment, this route of infection cannot be neglected for PCV-2 and should play a great role in the infectious process, especially in farrowing facilities where the contact structure is limited due to isolation in individual farrowing crates. The infectious potential of the environment within a farrowing crate, C, can then be expressed by the differential equation:

$$\frac{dC}{dt} = (1-r)\beta_1(\tau)I_S(t,\tau) - \mu C$$

with $I_S(t,\tau) = 0$ if the sow present in the farrowing crate is not infectious, $I_S(t,\tau) = 1$ if the sow is infectious and was infected τ time-units ago. r is a factor of reduction of infectiousness with time related to faecal shedding and μ corresponds to the daily death rate of the virus in the environment. Since the batch farrowing system allows for a down period between two successive batches for room cleaning and disinfection, a factor of reduced environmental infectious potential is added during this empty period.

Only a subclinical PCV2 infection is represented in the model. The disease (PMWS) possibly due to PCV2 in association with triggering factors is not represented, thus demographic processes (growth, mortality) are assumed to be unaffected by the PCV2 course of infection.

Salmonella epidemiological model

To model the infection of *Salmonella* in sows and pigs, animals are classified in the model according to their *Salmonella* health status: susceptible (S), seronegative shedder (I_-), seropositive shedder (I_+), and seropositive non-shedding carrier (C_+). A susceptible pig free of *Salmonella* (S) becomes shedder (I-) after ingestion of a sufficient quantity of *Salmonella*. After seroconversion, the pig is called the seropositive shedder (I_+) and becomes a seropositive carrying pig (C+) when the shedding stops. The shedding has been shown to be intermittent (Kranker et al., 2003), and the transition between the shedding and the carrying state can occur in both directions (Fig. 2) (Lurette et al., 2008b).

At each time step, the evolution of the number of pigs affected by a transition between health states is drawn from a binomial law. The transition between the status S and the status I_- is based on an indirect transmission. The probability of infection depends on the quantity of *Salmonella* in the room. This quantity is updated according to the quantity which survives from the time $t-1$ and the quantity shed by shedders (seropositve or not) in the room between time $t-1$ and time t. At each cleaning-disinfecting process, when a batch of pigs leaves room r, the *Salmonella* quantity in this room is updated:

$$Q(t,r)=(1-v^r)\,Q(t-1,r)\,,$$

with v^r the proportion of *Salmonella* infectious units eliminated by the cleaning-disinfecting process in room r ($v^r < 1$, under field conditions, this elimination process is never complete). The other transition probabilities depend on the durations in each health status following exponential distributions. We assume that demographic processes are not affected by the infection states of animals.

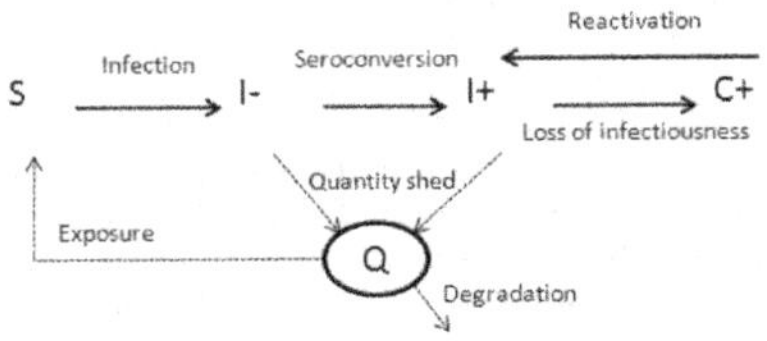

Fig. 2 Diagram of the *Salmonella* epidemiological model. S: Susceptible pig, I-: seronegative shedding pig, I+: seropositive shedding pigs, C+: seropositive carrying pig, Q: quantity of *Salmonella* in the rearing room.

In a first time, the adequacy of the zootechnical parameters from both population dynamics models is checked (Table 1).

Table 1. Main zootechnical parameters of IBM/day and Batch/week models describing the population dynamics within a farrow-to-finish pig herd

Parameter	Values
Number of batches of sows	7 batches
Interval of time between two consecutive batches	21 days
Number of sows in herd	166.9 sows (sd = 2.5)
Number of weaned piglets per litter	11.1 piglets (s.d = 0.09)
Annual culling rate	41.3% (s.d = 2.2)
Mortality rate (Weaning to slaughter)	7.2% (1.0)

IBM/day model: an individual-based model of pig herd dynamics with a discrete time step of one day; Batch/week model: a model of pig herd dynamics with a discrete time step of one week and the batch as the modelling unit

Then, the two population dynamics models were coupled, firstly with the PCV2 epidemiological model and, secondly, with the *Salmonella* epidemiological model. Epidemiological parameter values used were the same; they were only adapted to the representation level and the time step considered in each model of population dynamics. For instance, parameters given in day unit were adapted to the week unit.

Outputs compared

For the PCV2 models, the initial herd consisted of nulliparous sows in either state I or state R (same distribution as for replacement gilts). After a 10 year-long simulation, a stabilised herd had been obtained in terms of demography distribution. This stabilised herd was taken as the initial situation for simulations. One hundred repetitions of a 1-year long simulation were carried out. The output compared was the seroprevalence in a batch of piglets from birth to slaughterhouse delivery. This result is particularly relevant to follow up the PCV2 course of infection during pig growth because they could be compared with actual seroprevalence data obtained from a field study (Rose et al., 2003). The consistency between model outputs and field data was good.

For the *Salmonella* model, the seroprevalence in the initial herd was on average 10% in groups of delivered pigs. Four gilts are recruited at each reproduction cycle. Based on data from French supplier herds, the gilts are distributed in the four health states and the seroprevalence is exponentially distributed with a mean probability of 0.05 (Lejolivet, 2004). The results obtained from the batch/week model are obtained from 150 batches of pigs for 100 replications (i.e. 1500 batches). This number of replications allows us to obtain robust results. From the IBM/day model, results are obtained from the same number of batches. The first output is the mean prevalence of shedding (including pigs in states I– and I+) and of seropositive animals (including pigs in states I+ and C+) in a batch of pigs from birth until slaughterhouse delivery. The second outputs compared are the mean prevalence of shedding and the mean seroprevalence in groups of pigs delivered to the slaughterhouse. These results are particularly relevant for *Salmonella* study given its use in several control plans implemented in European countries (Mousing et al., 1997).

References scenarios are those obtained from the population dynamics model previously developed with the corresponding epidemiological model.

RESULTS

PCV2 spread

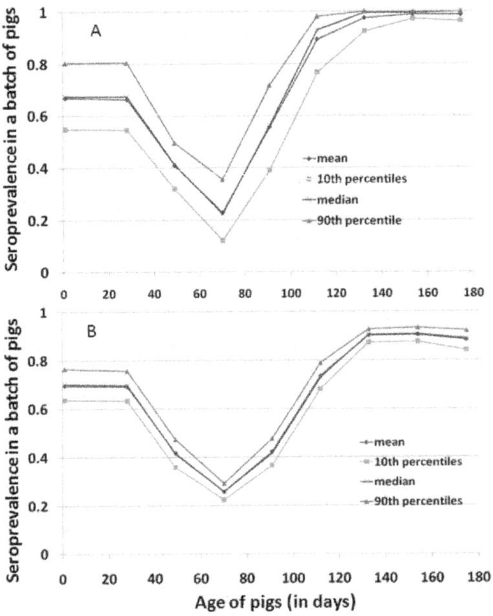

Fig. 3 PCV2 seroprevalence in batches of pigs from birth to slaughterhouse delivery. Results are obtained from 1500 batches. A - PCV2 spread using the IBM:day model ; B - PCV2 spread using a batch/week model.

The curve of the mean seroprevalence in a batch of pigs has a similar pattern for the two models used (Fig. 3 A - B). However, a difference between the two curves appears at the end of the pig growth (around 125 days). Actually, while the mean seroprevalence of the IBM/day model reaches almost 100% at 112 days and remains at this level until 176 days of age, the mean seroprevalence of the batch/week model attains only 85% at 133 days of age and, then, decreases between 150 and 176 days. At the end of the pig growth, the number of susceptible pigs is more numerous with the batch/week model. Moreover, the variability in the seroprevalence between batches differs for the two models. Actually, whatever the time step considered, this variability is lower for the model using the batch as a modelling unit and a time step of one week than for the other one.

Salmonella spread model

As for the previous pathogen tested, the mean seroprevalence curves are very close during the whole pig growth (data not shown). However, the mean seroprevalence is slightly higher for the IBM/day model than for the batch/week model. Although the difference between the two curves remains low, it reaches a maximum at the end of the pig growth, 27.6% versus 25.3 % for the IBM/day model and the batch/week model respectively. The same result is observed for the prevalence of shedding pigs. But, the difference is the lowest at the end of the finishing period (17.1% for the IBM/day model versus 17.8% for the batch/week model). Using the batch/week model leads to a break down of the curve at each room change. This break down is not observed with the IBM/day model at the entry in the post-weaning room and is one week later than the batch/week model at the entry in the finishing room.

As for the prevalences during pig growth, the distribution of the prevalences (shedding and seropositive pigs) in groups of delivered pigs are relatively close with the two population dynamics models (Fig. 4). In the distribution of the shedding prevalence, using the IBM/day model leads to obtain less groups with low prevalence than using the batch/week model. The highest difference is observed for the groups with prevalence between 5 and 10%. Same results are obtained for the seroprevalence, but the difference between the two distributions is milder.

Gain in terms of simulating time is significant (30 seconds instead of 3 minutes for a one-year simulation). For the same simulation duration, the number of batches run for the batch/week model is more than 10 times higher than for the IBM/day model.

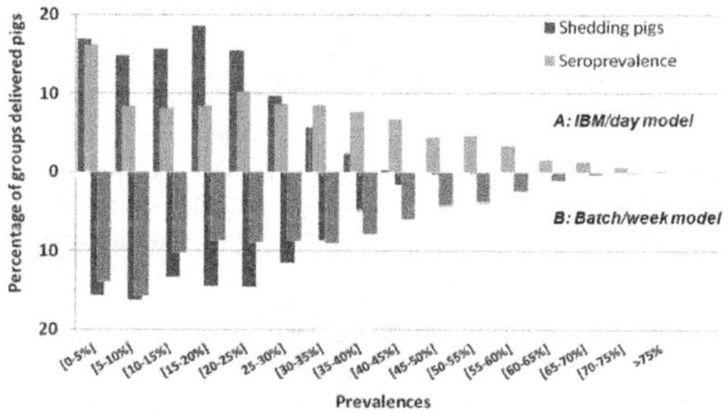

Fig. 5 Prevalence of shedder and of seropositive pigs in groups of delivered pigs. Results obtained from 1500 batches. A - *Salmonella* spread using an IBM/week model ; B - *Salmonella* spread using a batch/week model.

DISCUSSION

The aim of this study was to assess the relevance of the representation level of the population dynamics in the case of modelling epidemiology. Two different models describing the pigs' and sows' dynamics within pig herds were used (Andraud et al., 2007; Lurette et al., 2008a). The first one is an individual-based model with a time step of one day. The second is a compartmental model using the batch as the modelling unit and a time step of one week. Each of these models was combined with an epidemiological model representing the spread of two pathogens with drastic differences in transmission characteristics. The PCV2 is both directly and indirectly transmitted, with an important role of sows in the transmission process. The Salmonella are indirectly transmitted via the environment.

Even if differences in mean seroprevalence values remain low, these values are higher for the IBM/day model than for the batch/week model, for both PCV2 and Salmonella infections. It could be explained by the fact that the spread of the pathogen could be facilitated by taking into account both the within- and the between-herd spread instead of only the within room spread. This could also explain that, for both pathogen infections, the seroprevalence in a batch of pigs reach a maximum sooner with the IBM model than with the other one.

Using the same value for epidemiological parameters leads to slight differences both in mean seroprevalence values and in their variability. On the one hand, the PCV2 course of infection assessed through the age-related mean seroprevalence during the whole pig growth is close for the two models of population dynamics. However, the variability is lower when the modelling unit used is the batch and the time step is one week (instead of one day). It is possible that taking into account a weekly evolution of the system leads to a less accurate implementation of the time since-infection which seems to be a pivotal parameter in PCV2 transmission (Andraud et al., 2009). This representation level tends to homogenise the animal infection status within a batch. Moreover, the occupancy of one room, instead of the separation in several pens, could contribute to decrease the transmission rate variability within a batch as between-pen transmission was shown to be 10-fold lower than the within-pen one (Andraud et al., 2008).

Seroprevalence was shown to slightly decline after 160 days of age with the batch/week-based representation conversely to the IBM model. This decline might be due to the loss of immunity in several pigs beyond that stage because of the exponential distribution of durations in the batch/week model whereas a gamma distribution was taken for the durations of immunity in the IBM/day model which prevent from early escape from the R compartment. Further modelling studies are needed to improve the representation of the variability in the epidemiological parameter values for individuals forming a batch. This representation could, therefore, increase the variability in the seroprevalence results when using the batch/week model.

On the other hand, the use of batches as modelling units and week as time step is sufficient to account for the variability in the Salmonella spread within pig herds. Actually, the distributions of the prevalences (shedding and seropositive pigs) in groups of delivered pigs were very close for the two models developed, even if some slight differences appear for groups with low prevalence (especially between 5 and 10%). For this pathogen, the IBM/day model do not lead to increasing the variability. The batch representation level is particularly well adapted to assess the effect of control measures both on mean seroprevalence, and on low and high contaminated batches.

The gain in terms of simulation duration is not negligible here. Actually, a significant gain of time can lead to test a highest number of scenarios of control measures alone or in association. Moreover, given that the mean seroprevalences are very close for the two population dynamics models, we would expect the fastest model to be best suited for the assessment of the effect of control measures implementation on the mean comportment of the system. On the contrary, to assess the effect of control measures on extreme cases, such as slowly or highly contaminated batches, the use of the IBM/day model should be more efficient than the batch/week model. It could also be used to assess the effect of control measures implemented at the individual level, such as measures including cross-fostering. However, experimental or field data are generally obtained at the population level which can make the validation difficult at the individual level.

The use of herd models within a framework of connected herds through a complex network of relationships between these herds requires simple within-herd representations. To simplify such within-herds dynamics, the highest sources of variability need to be included in the parsimonious model. Even if IBM models are not well suited for such connective networks they might be helpful to preliminary identify the main sources of variability to be included in the final aggregate representation of the within-herd dynamics.

The study of two drastically different pathogens in pigs shows that depending on the pathogen considered and its infection characteristics, the modelling hypotheses can modify results of within-herd infection spread. This modification can then influence the interpretation from the simulated data of the potential efficiency of measures on this spread. A less specific representation level can be, however, border on the mean comportment of the system. The assessment of the efficiency of existing or possible control measures needs a large number of scenarios to be tested. Therefore, the modelling hypotheses have to combine a representation of the system the most accurate as possible with a minimal time of simulation. Individual-based models (IBM) with small time step and complex structure give a fine description of the dynamics of epidemics but are costly in computation time. Moreover, for stochastic models, the number of simulations needs to be dramatically increased to obtain robust results. Simplifying the population dynamics could be a good trade-off to optimise the use of the epidemiological model for scenarios assessment.

ACKNOWLEDGEMENTS

This study was funded by the INRA/AFSSA project "Santé animale et alimentation animale".

REFERENCES

Andraud, M., Leon, E.A., Pierre, J.S., Madec, F., Rose, N. (2007). A stochastic individual-based model representing population dynamics in a farrow-to-finish pig farm in order to assess the "sow effect" on an infectious process. Epidémiol. et santé anim. 51, 1-13.

Andraud, M. Grasland, B., Durand, B., Cariolet, R., Madec, F., Rose, N. (2009). Modelling the time-dependent transmission rate for Porcine Circovirus Type 2 (PCV2) in pigs by using data on serial transmission experiments. J. Roy. Soc. Interface. 230, 39-50.

Andraud, M., Grasland, B., Durand, B., Cariolet, R., Jestin, A., Madec, F., Rose, N. (2008). Quantification of porcine circovirus type 2 (PCV2) within- and between-pen transmission in pigs. Vet. Res. 39, article no. 43.

Keeling and Rohani, 2008. Modeling infectious diseases in humans and animals, Princeton University Press

Kixmöller, M., Ritzmann, M., Eddicks, M., Saalmüller, A., Elbers, K., Fachinger, V. (2008). Reduction of PMWS-associated clinical signs and co-infections by vaccination against PCV2. Vaccine 26, 3443-3451.

Kranker, S., Alban, L., Boes, J., and Dahl, J. (2003). Longitudinal study of *Salmonella enterica* serotype typhimurium infection in three Danish farrow-to-finish swineherds. Journal of Clinical Microbiology 41, 2282-2288.

Lejolivet A., (2004). Prévalence des salmonelles dans le schéma de sélection d'un groupement de producteurs de porcs, pratiques à risques et intervention sur l'excrétion, Veterinary thesis report, Nantes Veterinary School, France.

Lurette A., Belloc C., Touzeau S., Hoch T., Seegers H., Fourichon C. (2008a). Modelling batch farrowing management within a farrow-to-finish pig herd: influence of management on contact structure and pig delivery, Animal 2, 105–116.

Lurette, A., Belloc, C., Touzeau, S., Hoch, T., Seegers, H., Fourichon, C. (2008b). Modelling the *Salmonella* spread within a farrow-to-finish pig herd. Vet. Res. 39-49.

Mousing, J., Jensen, P. T., Halgaard, C., Bager, F., Feld, N., Nielsen, B., Nielsen, J. P. and Bech Nielsen, S. (1997) Nation-wide *Salmonella enterica* surveillance and control in Danish slaughter swine herds. Preventive Veterinary Medicine 29, 247-261.

Rose, N., Blanchard, P., Cariolet, R., Grasland, B., Amenna, N., Oger, A., Durand, B., Balasch, M., Jestin, A., Madec, F. (2007). Vaccination of Porcine Circovirus type 2 (PCV2)-infected sows against Porcine Parvovirus (PPV) and Erysipelas: Effect on Post-weaning Multisystemic Wasting Syndrome (PMWS) and on PCV2 Genome Load in the Offspring. J. Comp. Pathol. 136, 133-144.

Wearing, H.J., Rohani, P., Keeling, M.J., 2005. Appropriate Models for the Management of Infectious Diseases. PLOS Medicine, 2, 174.

WITHIN-HERD TRANSMISSION DYNAMICS OF PORCINE REPRODUCTIVE AND RESPIRATORY SYNDROME VIRUS (PRRSV) FOLLOWING SINGLE INTRODUCTION

C.M. EVANS*, G.F. MEDLEY, S.J. CREASEY AND L.E. GREEN

SUMMARY

A mathematical model of a farrow-finish pig herd was used to investigate the within-herd transmission dynamics of PRRSV and to test hypotheses for persistence and fadeout. Model parameters came from the literature and from pig PRRSV antibody data from a previous cross-sectional study of 103 pig herds. Likelihood profiles of the observational data were most probable when the transmission parameter and cross transmission terms between pigs were low. Maximum likelihood varied for different herds from the observational study, indicating differences in likely states of transmission dynamics. Following introduction of an infectious gilt in the model, fadeout of virus was likely within the breeding gilts and sows in approximately 75% of simulations. The probability of fadeout was significantly influenced by herd size, isolation measures and the contact structure of the herd, particularly between rearing pigs. Apparent instability, fadeout and reintroduction of virus are discussed, as well as the likely importance of metapopulation dynamics in persistence of the virus within pig herds.

INTRODUCTION

Porcine Reproductive and Respiratory Syndrome Virus (PRRSV) is a positive-sense single-stranded enveloped RNA virus (Wensvoort et al., 1991), which was first detected in North America in 1987 (Hill et al., 1990). Despite widespread attempts at control and elimination of the virus, PRRSV still remains a significant cause of reproductive disease (Hopper et al., 1992), pre-weaning mortality (Hopper et al., 1992) and respiratory disease (Drew, 2000) in pig herds.

When PRRSV first emerged in Denmark and the UK in 1992, the main route of introduction into commercial pig herds was the purchase of infected breeding females, aerial spread between neighbouring herds and the purchase of semen (Edwards et al., 1992, Mortensen et al., 2002).

Following introduction into a herd, the way a virus spreads between pigs is dependent on the contact structure, i.e., the type, intensity and frequency of contacts (Lurette et al., 2008). Fade out of an infectious disease from a herd is influenced by the contact structure between pigs within the herd as well as the number of susceptible and infectious individuals. For example, with few infectious individuals, fadeout may occur early after introduction of virus and with few susceptible individuals, fadeout may occur at the end of an outbreak. Susceptible pigs may enter a herd by birth, replacement, or following the decay of passive or active immunity. Piglets born to seropositive sows have passive immunity for up to 4-10 weeks of age in the field (Houben, et

* Charlotte Evans, Department of Biological Sciences, University of Warwick, Coventry CV4 7AL, United Kingdom. Email: C.M.Evans@warwick.ac.uk

al., 1995; Nodelijk, et al., 1997) and pigs can become seronegative 4.5-20 months after initial exposure (Yoon et al., 1995, Desrosiers et al., 2002). Since fadeout is influenced by the number of susceptible individuals, it will also be influenced by the herd size. An increased probability of fadeout in smaller herds has been reported for PRRSV (Nodelijk et al., 2000) and cross-sectional serological data suggest that fadeout of PRRSV may be common (Evans et al., 2008).

Although a within-herd model of PRRSV transmission has been published (Nodelijk et al., 2000), this excluded the contact structure of the pig herd with respect to age and reproductive status. Another model of a pig herd that investigated pig population dynamics included this structure (Lurette et al., 2008), but the influence on fadeout and persistence of an infectious disease was not investigated, particularly considering the role of the breeding herd and differences in isolation procedures.

Herd-level PRRSV antibody patterns and risks from a cross-sectional study of 103 pig farms with 50 pigs per farm were presented (Evans et al., 2008). Thirty four percent of herds were seronegative and 39% of positive herds had patterns that were indicative of fadeout of virus, where only breeding sows were seropositive. The herd characteristics that explained some of the between herd variability of PRRSV antibody in seropositive herds included purchasing practices, isolation facilities, herd size and pig density in the region.

A mathematical model of a farrow-finish pig herd was used to investigate the within-herd transmission dynamics of PRRSV. Model parameters are drawn from the literature and from the cross-sectional serological data. We use the model to investigate persistence and fadeout of infection and consider differences in isolation procedures, the contact structure within the herd and herd size. The observational data (previously described) are used to validate the model.

MATERIALS AND METHODS

Model structure

To investigate the within-herd transmission dynamics of PRRSV, a model of a farrow-finish pig herd was constructed. All code was written and run in MATLAB® (Version, 7.0, MatLab, The MathWorks, Natick, MA, USA). There are four main groups within the model: 1) sows with litters of piglets, 2) a rearing herd with pigs of 4-24 weeks of age, 3) a gilt house with young replacement breeding females and 4) a sow herd with gestating breeding female pigs.

Management cycles for each of the groups are depicted in Fig. 1. Arrows represent the movement of pigs of the same age and / or reproductive state between subsections of the herd at the end of each week. Individual batches of pigs remain together and their contact structures are explicitly modelled on the basis of their position within the cycles, described below.

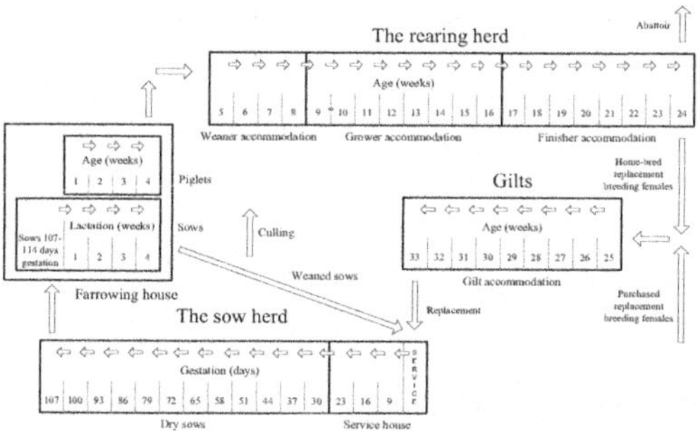

Fig. 1 The structure of the demographic assumptions within the mathematical model

Sows are moved to the farrowing house 1 week before they farrow and remain for five weeks. Piglets remain in the farrowing house until they are four weeks of age and then move to the rearing herd. The rearing herd consists of weaner (5-8 weeks of age), grower (9-16 weeks of age) and finisher (17-24 weeks of age) stages of production. Each week, 24 week old pigs are either selected as replacement stock or are 'sent' to an abattoir: all batches of rearing pigs consequently move up the rearing herd housing to occupy vacant pens and a batch of piglets enters the weaner accommodation. Gilts spend nine weeks in the gilt house and then join the sow group to replace sows that have been culled. Gilts enter the sow group at service (at approx. 231 days old), and are then defined as parity one sows. Sows spend four weeks in the service house, 12 weeks in the dry sow house and five weeks in the farrowing house. Sows are served 5 days after weaning and move to the farrowing house 7 days before farrowing (a gestation of 114 days). Sows go through this cycle six times before being culled. Sows of different parities of the same reproductive status are assumed to be housed together. Forty five percent of breeding sows are culled each year in the model (British Pig Executive, 2008). Sows are culled before service. The probability of a sow surviving a cull (p) is (1 – r) where the replacement rate (r) is 0.45. No parity 1 sows are culled. The longest period of time pigs can remain in the simulated herd is 1113 days (33 weeks when served, 21 weeks between consecutive services and six reproductive cycles before being culled).

<u>Modelling within-herd transmission dynamics</u>

A stochastic Susceptible-Infected-Recovered-Susceptible (SIRS) model is used to simulate the transmission dynamics of PRRSV within the herd. Pigs belong to one of the following states (defined below): 1) passively immune (M), 2) susceptible (S), 3) infected (and infectious) (I), 4) recovered and seropositive (immune and no longer infectious) (R_{pos}), 5) recovered and seronegative (susceptible to reinfection) (R_{neg}). Successive events control the transitions of pigs between the states with probabilities defined by specific rate parameters (Table 1). All parameters are treated as constant and all sojourn times are negatively exponentially distributed.

Table 1. Transitions of pigs between different epidemiological states in the model (the symbols are defined in the text)

Event	Rate	Outcome
Infection	$\frac{\beta SI}{N}$	S = S – 1 I = I + 1
Recovery	αI	I = I – 1 $R_{pos} = R_{pos}$ - 1
Loss of passive immunity	πM	M = M – 1 S = S + 1
Loss of active immunity	λR_{pos}	$R_{pos} = R_{pos}$ – 1 $R_{neg} = R_{neg}$ + 1
Reinfection of a recovered seronegative pig	$\frac{\beta R_{neg} I}{N}$	$R_{neg} = R_{neg}$ – 1 I = I + 1

The symbols are defined in the text.

In the model, the proportion of piglets born with passive immunity is equal to the proportion of infectious plus seropositive sows farrowing that week. The rate of loss of maternal immunity (π) is 6 weeks in the model.

Infection is density independent (i.e. transmission is assumed to not increase linearly with the density of pigs on the farm). The rate of infection in batch *i* is derived as a weighted sum of infection in all other groups (*j*) as:

$$\sum_j \frac{\beta(i,j)S(i)I(j)}{N(i)}$$

where $\beta(i,j)$ is the rate of transmission from infectious pigs in batch j to susceptible pigs in batch i (written as I(j) and S(i) respectively) and N(i) is the number of pigs in batch i. The β(i,j) are calculated from the relative transmission coefficients between pigs in the herd (described below) multiplied by an overall transmission coefficient.

Equal random mixing is assumed between pigs in the same pen (individual batches), within gestating sows and within maiden gilts. The transmission rate between pigs in pens that are closely situated to each other (including the weaner, grower and finisher pens within a building and between batches of sows in the service house) is reduced by 1×10^{-3}. Transmission between pigs in buildings that are closely situated to one another is reduced by 1×10^{-4}: that is batches of sows farrowing in the same week in the farrowing house, between maiden gilts and gestating sows, between maiden gilts / gestating sows and sows in the service house and between weaner, grower or finisher houses. Transmission between different sites within the herd, including the rearing herd, the farrowing house and the breeding herd is reduced by 1×10^{-6}.

Relative transmission coefficients are changed in the model to simulate differences in contact structure. When replacement gilts are not isolated, the relative transmission coefficient between maiden gilts and gestating sows is increased to one for equal random mixing. Increasing transmission coefficients between pens in individual houses within the rearing herd to 0.1 increases contact between rearing pigs, and increased contact between all pigs in the herd is achieved by increasing all transmission coefficients by a factor of 100 (up to a maximum of 1).

We assume a recovery rate of 56 days (α = 1/56d) (Terpstra et al., 1992, Nodelijk et al., 2000). After a mean duration of 9 months pigs become seronegative with rate λ = 1/252 days, and can be reinfected.

Experimental infection of sows on or after day 84 of gestation causes late-term abortions and the birth of stillborn and mummified pigs (Wensvoort et al., 1992, Kranker et al., 1998). Infection before this period has led to conflicting probabilities of *in utero* infection (Christianson, et al., 1992 and Kranker, et al., 1998). It is assumed that sows infected on or after week 12 of gestation (day 84) will have a 10% probability of aborting: the remaining 90% are assumed to farrow and give birth to 7 alive piglets and 4 piglets that are either born dead or die pre-weaning.

Model validation: The cross-sectional data

Cross-sectional serological profiles of 40 seropositive herds from a previous study (Evans et al., 2008) are used to validate the model. Nineteen bred their own replacement stock and the remaining 21 herds purchased replacement gilts. The herds are categorised by herd size into seven groups; 0-150, 151-300, 301-450, 451-600, 601-750, 751-900 and 1500 sows. Binomial probabilities of each of the cross-sectional serological profiles of the 40 herds are calculated, given the sensitivity and specificity of the ELISA and the seroprevalence of the different age groups from the model at 21 day intervals. This procedure is repeated for each run of the model and for seven herd sizes. Likelihood profiles are used to determine most likely transmission and cross-transmission coefficients and binomial probabilities of all cross-sectional serological profiles are used to validate patterns generated by the model.

Initial conditions and fadeout

The model is firstly run with no infection for 1000 weeks, ensuring demographic equilibrium. At the beginning of the simulation, one infectious gilt is introduced into the gilt house and all other pigs in the herd are susceptible. The model is run for 1200 days and is repeated 1000 times for each set of initial conditions which include differences in isolation, the contact structure of the herd and herd size.

Fadeout was assumed when the number of infectious pigs in the herd was zero.

RESULTS

Observational data

From the 40 observational herds, the median proportion of seropositive pigs was 0 for 8 week old pigs, 0.2 for 14 week old pigs, 0.4 for gilts, parity 1 and parity 2 sows, 0.6 for parity 3 sows and 0.4 for both parity 4 and parity 5 sows. Nineteen of the herds bred their own replacement stock and the remaining 21 herds purchased replacement gilts. 16/40 herds did not have any seropositive 8 or 14 week old pigs on the farm. Of the 24 herds that had seropositive youngstock, the median proportion seropositive was 0 for 8 week old pigs and 0.66 for 14 week old pigs.

Model validation

The likelihood profiles of the cross-sectional observational data were most likely (given the model outputs at 21 day intervals) when the transmission parameter and cross transmission terms between batches of pigs were low (data not shown). Likelihood profiles of the observational data, given the model outputs, also varied with time since introduction of virus, particularly during the early stages of the epidemic (Fig. 2). During the early stages of the epidemic, likelihood values either steadily increased initially post-introduction and then remained constant, or showed a marked peak soon afer introduction indicating that virus either persisted or faded out.

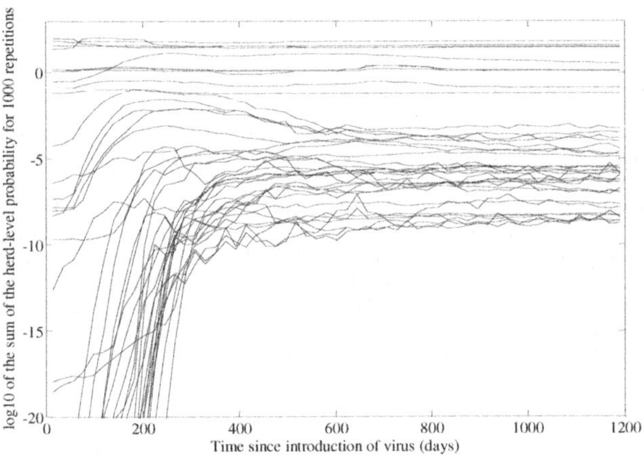

Fig. 2 Likelihood values of the model outcomes over time since introduction of virus for 40 seropositive herds, given their cross-sectional serological profiles and the model outputs at 21 day intervals

Transmission dynamics following introduction of virus

Using model parameter values that are most consistent and a herd size of 327 sows (the median herd size of herds in the previous study), fadeout occurred within 4 weeks in 21.9% of 1000 simulations. In approximately 50% of simulations (501/1000), fadeout of virus occurred before 63 days, corresponding to fadeout within the gilt group. If virus did not fadeout within the first 175 days, it was unlikely to fadeout within the simulated time. This corresponds with virus being unlikely to fadeout once it has reached the rearing pigs.

Isolation

When replacement gilts were not isolated from gestating sows before service, the probability of fadeout soon after introduction was lower (Fig. 3). 14.3% compared with 81.6% of simulations resulted in fadeout within 250 days when isolation was assumed.

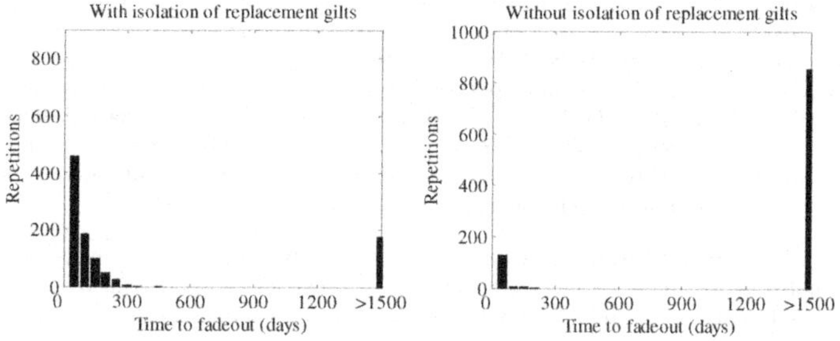

Fig. 3 Histograms of the time to fadeout of virus when the model is run for 1200 days, for 1000 simulations, for differences in isolation practices (herd size 327 sows)

Contact structure

The probability of persistence of virus for >1200 days increased from 17.6% to 23.8% when rearing pigs transmitted virus to one another with a probability of 10% (instead of 0.1%) (Fig. 4). The probability of persistence was 57.7% when cross transmission terms between all groups of pigs in the herd were increased 100 fold.

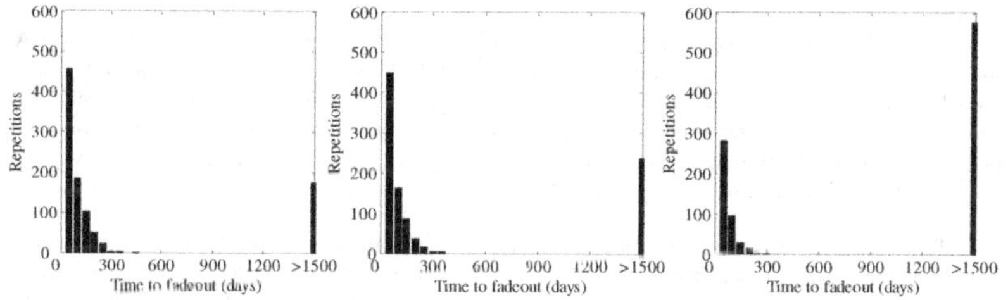

Fig. 4 Histograms of the time to fadeout of virus when the model is run for 1200 days, for 1000 simulations, for differences in the contact structure of the herd (herd size 327 sows)

Left: under normal conditions of the model (assuming a probability of contact between different batches of pigs within a single accommodation type of 0.1), middle: assuming 10% probability of transmission between batches of pigs within a single accommodation type, right: assuming a 100 fold increase in cross transmission between all pigs in the herd compared with normal conditions (as shown on the left)

The probability of persistence with herd sizes of 75, 226, 376, 526, 676 and 826 sows were 0.04, 0.17, 0.38, 0.22, 0.22 and 0.19 respectively (Figure 2). The median (range) time to fadeout for the different herd sizes was 44 (0-897), 44 (0-491), 40.5 (0-360), 35 (0-725), 34.5 (0-537), 40 (0-726) and 41.5 (0-364) respectively.

DISCUSSION

Serological profiles generated by the model were most consistent with the observational data at relatively low values of the transmission coefficient and at very low cross transmission values between groups within the herd. These low values suggest low transmissibility of PRRSV within a herd. Transmission to sentinel pigs over 1 - 2.5 metres has been demonstrated in field attempts (Wills et al., 1997, Otake et al., 2002), but transmission over longer distances, e.g. between barns connected via pipes have failed (Otake et al., 2002, Trincado et al., 2004). Another author has also reported that transmission of PRRSV is slow in naturally infected commercial herds, even within individual pens of pigs (Houben et al., 1995).

Following single introduction of virus, fadeout was likely to occur within the breeding herd and was unlikely once the virus spread to rearing pigs. Previous studies have also reported virus to not reach the rearing herd following initial introduction (Gordon, 1992).

Heterogeneities in serological profiles (from the observational data) and consequent differences in their likely state of transmission dynamics suggest that different herds may be at different stages of viral introduction, persistence and fadeout (Figure 2). These differences will generate differences in the proportion of susceptible and exposed pigs in the herd. In herds with large numbers of immune pigs, the probability of contact between infectious and susceptible pigs is lower. This makes the herd less susceptible to outbreaks of clinical disease. Herds with large numbers of susceptible pigs have been linked with outbreaks of clinical PRRS in a previous study (Dee et al., 1996) and may include those that are in the very later stages of fadeout or those at the beginning of an epidemic. Outbreaks in such herds may occur following introduction of virus, either from a different group within the herd or from another herd.

The availability of susceptible pigs in a herd is directly proportional to the herd size. An increased probability of persistence with increased herd size has been demonstrated in a previous mathematical modelling study for PRRSV (Nodelijk et al., 2000). In the current study, an increase in herd size was associated with a non-linear increase in the probability of persistence of virus. For herds larger than 376 sows, a further increase in herd size was not associated with an increase in the probability of persistence.

Observed heterogeneity in serology between herds (Evans et al., 2008) raises the possibility that between-herd transmission of PRRSV may be an important aspect of persistence in the national pig population. This may influence the validation analysis, since it was assumed that the serological profiles from the field study were generated as a result of a single introduction (and not multiple reintroduction) of virus.

If metapopulation effects are critical in the persistence of PRRSV in the national pig population, isolating replacement stock in appropriate facilities may be an effective way of reducing the probability of reintroduction, reported previously (Edwards et al., 1992, Evans et al., 2008). Since transmission in the model was more likely when the relative transmission coefficients between pigs were high, the segregation of pigs of different ages may reduce the spread of virus. Some authors have demonstrated elimination of PRRSV by only controlling replacement gilts coming into the herd (Dee et al., 1994). However, elimination of virus has failed in other studies when the rearing herd was only partially segregated compared with an all-in-all-out system (Fano et al., 2005). This may suggest that whilst reintroduction may be an important source of persistence, the contact structure of the herd, particularly the rearing herd, might be important in maintaining virus within that herd.

The model was constructed to represent a typical pig herd in terms of its structure and demography and whilst some necessary assumptions were made for purposes of simplicity, these may be more reasonable for some herds than others. In future research we intend to include non-routine movements of pigs as a consequence of infection-related returns to oestrus and / or abortions, as Lurette et al., (2008) have demonstrated the large impact that such movements can have within a herd. In addition, we will use the model framework to investigate the impact of PRRSV on production, and mitigation by different interventions, and further explore the metapopulation aspects of transmission dynamics.

ACKNOWLEDGEMENTS

We thank all the farmers and veterinarians who participated in the field study, and all field technicians and research staff involved in data collection and processing. We thank John Richardson (Intervet) and Tony Fowler (BPEX) for advice on the pig herd structure and assumptions. Charlotte Evans is in receipt of a case BBSRC studentship with industrial sponsorship from the British Pig Executive (BPEX).

REFERENCES

Christianson, W.T., Choi, C.S., Collins, J.E., Molitor, T.W., Morrison, R.B., Joo, H.S. (1992) Pathogenesis of Porcine Reproductive and Respiratory Syndrome Virus infection in mid-gestation sows and fetuses. Can. J. Vet. Res. 57, 262-268.

Dee, S.A., Joo, H.S., Pijoan, C. (1994) Controlling the spread of PRRS virus in the breeding herd through management of the gilt pool. Swine Health Prod. 3, 64-69.

Dee, S.A., Joo, H.S., Henry, S., Tokach, L., Park, B.K., Molitor, T., Pijoan, C. (1996) Detecting subpopulations after PRRS virus infection in large breeding herds using multiple serologic tests. Swine Health Prod. 4, 181-184.

Desrosiers, R., Boutin, M. (2002) An attempt to eradicate porcine reproductive and respiratory syndrome virus (PRRSV) after an outbreak in a breeding herd: Eradication strategy and persistence of antibody titers in sows. Swine Health Prod. 10, 23-25.

Drew, T.W. (2000) A review of evidence for immunosuppression due to Porcine Reproductive and Respiratory Syndrome Virus. Vet. Res. 31, 27-39.

Edwards, S., Robertson, J., Wilesmith, J., Ryan, J., Kilner, C., Paton, D.J., Drew, T.W., Brown, I., Sands, J. (1992) PRRS ("Blue-eared pig disease") in Great Britain. AASP Internaltional PRRS Symposium Edition 1992. 32-36.

Evans, C.M., Medley, G.F., Green, L.E. (2008) Porcine reproductive and respiratory syndrome virus (PRRSV) in GB pig herds: farm characteristics associated with heterogeneity in seroprevalence. BMC Vet. Res. 4, 48.

Fano, E., Olea, L., Pijoan, C. (2005) Eradication of porcine reproductive and respiratory syndrome virus by serum inoculation of naive gilts. Can. J. Vet. Res.-Rev. Can. Rech. Vet. 69, 71-74.

Gordon, S.C. (1992) Effects of blue-eared pig-disease on a breeding and fattening unit. Vet. Rec. 130, 513-514.

Hill, H. (1990) Overview and history of mystery swine disease (Swine Infertility Reproductory Syndrome). Proceedings mystery swine disease committee meeting, Denver, CO, 6 Oct. 1990.

Hopper, S.A., White, M.E., Twiddy, N. (1992) An outbreak of blue-eared pig disease (porcine reproductive and respiratory syndrome) in four pig herds in Great Britain. Vet. Rec. 131, 140-144.

Houben, S., van Reeth, K., Pensaert, M.B. (1995) Pattern of infection with the porcine reproductive and respiratory syndrome virus on swine farms in Belgium. Zentralblatt fur Veterinarmedizin. Reihe B. J. Vet. Med. B. 42, 209-215.

Kranker, S., Nielsen, J., Bille-Hansen, V., Botner, A. (1998) Experimental inoculation of swine at various stages of gestation with a Danish isolate of porcine reproductive and respiratory syndrome virus (PRRSV). Vet. Microbiol. 61, 21 - 31.

Lurette, A., Belloc, C., Touzeau, S., Hoch, T., Seegers, H., Fourichon, C. (2008) Modelling batch farrowing management within a farrow-to-finish pig herd: influence of management on contact structure and pig delivery to the slaughterhouse. Animal 2, 105-116

Mortensen, S., Stryhn, H., Sogaard, R., Boklund, A., Stark, K.D., Christensen, J., Willeberg, P. (2002) Risk factors for infection of sow herds with porcine reproductive and respiratory syndrome (PRRS) virus. Prev. Vet. Med. 53, 83-101.

Nodelijk, G., Van Leengoed, L.A.M.G., Schoevers, E.J., Kroese, A.H., De Jong, M.C.M., Wensvoort, G., Verheijden, J.H.M. (1997) Seroprevalence of porcine reproductive and respiratory syndrome virus in Dutch weaning pigs. Vet. Microbiol. 56, 21-32.

Nodelijk, G., De Jong, M.C.M., Van Nes, A., Vernooy, J.C.M., Van Leengoed, L.A.M.G., Pol, J.M.A., Verheijden, J.H.M. (2000) Introduction, persistence and fade-out of porcine reproductive and respiratory syndrome virus in a Dutch breeding herd: A mathematical analysis. Epidemiol. Infect. 124, 173-182.

Otake, S., Dee, S.A., Jacobson, L., Pijoan, C., Torremorell, M. (2002) Evaluation of aerosol transmission of porcine reproductive and respiratory syndrome virus under controlled field conditions. Vet. Rec. 150, 804-808.

Terpstra, C., Wensvoort, G., Van Leengoed, LAMG. (1992) Persistence of Lelystad virus in herds affected by porcine epidemic abortion and respiratory syndrome. Proceedings of 12th International Pig Veterinary Society Congress, The Hague, The Netherlands., 118.

Trincado, C., Dee, S., Jacobson, L., Otake, S., Rossow, K., Pijoan, C. (2004) Attempts to transmit porcine reproductive and respiratory syndrome virus by aerosols under controlled field conditions. Vet. Rec. 154, 294-297.

Wensvoort, G., Terpstra, C., Pol, J., ter Laak, E., Bloemraad, M., De Kluijver, E.P., Kragten, E., van Buiten, L., Den Besten, A., Wagenaar, F., Broekhuijsen, J., Moonen, P.L.J.M., Zetstra, T., de Boer, E., Tibben, H., De Jong, M.F., P., v.t.V., G.J.R., G., van Gennep, J., Voets MTh, Verheijden, J.H.M., Braamskamp, J. (1991) Mystery swine disease in the Netherlands: the isolation of Lelystad virus. Vet. Quart. 13, 121-130.

Wills, R.W., Zimmerman, J.J., Swenson, S.L., Yoon, K.J., Hill, H.T., Bundy, D.S., McGinley, M.J. (1997) Transmission of PRRSV by direct, close, or indirect contact. Swine Health Prod. 5, 213-218.

Yoon, K.J., Zimmerman, J.J., Swenson, S.L., McGinley, M.J., Eernisse, K.A., Brevik, A., Rhinehart, L.L., Frey, M.L., Hill, H.T., Platt, K.B. (1995) Characterization of the humoral immune response to porcine reproductive and respiratory syndrome (PRRS) virus infection. J. Diagn. Invest. 7, 305-312.

NETWORK ANALYSIS

HERD CONTACT STRUCTURE BASED ON COMMON WATERING AND GRAZING POINTS IN THE HIGHLANDS OF ETHIOPIA

A. WARET-SZKUTA*, A. ORTIZ-PELAEZ, F. ROGER, D. U. PFEIFFER AND F. J. GUITIAN

SUMMARY

Little is known about the contact structure of the farming population in developing countries which is expected to be complex and heterogeneous as a result of the need for continuous adaptation to variable environmental conditions.

The use of shared common water (WP) and grazing points (GP) at two different levels of administrative aggregation (village and *kebelle*) was explored, by means of a questionnaire survey in the Bassona region (*wereda*) of the highlands of Ethiopia, as a potential risk factor for pathogen transmission. Several symmetric binary networks based on villages linked through common WP and GP were built and described. Random permutation tests and quadratic assignment procedure (QAP) were applied to test the association between network parameters and village attributes.

The findings from this study should be taken into consideration in the design of surveillance and control activities for infectious diseases such as *Peste des Petits Ruminants* (PPR).

INTRODUCTION

Ethiopia has the largest livestock population in Africa and is ranked 9th in the world. The livestock sub-sector accounts for 40% of the agricultural gross domestic product (GDP) and 20% of the total GDP without considering the livestock contribution in terms of traction power, fertilizing and means of transport. In 2006, the sheep and goat populations were estimated to be 20.7 million and 16.4 million, respectively (CSA, 2006). Sheep and goats make up 25% of meat consumption within the country, with the production surplus mainly being exported as live animals (Alemayehu et al., 1991). Both species also supply half the domestic needs in wool, and about 40% of skins and 92% of the value of hides and skin are exported (ILCA, 1993). The annual production of sheep and goat meat is estimated as 56,560 and 28,650 tonnes, respectively.

The very diverse geography/geology of the country defines several geoclimatic zones. The central part is characterized by a mountainous range that covers half of the territory. It is a zone of highlands ranging from 2,300 to 3,500m in altitude called *Dega*, surrounded by a temperate transition zone between 1,500 and 2,300m called *Woinadega* that dives into the central Rift

* Agnès Waret-Szkuta, Royal Veterinary College, London, AL9 7TA UK and CIRAD, Montpellier, 34398 Cedex 5, France. Email: awaret@rvc.ac.uk

Valley towards the south west. East, the tectonic deflection opens on the lowland areas *Bereha* and *Kola* (0 to 1,200m), zones of pastoral nomadic livestock husbandry (Anon., 1973).

The climate is characterized by a long rainy season called *Meher* from June to September representing around 75% of the annual rainfall and a short rainy season called *Belg* from February/March to April/May. The dry season takes place from October to January. The minimum average monthly temperature ranges from 2°C in November to 8°C in August and the maximum from 18°C in September to 23°C in June (Larbodière, 1995). The strong rainfalls, often involving snow and hail during *Meher*, together with the low temperatures at the beginning of the long dry season, are an important constraint for agriculture and livestock production. At the end of the dry season, the lack of water in some locations can be a major problem.

Around half of the small ruminants in Ethiopia are found in the highlands with a population composed mainly of sheep. Production systems of goats are not well documented in that region but usually follow the same pattern as those of the sheep where they exist. Traditional farmers mainly raise goats and other livestock in addition to agricultural activity. The mixed livestock-agriculture system, with small herds that prevail in the highlands contrasts with the pastoral system found in the Lowlands, where larger flocks/herds can be found (Tibbo, 2006). Mixing of animals belonging to different farmers from the village is a common practice (90%) but most of them (80%) stop this practice during the long rainy season (Larbodière, 1995). Grazing, for example, is communal during the dry season and separate during the rest of the year with owners grazing the animals on their own land. Shepherded mainly by children, small ruminants graze some distance away from the village in zones of intense cropping activities. The process of "villagisation" during the mid-80's in Ethiopia has pushed farmers away from their plots of land (Luling V., 1986).

Little is known about the contact structure of the farming population in developing countries, which is expected to be complex and heterogeneous due to the need for continuous adaptation to variable environmental conditions. Management practices that favour contacts between animals from different origins in regions situated between the two parallels of 40° latitude north and south, are often used to explain the persistence of a number of directly transmitted diseases. Mixing at watering points and grazing points has been identified as a key factor for transmission of diseases like rinderpest, Peste des Petits Ruminants (PPR) and foot and mouth disease (FMD) (Lefevre et al., 2003). Social network analysis (SNA) can help describe the topology of the contact structure of livestock populations and understand the impact of network structures on the potential routes of transmission of infectious diseases provided that the nature of the links relates to known risk factors of disease transmission. Previous studies have shown the implications of such structures of the efficacy of surveillance and control programs (Woolhouse et al., 2005 ; Kiss et al., 2006).

The aim of this study was to describe and compare the contact networks created by sharing of small ruminants' watering and grazing points in a region (*wereda*) of the highlands in Ethiopia at different levels (*kebelle*, villages) and to discuss the implications of such structures for the design of surveillance and control activities.

MATERIALS AND METHODS

Study site and sampling method

The study area was the Bassona werena *wereda* which covers 102,035Ha in the central part of Ethiopia (Fig. 1). It was a convenient study area due to its proximity to Addis Abeba (130 Km. north east), and the availability of baseline production information from previous field studies (Alemayehu et al., 1991 ; Larbodière, 1995). The study area was the result of grouping the two different agro-ecological settings found in the highlands: *Dega* from 2300 meters above sea level (masl) to 3500masl (52%) and *Woina Dega* from 1500masl to 2300masl (48%). Administratively, the study area includes 29 *kebelles*, of which ten were purposively selected based on accessibility criteria. Of them the 2 located further away from Debre Berhan town were selected for the pilot study. Within the other 8 *kebelles*, 80 villages were randomly selected: 10 villages in 6 *kebelles*, 11 in 2 *kebelles* and 8 in one *kebelle*.

In each village, 10 small ruminant owners were selected in a systematic way for individual interviews. The interviewer started from the centre of the village selecting for interview every second owner on a straight imaginary line heading north, then moved to west, south and finally east until 10 small ruminant owners were identified. The dispersion of the households around the village was assumed to be sufficient for most of the directions to be covered and the sample to be representative and random. The subset of the questionnaire relating to watering and grazing points was administered to a group of children in each of the 80 villages, given their role in taking the animals out for grazing. In order to increase the reliability and validity of the answers, all available children from the village were gathered in the evening of the day of the visit.

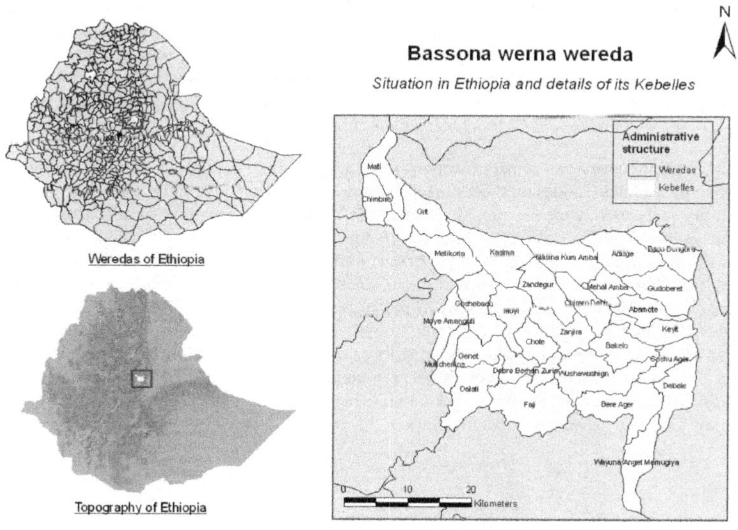

Fig. 1 Study site, location in Ethiopia and topography

Field data collection

Two questionnaires (one for the individual animal owners and another for the group of children) were designed and piloted, together with the sampling method described above, in the 2 most remote *Kebelles* of the 10 that were randomly selected. The owner questionnaire was administered to individual owners and included questions on flock/herd size and species composition, the possibility of *Rebi* practice (keeping animals of other owners in return, for example, for newborn lambs/kids), number and origin of the animals kept and period during which *Rebi* is practiced (long rainy season, short rainy season, long dry season, short dry season). The children questionnaire was filled in during the meeting with the group of children, when they were asked the names and time of use of the grazing and watering points (long rainy season, short rainy season, long dry season, short dry season). The questionnaires were administered by 3 interviewers (two of them being trained by the first one) from February to March 2007. During the visit, the GPS location was recorded for each village, along with the total number of households in the village and the number of households raising small ruminants.

Data management and analysis

The results of the questionnaire were entered into Microsoft Excel 2003 (Microsoft Corporation) and general descriptive statistics and t-tests were calculated using SPSS for Windows version 15.0 (SPSS Inc.). For t-tests, homogeneity of variance was assessed based on Levene's test for equality of variance. Statistical comparisons used $\alpha = 0.05$ (two-sided).

Network data were entered as matrices using Microsoft Excel 2003 (Microsoft Corporation). Several symmetric binary networks were built with all the studied *kebelles* and villages as nodes and the ties: "sharing waterpoints", "sharing grazing points", and the correspondent valued networks with the links being: "the number of shared water points", "the number of shared grazing points". Moreover for each individual *kebelle* two symmetric binary networks were created with nodes being villages and ties: "sharing waterpoints", "sharing grazing points". Networks were also constructed by season (long dry season, short dry season, long rainy season, short rainy season) with villages as nodes and "sharing waterpoints", "sharing grazing points" as ties.

For each network the density (proportion of all possible ties that are actually present), and number of isolates (nodes not connected to any other) were obtained. For each node, two centrality measures were extracted: degree, defined as the number of alternative sharing villages/*kebelles* and betweenness, defined as the frequency with which a node falls between pairs of other nodes on the geodesic (shortest) path connecting them divided by the maximum value it can have in the network (Freeman, 1978/9). Bootstrap paired sample t-tests were applied to test for differences in the probability of ties of two classes using 10,000 random permutations per test (Hanneman, 2005). The quadratic assignment procedure (QAP) correlation function in Ucinet (www.analytic-tech.com) was used to calculate the correlation between two matrices, using the Jaccard coefficient after 5000 permutations (Hanneman, 2005). Statistical tests of network data were conducted using UCINET 6.182 and visualization of the networks with Netdraw v2.074 (www.analytic-tech.com/).

RESULTS

Questionnaire results

Data from 80 villages were collected ranging from 2655masl to 3336masl of altitude. On average 82% of the households in the villages investigated had small ruminants. Locations of the investigated *kebelles* and villages are shown in Fig. 2.

The villages had on average 28 households with small ruminants (range= 11-47) and the average flock had 11.5 sheep (range= 0 -63) and 1 goat (range=0-39). Sixty-nine (76%) of villages had households rearing both sheep and goats, nine (21.3%) had only sheep and the information was missing in 2 villages (2.5%). Villages keeping both species were situated significantly higher in altitude than the villages with only sheep (t-test for independent samples, $P<0.001$). In 27% of the villages interviewed at least one owner declared practicing *Rebi.*

During the interviews in the villages, 154 watering points and 208 grazing points along with their period of use were identified. Two subgroups could be distinguished based on the geographical position in the *wereda* and altitude: one located west of the *wereda* including 3 *kebelles* (Goshebado, Angolela, Birbisa) with a mean altitude of 2772 masl and the other east of the *wereda* including 5 *kebelles* (Abamote, Keyit, BereAger, Gudoberet, Debele) with a mean altitude of 3108 masl (t-test for independent samples, $P<0.001$).

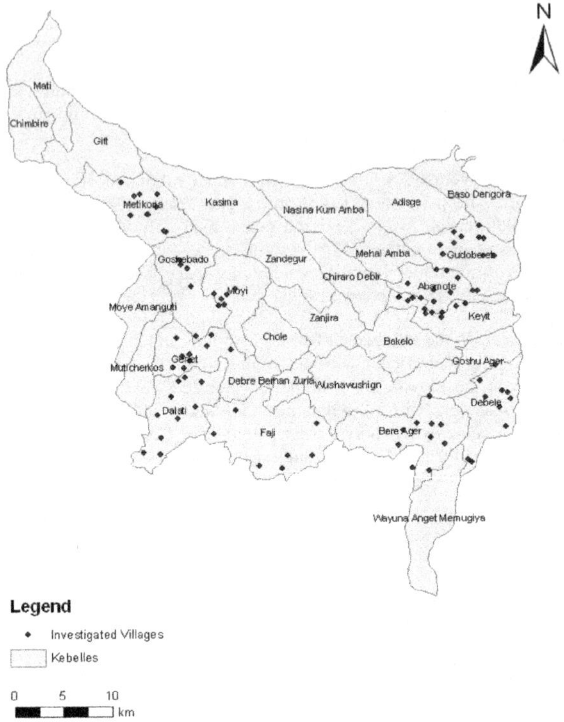

Fig. 2 Map of Bassona werana *wereda* showing the administrative boundaries of all *kebelles* and the locations of the interviewed villages

<u>Network results</u>

<u>At *kebelle* level</u>

The networks with *kebelle* as nodes and links based on "sharing grazing points" or "sharing watering points" show no isolates among their 8 nodes (Fig.3 and 4). The average degree of the nodes (number of *kebelles* each *kebelle* is linked to) in the grazing point network (6) is the result of relatively homogenous values for each of the nodes (*kebelle*). This is much higher than the same measure in the watering points network (2.7) where there are 2 pendants (nodes tied to the group by only one connection) and a maximum average degree of the nodes of 5, as shown in Table 1. Betweenness of each node was very variable in the watering point network ranging from 0 to 6.67 and being null for three nodes: Abamote, Birbisa and Debelle. In the grazing point network, half of the nodes (4) had a betweenness of 0.167 and the other half a betweenness of 0.333. The two networks had a high density (93% of the ties being present in the grazing and 46% in the watering point network) showing great connectivity. The density of the grazing point network (0.93) was also significantly higher than the density of the watering point network (0.46) (bootstrap paired sample T-test, P<0.001).

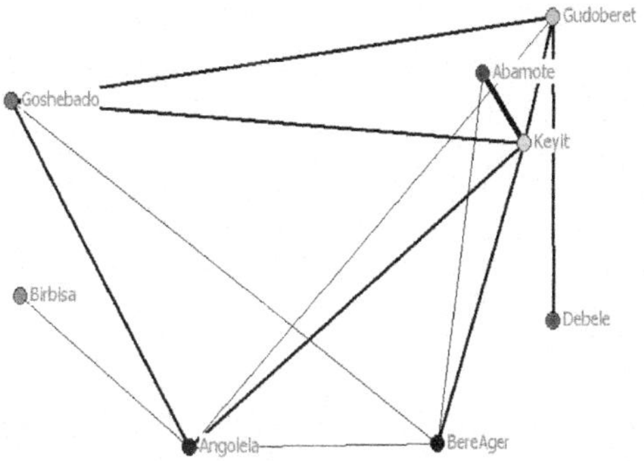

Fig. 3 Watering points network [*Kebelles* (nodes) have been dragged and dropped into their relative geographical positions. The properties of the lines have been changed so that the thicker the line the more numerous are the common watering points]

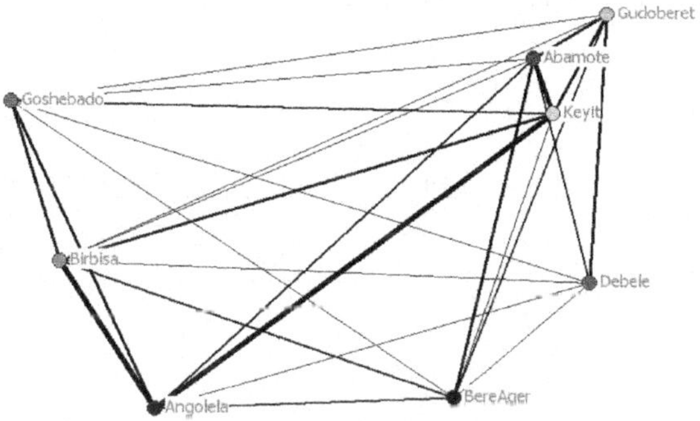

Fig. 4 Grazing points network [*Kebelles* (nodes) have been dragged and dropped into their relative geographical positions. The properties of the lines have been changed so that the thicker the line the more numerous are the common grazing points]

The QAP correlation coefficient (0.467, P-value=0.013) indicates that there is a correlation between contacts due to grazing and watering points.

Table 1. Degree and node betweenness of the watering and grazing point networks with node=*kebelle*

	WATERING POINTS		GRAZING POINTS	
Kebelle	*Degree*	*Node Betweenness*	*Degree*	*Node Betweenness*
Abamote	2	0	6	0.33
Angolela	4	6.67	6	0.17
BereAger	2	1.5	7	0.33
Birbisa	1	0	7	0.33
Debelle	1	0	6	0.17
Goshebado	4	0.67	5	0.33
Gudoberet	3	6	5	0.17
Keyit	5	4.2	6	0.17

At village level

Focus on villages grouped by *kebelle*: A network was created for each *kebelle* with villages included in the study (10 villages for 6 *kebelles* of the study, 11 villages for 2 *kebelles* and 8 villages for one *kebelle*) as nodes and ties being "sharing watering points" or "sharing grazing points". Table 2 presents a summary of the results found for the extracted parameters for each of the eight networks that were built.

Table 2. Density, isolates, mean degree of nodes and betweenness (overall centralization index) considering each *kebelle* separately, nodes being villages.

	WATERING POINTS				GRAZING POINTS			
Kebelle (no. of villages)	*Density (%)*	*No. of isolates*	*Mean d° of nodes*	*between -ness (%)*	*Density (%)*	*No. of isolates*	*Mean d° of nodes*	*between -ness (%)*
Abamote (10)	11	3	1	0	8.9	4	0.8	8.33
Angolela (10)	33.3	0	3.4	21.91	11.1	4	1	5.56
BereAger (11)	7.3	7	0.8	4.44	14.5	4	1.45	20.89
Birbisa (10)	40	2	4.4	27.78	31.1	1	2.8	39.2
Debelle (11)	5.5	6	0.6	2.22	14.5	5	1.45	8
Goshebado (10)	11	4	1	5.56	28.9	0	2	26.54
Gudoberet (8)	4	6	0.25	0	22.2	0	1.5	4.76
Keyit (10)	11.1	5	1.4	10.19	20	1	1.8	20.68

The quantitative structure of the networks was very variable considering their links through watering or grazing points.

For the links through watering points, the number of isolates varied from 0 to 7 (median=4.5). Amongst the grazing point networks the number of isolates ranged from 0 to 5 (median=2.5).

The mean degree of the nodes (villages linked to other villages inside each *kebelle*) was very variable in each of the networks although there were no isolates. The degree was more variable in the networks with "sharing watering points" as ties. The highest value for the degree of the nodes was found in Birbisa *kebelle* where villages were on average linked to 4.4 other villages of the same *kebelle* by means of watering points.

In general, the density was higher in the grazing point networks compared to the watering point networks although the highest values were found in one of the watering point networks (density of 40% for Birbisa with links "sharing watering points"). The overall centralization index (betweenness) was higher in the grazing points than the watering points network for each of the *kebelles* except one (Angolela).

All villages considered as nodes: The two networks considered here were built considering all studied villages as nodes and ties based on "sharing watering points" or "sharing grazing points". The size of both networks was 80 nodes (corresponding to the 80 villages interviewed during the study). Table 3 summarises the findings for the number of isolates, the density, the degree (range, average and median) and the network centralization index (betweenness) for the two networks considered.

Table 3. Isolates, density, degree (including average and median) and betweenness (overall centralization index) considering the networks of all villages interviewed (nodes), ties being "sharing watering points" and "sharing grazing points", respectively.

	NUMBER OF ISOLATES	DENSITY	DEGREE RANGE OF NODES	AVERAGE DEGREE	MEDIAN DEGREE	BETWEEN-NESS
Watering points	20	2.6%	0-11 (Dalati)	2.9	2.5	2.74%
Grazing points	11	5.7%	0-22 (Dibut)	4.8	3	14.72%

Both networks showed low connectivity (density 2.6% and 5.7% respectively). The number of isolates when "sharing watering points" was considered as ties was almost double when compared to the number of isolates considering "sharing grazing points" as ties. On average villages were linked to 2.9 other villages by means of watering points (median=2.5 ; range: 0-11) and 4.8 other villages via grazing points (median 3; range=0-22). The betweenness was much higher in grazing (14.72%) compared to watering point networks (2.74%).

The significant difference in density observed at *kebelle* level was confirmed at village level (P-value<0.001), with the density of the grazing network being higher than the density of the watering point network.

The QAP correlation coefficient (0.259, P-value=0.000) also confirmed even more strongly that villages having contacts through sharing of grazing points were more likely to also share watering points.

The mean degree of single-species villages (lower in altitude) was significantly higher than the mean degree of multi-species villages when considering edges being watering points (difference in means=-2.745, P-value<0.001). However, no difference was found for grazing points (difference in means=-0.022, two-tailed P-value=0.99).

Each of the two networks with villages as nodes (considering "sharing grazing points" and "sharing waterpoints", respectively) were then split into two networks in order to take into account the seasonality of the links between villages (rainy season and/or dry season). Table 4 reports the resulting number of isolates, density, degree (average and median) and betweenness values during the rainy and dry season of these networks.

Isolates were more numerous for the rainy season networks considering both watering or grazing points as ties; the density was lower and betweenness higher. Although the average degree was higher during the rainy season compared to the dry season when considering watering points, it was the opposite when looking at the grazing points, with degree being more variable during the rainy season.

Table 4. Descriptive network parameters using villages as nodes and "sharing watering points" or "sharing grazing points" as links and taking into account seasonality (rainy season ; dry season)

LINKS	SEASON	NO. OF ISOLATES	DENSITY (%)	AVERAGE DEGREE (%)	MEDIAN DEGREE (%)	BETWEENNESS (%)
"sharing WP"	Rainy	30	2.3	3.1	1.3	1.6
	Dry	24	2.6	2.6	2.5	2.3
"sharing GP"	Rainy	19	4.5	3.58	2	42.4
	Dry	11	5.1	4	3	58.3

The density of the watering point network during dry season was significantly higher than during rainy season (difference in density=0.0035, Bootstrap t-test two-tailed P-value=0.04). The two networks were significantly correlated (QAP correlation coefficient=0.906; P-value<0.001) so that villages sharing watering points during the rainy season are more likely to share them during the dry season.

When comparing the grazing point networks, the difference in density between the dry and rainy season was not significant (P=0.22), with both networks also strongly correlated (QAP correlation coefficient=0.77; P-value<0.001).

Comparing the 2 village groups identified based on altitude, villages situated east of the *wereda* (higher in altitude) were less likely to share watering points than villages situated west of the *wereda*. The average degree for the western village group being significantly higher than for the eastern (difference in means=-2.387, P-value<0.001). No difference was found for grazing points (difference in mean degree=-0.227; two tailed P-value=0.83).

DISCUSSION

The aim of this study was to describe and compare the networks created by sharing of small ruminants watering and grazing points at different administrative levels in the highlands of

Ethiopia, as a potential risk factor for pathogen transmission. To our knowledge it is the first field study of this type designed in Sub-Saharan Africa with this objective. It is acknowledged that the purposive selection of *kebelle* within the *wereda* may have resulted in some degree of bias. However, it is unlikely that this will have affected the biological relevance of the conclusions from this work.

The random permutations tests performed take into account that the "observations" in network data are not "independent" samples from a population. Through "boot strapping" and permutations the sampling distribution of required statistics can be directly calculated from the observed networks by using random assignment across thousand of trials under the assumption that null hypotheses are true. For instance, these procedures allow the boostrap paired sample t-tests to compare the differences in probability of a tie between two classes (Hanneman, 2005).

Although the questionnaires were administered once at the beginning of the rainy season, seasonal variation patterns (crucial areas where farmers are dependant upon natural resources which are variable in time) could also be addressed when analysing retrospective questions. Results obtained regarding the small ruminant population structure and management practices were similar to those reported 15 years ago (Larbodière, 1995).

Despite grazing points being more abundant than watering points, they appeared to provide more contact opportunities for animals from different *kebelles* and villages. Expansion of cultivated land forcing farmers to increase mobility when searching for grazing points shared by multiple villages could explain this result. This effect was stronger in villages located in highland areas which tend to be more isolated and rear mixed flocks of sheep and goats. Only-sheep villages share on average 4.4 watering points compared to 1.6 among mixed-flock villages ($P<0.001$). As expected the watering point network is more dense during the dry season when some of the WP become unavailable.

There was great variability in the contact structure of the selected villages within *kebelles* for both networks in terms of the number of isolates, degree and average betweenness, this variability being higher in the grazing point networks for each *kebelle*. Betweenness can be interpreted as providing an indication of the extent to which a node facilitates the transmission of an infectious agent amongst members of the network (Borgatti, 1995). Betweenness was higher for nodes linked by grazing than by watering points, and very variable, potentially as a result of differences in the size of the grazing points or their ownership characteristics (private or communal). Although values of betweenness are high when considering villages as nodes, the values are very low when using *kebelle*, suggesting that the more detailed contact structure based on villages may be more appropriate for this type of study.

Grazing points appear to be the most important contact point for livestock among small farming systems in the highlands of Ethiopia at the village and aggregated *kebelle* scale. Contrary to the common assumption that congregation of livestock at watering points is critical for the potential transmission of infectious diseases, the results from the current study suggest that interventions associated with shared grazing areas in the Ethiopian highlands may also be important for the contact between flocks. The connectedness of the contact networks depends on the husbandry and altitude which defines two distinctive regions within the study area. Rotation of the areas used for common and individual grazing in the highlands and the relatively small size of the current study compared with the diversity and size of the country advises to caution when drawing generalised conclusions from this work. But, perhaps increased awareness of farmers and veterinary services of the potential for disease transmission while using shared grazing areas as well as a reasoned management of the grazing rotation may help the control and prevention of infectious diseases amongst small ruminants in the highlands of Ethiopia.

If grazing and watering points are to be considered when designing surveillance and control activities, it is also recommended that a better understanding of contact structure through markets be obtained.

ACKNOWLEDGEMENTS

The questionnaire was prepared by the first author then translated in Amharic in Ethiopia and double checked by an Ethiopian MSc student in England for validation.

This study was carried out as part of the EU funded INCO-CT-2004-003670 RP/PPR MARKVAC project.

REFERENCES

Alemayehu, Z. and Fletcher, I. (1991). Small ruminants productivity in the central Ethiopia mixed farming systems. Addis Ababa: IAR (Institute of Agricultural Research).

Anonymous (1973). Grand Atlas du continent Africain. Paris: Edition Jeune Afrique.

Borgatti, S.P. (1995). Centrality and AIDS. Connections 18(1), 112-115.

CSA (Central Statistical Agency) (2006). Agricultural sample survey 2005/2006 [1998 E.C.], Report on livestock and livestock characteristics. Statistical bulletin n°361 Volume II. Addis Abeba.

Freeman, L.C. (1978/9). Centrality in social networks conceptual clarification. Social Networks 1, 215-239.

Hanneman, R.A. and Riddle, M. (2005). Introduction to Social Network Methods. University of California Riverside, Riverside, CA.

ILCA (International Livestock Center for Africa) (1993). Handbook of African Livestock Statistics. Addis Ababa.

Kiss, I.Z., Green, D.M., Kao, R.R. (2006). Infectious disease control using contact tracing in random and scale-free networks. Journal of the Royal Society Interface 3, 55-62

Larbodière, L. (1995). Enquête productivité en élevage ovin traditionnel dans la region de Debre Berhan (Ethiopie). Mémoire de stage de DESS Production animales en régions chaudes, Cirad-emvt, Montpellier, France, 86p.

Lefevre, P.C., Blancou, J. and Chermette, R. (2003). Principales maladies infectieuses et parasitaires du bétail. Europe et régions chaudes. Tome 1. Généralités, Maladies virales. Chapitre 4 : Particularités épidémiologiques des régions chaudes (Lefevre PC, Blancou J.) p.47-54. Ed, Lavoisier, Paris.

Luling, V. (1986). Ethiopia: Resettlement, Villagisation and the Ethiopian People. International Work group for Indigenous Affairs, Copenhagen, Danemark, 47, 27-39

Tibbo, M. (2006). Productivity and Health of Indegenous Sheep breeds and crossbreds in the Central Ethiopian Highlands. *PhD Thesis*. Swedish University of Agricultural Sciences, Uppsala.

Woolhouse, M.E.J., Shaw, D.J., Matthews, L., Liu, W.C., Mellor, D.J., Thomas, M.R. (2005). Epidemiological implications of the contact network structure for cattle farms and the 20-80 rule. Biol. Lett. UK, 1, 350-352.

CONSEQUENCES OF NETWORKS IN EPIDEMIOLOGICAL PREDICTIONS OF FMD

T. LYYTIKÄINEN*, E.R. KALLIO, L. SAHLSTRÖM AND T. VIRTANEN

SUMMARY

The Finnish FMD Monte Carlo simulation model was applied to estimate the spread of FMD among Finnish pig farms. Estimates were then compared to estimations from a model where information on contact farms was ignored (random network simulation). Both model approaches gave roughly similar results for the average epidemic size in the country. However, the worst case estimate for the country was three times higher by random network simulation. Model outcomes also differed when the outcomes of the two models were compared at the farm level. Based on the model iterations, the average epidemic size by random network simulation was different from the value from the structured network simulation for 40 % of farms when they acted as the primary infected farm. The results of the study highlight the importance of the structured network information when worst case scenarios or farm specific estimates are predicted.

INTRODUCTION

Foot-and-mouth disease (FMD) is a highly contagious viral disease of cloven-hoofed animals, which causes painful vesicles and lesions in the animals. FMD causes significant economic losses although the mortality rate in adult animals is low. To halt the spread of the infection, all infected or in-contact susceptible animals are culled. FMD may spread by direct contact between animals, indirectly via fomites and through airborne transmission (e.g. Sutmoller et al., 2003).

The outbreaks of infectious diseases of domestic animals, such as FMD, are partly dependent on the number and the type of contacts the first infected (primary) farm has during the period of time for which the disease is infectious but not yet detected. Farms are connected to each other via different kinds of contacts, which together result in networks in which contagious diseases are spread. Hence, the properties of the first infected farm are not the only determinants of the epidemiological consequences; the other farms that take part in the network also have an influence on the magnitude of the outbreak. Consequently, the outcome is a combination of the properties of the primary farm and the properties of those farms which are connected to it.

Network analysis has produced a new way to incorporate heterogeneity into the epidemiological predictions of disease spread (Barthélemy et al., 2004; Barthélemy et al., 2005; Crepey et al., 2006; Colizza et al., 2006; Masuda & Konno, 2006; Meyers et al., 2006; Kenah & Robins, 2007). The employment of network analyses has also recently increased in animal

* Tapani Lyytikäinen, Finnish Food Safety Authority (Evira), Risk Assessment Unit, Mustialankatu 3, 00790 Helsinki, Finland. E-mail: tapani.lyytikainen@evira.fi

disease epidemiology. After the FMD outbreak in the UK in 2001, networks have been studied as one of the reasons of rapid escalation of the disease (Shirley & Rushton, 2005). Several models and descriptive studies of the 2001 epidemic have been published (Ferguson et al., 2001; Gibbens & Wilesmith, 2002; Kao, 2002; Lawson & Zhou, 2005; Chowell et al., 2006). Some of the studies have also applied models using network descriptions (Morris et al., 2001; Stevenson, 2003; Green et al., 2006; Kao et al., 2006). Network studies and epidemiological models have also been applied for predictive purposes in other countries (e.g. Bigras-Poulin et al., 2007; Tildesley & Keeling, 2008).

Network structures have two distinct topologies: spatial (space) and temporal (time). In epidemiology, most of the work has been concentrated on spatial topology, by using a fixed temporal topology, in other words using static network descriptions (e.g. Kao et al., 2006). Recently, dynamic networks have also been applied (Heath et al., 2008), where temporal characteristics, e.g. the sequences of events within the network will influence the potential outcome.

In theory, the complete network model (i.e. including both spatial and temporal topologies) would be the closest model to the real world and could be regarded as a "golden standard" for modelling the spread of infectious animal diseases. Network models require more data than other types of models; a list of events, sources, targets and times. This may cause problems because such data are rarely available. The construction of the network and data collection becomes especially difficult when the disease can spread by several routes such as in FMD, when there are several operations to model and data sources are scattered. These difficulties mean that it is worth considering whether or not the development of a network model is justified.

The aim of this study is to estimate whether detailed information of spatial and temporal networks would improve the assessment of the spread of infectious disease. A detailed, structured network model was applied to simulate the spread of FMD within the pig population in Finland. A structured network simulation model which contains detailed description of the operations and networks of Finnish pig production, was applied in the study. The model has been used previously in risk classification of Finnish pig farms and estimation of economical consequences of the disease (Lyytikäinen & Kallio, 2009; Niemi et al., 2008). The outcomes of the simulation model were compared to a model with less information: target farms were selected randomly from the Finnish pig farm population. The probability and magnitude of an epidemic outbreak were studied both by a random network model and by a structured network model.

MATERIALS AND METHODS

The Finnish Monte Carlo simulation model was employed to study the spread of FMD among pig farms in Finland and is described in more details in Lyytikäinen & Kallio (2009). The structured network model resembles several other simulation models that have been applied to study the relationship between the spread of FMD and production structures or control policies, such as Interspread plus, InterFMD and NAASDM (Sanson, 1993; Mourits et al., 2002; Harvey et al., 2007; Schley, 2007; Velthuis & Mourits, 2007). All these models use the concept of transmission probabilities and contacts to estimate the number of infections.

The structured network model contains information about the frequency of potential contacts and potential targets of contacts in time and space. The structured model directly uses an animal registry database as a description of the animal transportation network. Spatiality and temporality in animal transportation is defined by the registry but indirect contacts by animal transportation vehicles are constructed indirectly by a three mode network (in other words connected indirectly by two separate factors), where farms are linked by sharing the same vehicle during the same day. The identities of the farms, which are visited by a certain vehicle in a day, are known but the order of the visits is not known. Similarly, the transportations to slaughter are linked in the model by sharing the same transport day and the same slaughterhouse. The static component of neighbouring farms is constructed directly by farm location. Other parts of networks are constructed by 2-mode networks connected by a separate factor, where the temporal component is described by a Poisson process. For instance visitors like veterinarians and AI technicians are spatially linked with their operational regions (Table 1).

The Monte Carlo simulation model was developed in the Matlab 7.3 (Mathworks Inc., MA, USA) environment. The Econometrics toolbox (Le Sage, 2002) was used to generate random variables. Events were simulated on a daily basis: the first simulation day represents the infection day of the primary farm.

The simulation was started separately from each of the Finnish pig farms. The first farm of each iteration is defined as a primary infected farm. The source of the infection at the primary infected farm is assumed to be unknown. In order to create an epidemic, the primary infected farm must infect at least one other farm. The other infected farms can then induce further infections during their infective period. The infective period starts 7 days after the infectious contact and continues for 3 weeks without restrictive measures (see below for restrictive measures). Transmission is possible when a susceptible farm receives at least one infective contact. Several categories of contacts are included in the model: receiving live pigs (high risk contact), a visit by a livestock transportation vehicle or person visiting animal holdings (medium risk contact), a person visiting at the farm (low risk contact), having an infected farm within 1.5 km, and having an infected farm within 1.5 and 3 km. The two last contact types include the so-called neighbourhood transmission, where the vector is unknown. Each of the contact types has a different transmission probability that defines the probability of initiating an infection (Lyytikäinen & Kallio,2009).

Table 1. Data and processes used for the structured model of the Finnish pig production network.

Vector	Incident leading to transmission of infection	Spatiality of network	Temporality of network	Connection rule
Pig	Transportation of live pigs between farms	Animal movement registry	Animal movement registry	Historical, year 2006, animals are transported between farms
Vehicle	Vehicle transporting pigs between farms	Animal movement registry	Animal movement registry	Historical, year 2006, same transportation vehicle
Vehicle	Vehicle transporting pigs to slaughter	Animal movement registry	Animal movement registry	Historical, year 2006, same slaughterhouse and day of slaughter
Person	Visit to the production unit	Depending on the operational region of the visitor	Simulated Poisson process	Same operational region as infected farm
Person	Visit without entering the production unit	Depending on the operational region of the visitor	Simulated Poisson process	Same operational region as infected farm
Person	Substitute	Depending on the operational region of the visitor	Simulated binomial process	Same operational region as infected farm
Person	Culling of pigs	Depending on the operational region of the visitor	Conditional to detection, uniformly distributed lag	Same operational region as infected farm
Unknown	Neighbouring pig farms within 1.5 km	Farm registry	No temporal events – static	Proximity as given
Unknown	Neighbouring pig farms within 1.5-3 km	Farm registry	No temporal events - static	Proximity as given

In the model, it is assumed that the first detection takes place at the primary infected farm and by the farmer. Thereafter, detecting the infection at a farm may occur in several ways. It can be done by the farmer, by contact tracing, by routine screening (clinical and/or serological) in restriction zones (a protection zone of 3 km, and a surveillance zone between 3 and 10 km) around the infected farms. On farms where the disease has been confirmed pigs are culled and the animal holdings are cleaned and disinfected. For most contact types the infective period ends on the day when restrictive measures are lifted. The infective period of neighbourhood spread ends when the farm is initially cleaned. For the farms in the restriction zones, the contacts are limited and the farmers are obliged to inform the officials of any signs of disease. All pig farms in the protection zones are visited by a screening team within one week. Serological screenings in the protection zones are performed 30 days, and clinical screenings in the surveillance zones are performed 20 days after the last confirmed infected premises in the zone has been initially cleaned. The restrictive measures are applied to the traced contact farms. These farms are visited for clinical inspection within one week from tracing. The iteration is terminated when all infected farms are detected and cleaned and no new infections are occurring.

Simulations

The simulations were started on three dates: 01/01/06 (day 0), and 90 and 180 days later. On each day, 300 000 iterations were performed, which means that every farm acted as the primary farm in approximately 93 iterations per starting date (all together 279 iterations per farm). Because the primary farms were selected randomly, the number of iterations per primary farm varied within a date and also between the starting dates.

The simulation with a structured network (n=900000) was started from each pig farm in the country (n=3228) separately to define the size of an epidemic outbreak. Another simulation (n=900000) was performed to estimate the predictions without network information but with the same number of contacts (random network) (Fig. 1). The latter simulation corresponded to a situation where spatial network information is missing. Ignoring spatial network information also breaks potential spatio-temporal correlations.

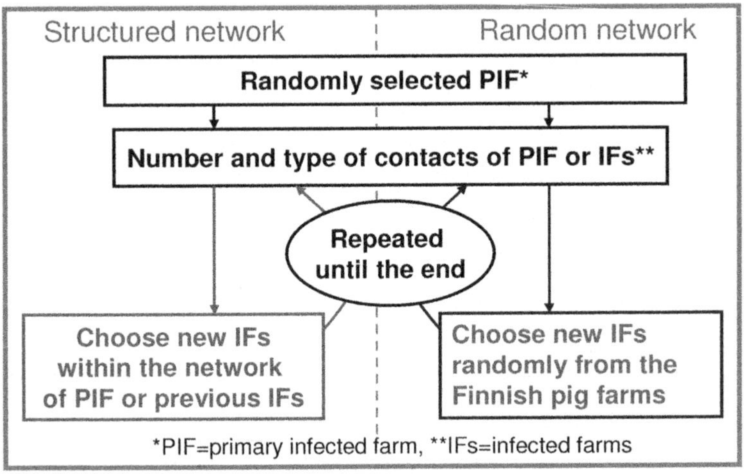

Fig. 1 Schematic diagram showing the difference between the two studied simulation strategies.

The output of the simulations consisted of the number of infected farms at the end of each iteration, the date of infection at a farm, the identity of the infected farms and the identity of the farm which was the source of infection and the type of contact which initiated the infection.

Outcomes of the simulations

Farm specific outcomes were calculated separately for each farm applying the iterations when it acted as the first infected farm in the country (primary infected farm). Relevant variables for risk assessment were selected to be studied: the probability and magnitude of a non-beneficial event. Two different magnitude estimates are useful in infectious animal disease risk assessment: the expected and the worst case scenario value of the outcome.

The probability of the epidemic outbreak was calculated for each farm based on those iterations where a particular farm acted as the primary infected farm. The average, the maximum and the standard deviation of the epidemic size were calculated for each farm based on the iterations that produced new infection(s). Estimates for the whole country were calculated from farm specific estimates.

Comparison of outcomes by structured and random network

Outcomes of the two simulations for each farm were compared to identify the farms whose ability to spread the disease was statistically significantly altered by ignoring the network information. The estimates were compared using a non-parametric bootstrapping method with replacement. Estimates from both simulations were resampled 1000 times from those iterations which were started from a certain farm and the probabilities that the estimates were different were calculated according to those 1000 comparisons.

Comparisons were performed on the average, the maximum and the standard deviation of the epidemic size. The maximum and the standard deviation comparisons should be considered as indices of a worst case scenario while the average epidemic size is obviously indicating the expected size of an epidemic outbreak when the outbreak has been started at a certain farm.

Farms were classified into three groups according to the estimated probability by bootstrapping. If bootstrapping indicated that the probability estimate by the random network was either higher or lower than the estimate from the structured network simulation for the same farm (P>0.95), the farm estimate was classified as either over- or under-estimation, respectively. Otherwise the result of an estimate was considered as equal.

RESULTS

Country level predictions

The size of the epidemics differed between the random and structured networks. The random networks caused on average a 6% larger expected epidemic size in the country (average number of infected farms 4.20 vs. 4.45). The maximum epidemic size in the country based on the random network simulation was 2.99 times larger than that found using the structured network model (568 vs. 190).

Farm level predictions

The pre-requirement for a comparison between the outcomes of the structured and the random network simulations is that the probability of an epidemic outbreak at the farm level is equal in both simulations. The epidemic outbreak probability (mean=0.66, std=0.27) was similar in both simulations and farm specific probabilities were closely correlating with each other

(Spearman r=0.99). The regression slope of the epidemic outbreak probability between the structured and random network simulations did not deviate from 1 (0.97; 95% CI ± 0.04) and the intercept was zero (0.00, 95% CI ±0.04), indicating that the simulation results in this sense were equal. In both cases, the relationship between the probability of an epidemic outbreak and the average epidemic size was non-linear and showed a similar pattern (Fig. 2a and b).

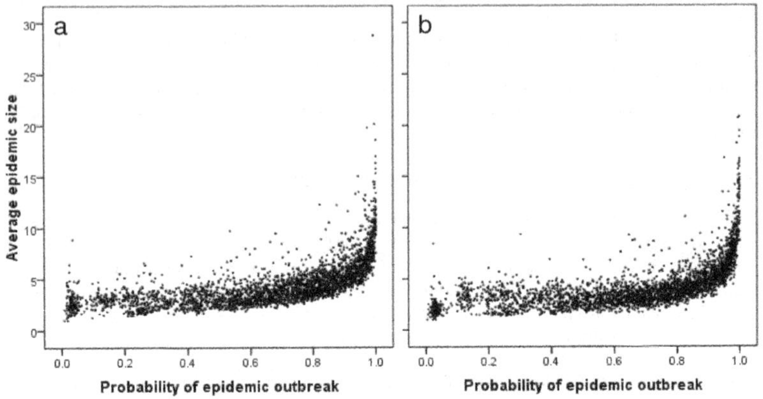

Fig. 2a and b The relationship between the probability of an epidemic outbreak and the average epidemic size when simulated by a random network (a) and by a structured network simulation (b). Each dot represents the averaged outcome for a certain Finnish pig farm (n=3228) when it acted as the primary infected farm.

The farm specific average epidemic sizes, outcomes of the structured and random simulations, were strongly positively correlated (Spearman r=0.79, P<0.001, Fig. 3a). The correlation indicates that approximately 62 % of the epidemic outcome is defined solely by the contact patterns of a primary infected farm and by the average contact patterns in the country. The farm specific maximum epidemic size was on average 1.84 times larger using the random network than that obtained by using the structured network model. The maximum epidemic size values given by the two approaches were positively correlated (Spearman r=0.50, P<0.001, Fig. 3b). The standard deviation of epidemic size was also typically larger in the random simulation.

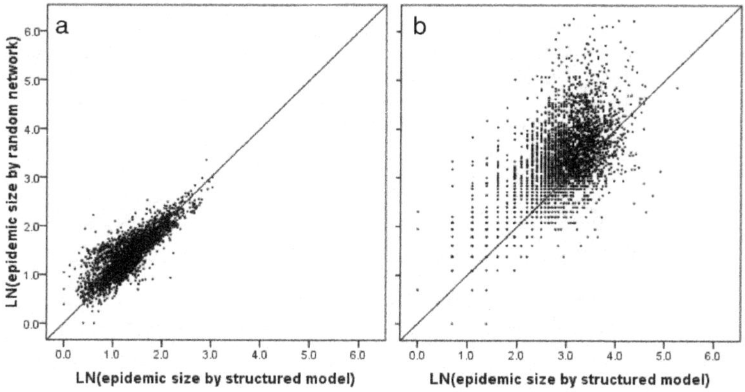

Fig. 3a and 3b Average (a) and maximum (b) epidemic size for Finnish pig farms by the structured model and the random network simulation. Each dot represents the outcome of a certain Finnish pig farm (n=3228) as a primary infected farm. The lines represent a slope of 1.

The relationship between the average epidemic sizes for an individual farm varied strongly among Finnish pig farm populations. Some farms created larger epidemics when the structured network information was used (Table 2), while the others spread disease less efficiently when the network information was applied. However, most of the farms (60%) presented a similar average epidemic size in both simulations (Table 2). The maximum epidemic size and standard deviation were more often larger than the average epidemic size (Table 2) as the random network produced larger maximum and standard deviation of epidemic size. The random network simulation overestimated the outcomes; both maximum and standard deviation were on average over 2 times larger than the outcomes from the structured network simulation.

Table 2. Simulated outcomes at the farm level. The random network simulations are compared with the structured model. When a simulation is run randomly (without using the network information) it can result in either under- or overestimations when compared to the results of a structured network.

		Outcomes by random network		
		Underestimates	Equals	Overestimates
Mean number of IF	%	13.8	60.0	26.2
Random/structured model	mean (std)	0.78 (0.08)	1.02 (0.14)	1.50 (0.37)
Maximum number of IF	%	3.7	61.1	35.3
Random/structured model	mean (std)	0.57 (0.15)	1.42 (0.96)	2.88 (1.98)
Standard deviation of IF	%	3.1	55.1	41.8
Random/structured model	mean (std)	0.61 (0.16)	1.22 (0.59)	2.23 (1.27)

IF =number of infected farm in an epidemic outbreak

The potential of a primary farm to promote an epidemic outbreak had an impact on the difference between the structured and random network simulations. The proportion of simulations where both the structured and random networks gave equal predictions of the average epidemic size declined along with the increasing probability of epidemic outbreak. Underestimation by the random network simulation was clearly more frequent when the epidemic outbreak probability of the primary farm was over 0.95. On the contrary, the overestimation by the random network simulation was most frequent when the probability of epidemic outbreak was between 0.5 and 0.95 (Table 3).

Table 3. Relationship between the probability of inducing an epidemic and the percentage of farms in each estimation category.

Probability of a primary farm inducing an epidemic outbreak	**Percentage of farms in different estimation categories**			
	Under-estimates (%)	Equals (%)	Over-estimates (%)	Total (n)
0.00 – 0.25	12.9	74.5	12.6	365
0.25 – 0.50	11.6	67.8	20.6	475
0.50 – 0.75	9.9	59.8	30.3	881
0.75 – 0.95	10.8	56.0	33.2	1116
0.95 – 1.00	34.9	49.0	16.2	390

DISCUSSION

The results from this study highlight the importance of detailed information on the network structure to study the spread of infectious diseases in pig production. This may be important for farm risk classification purposes as well as for the development of predictive models on the transmission of diseases between farms. The network structure in pig production seemed to suppress the potential magnitude of epidemic outbreaks. However, there were still a large number of farms which were connected to each other in a way that amplify the expected magnitude of an epidemic outbreak.

The random network simulation model in our study is essentially a scrambled version of the structured network model which does not take into account any detailed information about the production structure in Finland on farm level. The random network sampling assumes that farms are located within equal distances. In the random network simulation production related movements have no spatial structures: distances are ignored in animal transportation, as are movements of various people. In addition, the random model also ignores all temporal information such as the synchronization of production cycles of connected farms. Both models should give equal results only if the incorporated network information is essentially random and does not add any value on modelling.

Surprisingly, the average epidemic size at the country level was according to our simulations almost the same with or without the network information. Therefore it may be concluded that for country level average epidemic size estimation, inclusion of detailed network information improves estimates only slightly. This result applies if models and network structures used in the comparison are roughly similar as used in this study. If potential networks are larger, for instance because of a more spatially concentrated production, more farms or the infective period is longer, differences between structured and random network simulations could be larger with respect to average epidemic size. If the purpose is to estimate some outcomes other than the average epidemic size in the country, efforts to gather and incorporate network related information might improve estimates.

Using the information of the network structure is important in estimating the worst case scenarios for the country. Lack of network information could generate a three times overestimated worst case scenario. This result is consistent with the study of Eames (2008) where he showed that regular contacts tend to limit the size of an epidemic outbreak in clustered populations. If the aim of the simulation is to estimate the need for resources, this may lead to some unnecessary costs due to scaling up of the requirements. However, for the sake of practical disease eradication and preventive purposes, it is clear that overestimation of the worst case scenario is far more safe than underestimation. Nevertheless, the magnitude appeared to be so elevated that it is not practically sensible to apply random network simulations to estimate the worst case scenario for the country.

Network related information was more important at the farm level than for the country level estimates. Only 60 % of farm specific average epidemic sizes were estimated similarly using both the random network and the structured network simulations. By ignoring network information and using only the properties of the primary infected farms in the simulation, it might be possible to identify high risk pig farms whose ability to promote epidemic outbreak is directly related to their frequent contacts. Other farms, which are efficient spreaders indirectly due to the properties of the farms they are connected with, could be identified only by studying or simulating consequences of network information. For farm level predictions it is more sensible to apply structured network simulations, which have wider applicability than random network simulations.

The maximum epidemic size and standard deviation at the farm level were overestimated for a large number of farms (35-40 %) by random network simulation, which also is consistent with the results of Eames (2008). The results could be expected because all regularities of contacts due to production structures are lost in randomization and contacts may reach completely different farms than in reality. In practice, this means that if the identity of the primary infected farm and farm related network structure are applied in the estimation, in one third of the cases, uncertainty of an outcome and the worst case scenario is approximately halved.

Some of the farms (13.7 %) appeared to possess a higher risk than could be expected directly by studying their contact frequencies - namely the farms whose estimates were underestimated by the random network model. It was alarming that underestimations were more common among farms, which had the highest probability of causing epidemic outbreaks. This can lead to downscaled preventive measures. Underestimation also has non-beneficial side-effects to risk classification of farms, as only part of the members of the highest risk group could be identified by using the properties of the primary infected farm. A similar result has been achieved earlier when it was attempted to predict risk classes solely by the properties of the farm (Lyytikäinen & Kallio, 2009). This leads to a conclusion that inclusion of more farm related details alone would not improve predictive risk classification, but the improvement is obvious when the network properties are also applied.

The studied structured model is partly incomplete as temporal topology is only partially defined and parts of spatial networks are indirectly formed using operational regions to bond farms as 2-mode networks. It can be expected that a complete network model would deviate even more from the results of the random network model. One limitation of the structured network model is that autocorrelation of events on the farm is not fully described as there is generally no cohesive information on at what point in time there are visitors on the farm. This leads to underestimations of spatio-temporal relationships. If sequences of different events could be described fully at the farm level, it would modify further the outcomes of the simulation and make the distinction of structured and random network models even more obvious.

If farm level information is applied to estimate the potential outcome of an ongoing epidemic outbreak and the primary infected farm is already identified, structured network information would give better estimates than random networks. Nevertheless, to apply structured network information for ongoing epidemics would require that information could be used in real-time. Animal movement registries and farm registries would in theory enable real-time predictions. If most of the information is concentrated in central registries, the development of real-time predictions could be possible. Benefits of this approach should be assessed for risk management purposes.

ACKNOWLEDGEMENTS

The research is partially funded by the National Agricultural Development Fund (MAKERA).

REFERENCES

Barthélemy, M., Barrat, A., Pastor-Satorras, R. and Vespignani, A. (2004). Velocity and hierarchical spread of epidemic outbreaks in scale-free networks. Phys. Rev. Lett. 92, 1-4

Barthélemy, M., Barrat, A., Pastor-Satorras, R. and Vespignani, A. (2005). Dynamical patterns of epidemic outbreaks in complex heterogeneous networks. J. Theor. Biol. 235, 275-288

Bigras-Poulin, M., Barford, K., Mortensen, S. and Greiner, M. (2007). Relationship of trade patterns of the Danish swine industry animal movements network to potential disease spread. Prev. Vet. Med. 80, 143-165

Chowell, G., Rivas, A.L., Hengartner, N.W., Hyman, J.M. and Castillo-Chavez, C. (2006). The role of spatial mixing in the spread of foot-and-mouth disease. Prev. Vet. Med. 73, 297-314

Colizza, V., Barrat, A., Bathélemy, M. and Vespignani, A. (2006). The role of the airline transportation network in the prediction and predictability of global epidemics. PNAS 103, 2015-2020

Crepéy, P., Alvarez, F.P. and Barthélemy, M. (2006). Epidemic variability in complex networks. Phys. Rev. E 73, 1-7

Eames, K.T.D. (2008). Modelling disease spread through random and regular contacts in clustered populations. Theor. Pop. Biol. 73(1), 104-111

Ferguson, N.M., Donnelly, C.A. and Anderson, R.M. (2001). The Foot-and-Mouth epidemic in Great Britain: Pattern of spread and impact of interventions. Science 292, 1155-1160

Gibbens, J.C. and Wilesmith, J.W. (2002). Temporal and geographical distribution of cases of foot-and-mouth disease during the early weeks of the 2001 epidemic in Great Britain. Vet. Rec. 151, 407-412

Green, D.M., Kiss, I.Z. and Kao, R.R. (2006). Modelling the initial spread of foot-and-mouth disease through animal movements. Proc. R. Soc. B. 273, 2729-2735

Harvey, N., Reeves, A., Schoenbaum, M.A., Zagmutt-Vergara, F.J., Dube, C., Hill, A.E., Corso, B.A., .McNab, W.B., Cartwright, C.I. and Salman, M.D. (2007).The North American Animal Disease Spread Model: A simulation model to assist decision making in evaluating animal disease incursions. Prev. Vet. Med. 82, 176-197

Heath, M.F., Vernon, M.C. and Webb, C.R. (2008). Construction of networks with intrisic temporal structure from UK cattle movement data. BMC Vet. Res. 4:11. http://www.biomedcentral.com/1746-6148/4/11

Kao, R.R. (2002). The role of mathematical modelling in the control of the 2001 FMD epidemic in the UK. Trends Microbiol. 10(6), 279-286

Kao, R.R., Danon, I., Green, D.M. and Kiss, I.Z. (2006). Demographic structure and pathogen dynamics on the network of livestock movements in Great Britain. Proc. R. Soc. B. 273, 1999-2007

Kenah E. and Robins J.M. (2007). Network-based analysis of stochastic SIR epidemic models with random and proportionate mixing. J. Theor. Biol. 249, 706-722

Lawson, A.B. and Zhou, H. (2005). Spatial statistical modelling of disease outbreaks with particular reference to the UK foot and mouth disease (FMD) epidemic of 2001. Prev. Vet. Med. 71, 141-156

Le Sage, J.P. (2002). Econometrics toolbox. http://www.spatial-econometrics.com/

Lyytikäinen, T. and Kallio, E. (2009). Risk categorisation of Finnish pig farms by simulated Foot and mouth disease spread. Prev. Vet. Med., accepted

Masuda, N. and Konno, N. (2006). Multi-state epidemic processes on complex networks. J. Theor. Biol. 243, 64-75

Meyers, L.A., Newman, M.E.J. and Pourbohloul, B. (2006). Predicting epidemics on directed contact networks. J. Theor. Biol. 240, 400-418

Morris, R.S., Wilesmith, J.W., Stern, M.W., Sanson, R.L. and Stevenson, M.A. (2001). Predictive spatial modelling of alternative control strategies for the foot-and-mouth disease epidemic in Great Britain, 2001. Vet. Rec. 149, 137-144

Mourits, M.C.M., Nielen, M. and Léon, C.D. (2002). Effect of control measures on the course of simulated foot and mouth disease epidemics started on different farm types in various Dutch areas. *In* Proceedings of Society for Veterinary Epidemiology and Preventive Medicine, Cambrigde, UK, pp.190-200

Niemi, J.K., Lehtonen, H. , Lyytikäinen, T. and Kallio, E. (2008). Market implications of FMD epidemics in the Finnish pig sector: Does market structure matter? XIIth Congress of the European Association of Agricultural Economists EAAE 2008 Congress, Ghent, Belgium August 26-29, 2008, poster

Sanson, R.L. (1993). The development of decision support system for an animal disease emergency. Ph.D. Thesis, Massey University, Palmerston North, New Zealand, 264 p

Schley, D. (2007). Recommendations for enhancing confidence in epidemiological models of Foot-and-mouth disease. 37th general session of the European commission for the control of foot-and-mouth disease. 1-17

Shirley, M.D.F. and Rushton, S.P. (2005). Where disease and networks collide: lessons to be learnt from a study of the 2001 foot-and-mouth disease epidemic. Epid. Infect. 133, 1023-1032

Stevenson, M.A. (2003). The spatio-temporal epidemiology of bovine spongiform encephalopathy and foot-and-mount disease in Great Britain. Ph.D. Thesis. Institute of Veterinary, Animal and Biomedical Sciences, Massey University, Pelmmerston, New Zealand. 249p

Sutmoller, P., Bartelling, S.S., Olascoaga, R.S. and Sumption, K.J. (2003). Control and eradication of foot-and-mouth disease. Virus Res. 91, 101-144

Tildesley, M.J. and Keeling, M.J. (2008). Modelling foot-and-mouth disease: A comparison between the UK and Denmark. Prev. Vet. Med. 85, 107–124

Velthuis, A.G.J. and Mourits, M.C.M. (2007). Effectiveness of movement prevention regulations to reduce the spread of foot-and-mouth disease in the Netherlands. Prev. Vet. Med. 82, 262-281

Society for Veterinary Epidemiology and Preventive Medicine

PAST VENUES AND ORGANISERS OF ANNUAL MEETINGS

Year	Venue	Organiser(s)
1983	Southampton	Davies & Thrusfield
1984	Edinburgh	Thrusfield
1985	Reading	Thrusfield
1986	Edinburgh	Thrusfield
1987	Solihull	Thrusfield
1988	Edinburgh	Thrusfield
1989	Exeter	Howe
1991	London	Jones
1992	Edinburgh	Thrusfield
1993	Exeter	Howe
1994	Belfast	Menzies
1995	Reading	Paterson
1996	Glasgow	Reid
1997	Chester	Clarkson
1998	Ennis, Eire	Collins
1999	Warwick	Green
2000	Edinburgh	Thrusfield & Mellor
2001	Noordwijkerhout, The Netherlands	van Klink
2002	Cambridge	Wood & Newton
2003	Warwick	Green
2004	Martigny, Switzerland	Stärk
2005	Nairn	Gunn
2006	Exeter	Peeler
2007	Dipoli, Finland	Virtala & Alban
2008	Liverpool	Pinchbeck & Robinson
2009	London	Pfeiffer

PAST PRESIDENTS

1982-'83	G. Davies
1983-'84	P.R. Ellis
1984-'85	G. Gettinby
1985-'86	R.W.J. Plenderleith
1986-'87	M.V. Thrusfield
1987-'88	K.S. Howe
1988-'89	A.M. Russell
1989-'90	S.G. McIlroy
1990-'91	J.E.T. Jones
1991-'92	J.M. Booth
1992-'93	E.A. Goodall
1993-'94	R.G. Eddy
1994-'95	J.T. Done
1995-'96	G.J. Gunn
1996-'97	M.S. Richards
1997-'98	J.D. Collins
1998-'99	F.D. Menzies
1999-'00	K.L. Morgan
2000-'01	S.W.J. Reid
2001-'02	A.D. Paterson
2002-'03	L.E. Green
2003-'04	J.L.N. Wood
2004-'05	E.G.M. van Klink
2005-'06	D.J. Mellor
2006-'07	E. J. Peeler
2007-'08	J. R Newton

EXECUTIVE COMMITTEE 2008-2009

L. Alban (President), J.R. Newton (Senior Vice- President), D.U. Pfeiffer (Junior Vice-President), T.D.H. Parkin (Honorary Secretary), L.A. Kelly (Honorary Treasurer), C. Fourichon, T. Martinez, K. Mintiens, S. More, K. Verheyen.

Honorary Auditors: Dominic Mellor & Fraser Menzies

LIFE MEMBERS

J.M. Booth, M.J. Clarkson, J.D Collins, G. Davies, J.T. Done, R.G. Eddy, P.R. Ellis, E.A. Goodall, M.E. Hugh-Jones, A.M. Russell, M.V. Thrusfield

PLENARY TALKS

Year	Gareth Davies Lecture	Conference Opening Plenary
2009	Jørgen Westergaard The interaction between veterinary science, legistlation and management in animal disease control in the European Union	Katharina Stärk Food safety challenges in a global market – are we ready?
2008	Paul Fine Infectious disease eradication – meanings and implications	Kenton Morgan For the benefit of Mr Kite
2007	Yrjö Gröhn Food supply veterinary medicine: Modelling of production, health and food safety	Laura Green Improving Animal Health
2006	David Galligan From partial budgets to real options - concepts in animal health economics	Nigel French Understanding human exposure to zoonoses from food and the environment: The application of molecular tools and modeling
2005	Bill Reilly: From TB to VTEC: The changing epidemiology of foodborne zoonoses	Simon More: Towards eradication of bovine tuberculosis in Ireland: A vritical review of progress
2004	Ulrich Kihm: BSE and the stable to table concept	Gary Smith: Spatial models of infectious disease in the USA: a crisis of conference and confidentiality
2003	Sir David Cox: The current state of statistical science	Ynte Schukken: Molecular and mathematical epidemiology of bovine mastitis
2002	George Gettinby: Informatics and epidemiology – the first 400 years	Bryan Grenfell: Deterministic and stochastic influences on the dynamics and control of infectious diseases
2001	Will Houston: Science politics and animal health policy: epidemiology in action	Mart de Jong: Design and analysis of transmission experiments
2000	Jim Scudamore: Surveillance – past, present and future	Dirk Pfeiffer: Spatial analysis – a new challenge for veterinary epidemiologists

1999	Aalt Dijkhuizen: The 1997/98 outbreak of classical swine fever in the Netherlands: lessons learned from an economic perspective	Mark Woolhouse: Understanding the epidemiology of scrapie
1998	Wayne Martin: Art, science and mathematics revisited: the role of epidemiology in promoting animal health	-

SOCIETY FOR VETERINARY EPIDEMIOLOGY AND PREVENTIVE MEDICINE

APPLICATION FOR MEMBERSHIP

Name ....

Address ....

....

....

....

Telephone: ....

Fax: ....

E-mail:..

Signed .... Date ....

Please enclose the membership fee (£20 sterling) along with this application form. Overseas members without British bank accounts are requested to pay 2 - 3 years in advance. Cheques should be in £ sterling and drawn from a British bank. British members should pay future dues by standing order (forms are available from the Secretary or Treasurer). Payment can also be made by credit card; the appropriate form is available from the Society's web site, http://www.svepm.org.uk/, or from the Secretary or Treasurer.

Please send this form to the Society's Treasurer:

Dr Louise Kelly
Department of Statistics and Modelling Science
University of Strathclyde
Glasgow
G1 1XH

TEL +44 (0) 141 548 3659
FAX +44 (0) 141 552 2079
Email: louise@stams.strath.ac.uk

Please turn over

INTEREST GROUPS

Please tick appropriate boxes to indicate your interests:

- ☐ Analytical Epidemiology (Observational Studies)
- ☐ Quantitative Epidemiology & Statistical Techniques (Incl. Statistical/Mathematical Modelling)
- ☐ Herd/Flock Level Disease Control Strategies
- ☐ National/International Disease Control Policy
- ☐ Sero-Epidemiology
- ☐ Herd Health and Productivity Systems
- ☐ Disease Nomenclature and Epidemiological Terminology
- ☐ Economic Effects of Disease on Animal Production
- ☐ Veterinary Public Health and Food Hygiene
- ☐ Computing, including data logging
- ☐ Computer Programming *per se*
- ☐ Population and Animal Disease Databases
- ☐ Information System Design
- ☐ Geographical Information Systems (GIS)
- ☐ Risk Analysis

CONSTITUTION AND RULES

NAME

1. The society will be named the Society for Veterinary Epidemiology and Preventive Medicine.

OBJECTS

2. The objects of the Society will be to promote veterinary epidemiology and preventive medicine.

MEMBERSHIP

3. Membership will be open to persons either actively engaged or interested in veterinary epidemiology and preventive medicine.
4. Membership is conditional on the return to the Secretary of a completed application form and subscription equivalent to the rate for one calendar year. Subsequent subscriptions fall due on the first day of May each year.
5. Non-payment of subscription for six months will be interpreted as resignation from the Society.

OFFICERS OF THE SOCIETY

6. The Officers of the Society will be President, Senior Vice-President, Junior Vice-President, Honorary Secretary and Honorary Treasurer. Officers will be elected annually at the Annual General Meeting, with the exception of the President and Senior Vice-President who will assume office. No officer can continue in the same office for longer than six years.

COMMITTEE

7. The Executive Committee of the Society normally will comprise the officers of the Society and not more than four ordinary elected members. However, the Committee will have powers of co-option.

ELECTION

8. The election of office bearers and ordinary committee members will take place at the Annual General Meeting. Ordinary members of the Executive Committee will be elected for a period of three years. Retiring members of the Executive Committee will be eligible for re-election. Members will receive nomination forms with notification of the Annual General Meeting. Completed nomination forms, including the signatures of a proposer, seconder, and the nominee, will be returned to the Secretary at least 21 days before the date of the Annual General Meeting. Unless a nomination is unopposed, election will be by secret ballot at the Annual General Meeting. Only in the event of there being no nomination for any vacant post will the Chairman take nominations at the Annual General Meeting. Tellers will be appointed by unanimous agreement of the Annual General Meeting.

FINANCE

9. An annual subscription will be paid by each member in advance on the first day of May each year. The amount will be decided at the annual general meeting and will be decided by a simple majority vote of members present at the Annual General Meeting.

10. The Honorary Treasurer will receive, for the use of the Society, all monies payable to it and from such monies will pay all sums payable by the Society. He will keep account of all such receipts and payments in a manner directed by the Executive Committee. All monies received by the Society will be paid into such a bank as may be decided by the Executive Committee of the Society and in the name of the Society. All cheques will be signed by either the Honorary Treasurer or the Honorary Secretary.
11. Two auditors will be appointed annually by members at the Annual General Meeting. The audited accounts and balance sheet will be circulated to members with the notice concerning the Annual General Meeting and will be presented to the meeting.

MEETINGS

12. Ordinary general meetings of the Society will be held at such a time as the Executive Committee may decide on the recommendations of members. The Annual General Meeting will be held in conjunction with an ordinary general meeting.

GUESTS

13. Members may invite non-members to ordinary general meetings.

PUBLICATION

14. The proceedings of the meetings of the Society will not be reported either in part or in whole without the written permission of the Executive Committee.
15. The Society may produce publications at the discretion of the Executive Committee.

GENERAL

16. All meetings will be convened by notice at least 21 days before the meeting.
17. The President will preside at all general and executive meetings or, in his absence, the Senior Vice-President or, in his absence, the Junior Vice-President or, in his absence, the Honorary Secretary or, in his absence, the Honorary Treasurer. Failing any of these, the members present will elect one of their number to preside as Chairman.
18. The conduct of all business transacted will be under the control of the Chairman, to whom all remarks must be addressed and whose ruling on a point of order, or on the admissibility of an explanation, will be final and will not be open to discussion at the meeting at which it is delivered. However, this rule will not preclude any member from raising any question upon the ruling of the chair by notice of motion.
19. In case of an equal division of votes, the Chairman of the meeting will have a second and casting vote.
20. All members on election will be supplied with a copy of this constitution.
21. No alteration will be made to these rules except by a two-thirds majority of those members voting at an annual general meeting of the Society, and then only if notice of intention to alter the constitution concerned will have appeared in the notice convening the meeting. A quorum will constitute twenty per cent of members.
22. Any matter not provided for in this constitution will be dealt with at the discretion of the Executive Committee.

April, 1982
Revised March, 1985; April, 1988; November 1994
Corrected January 1997; April 2002